Re-entrant Arrhythmias

Mechanisms and Treatment

Re-entrant Arrhythmias

Mechanisms and Treatment

Edited by

Henri E. Kulbertus

Division of Cardiology and Electrocardiology
Institute of Medicine
University of Liege

University Park Press
Baltimore

Published in USA and Canada by
University Park Press
Chamber of Commerce Building
Baltimore, Maryland, 21202, USA

Published in the UK by
MTP Press Limited
St Leonard's House
Lancaster
England

Library of Congress Cataloging in Publication Data
Main entry under title:

Re-entrant arrhythmias.

   Proceedings of a symposium held in Liege, Belgium at the
University of Liege, Sept. 27–29, 1976.
   1. Arrhythmia—Congresses. I. Kulbertus, Henri.
[DNLM: 1. Arrhythmia—Physiopathology—Congresses.
2. Arrhythmia—Therapy—Congresses. WG 330 R 327 1976]
RC685.A65R43   616.1′28   77–7599
ISBN 0-8391-1120-7

Printed in Great Britain

Preface

'It seems then that the reciprocating rhythm may reasonably be regarded as due to a circulating excitation. The circumstances under which the phenomenon made its appearance was such as to produce the favourable conditions of slow conduction and short refractory period. By its continuance, the circulating rhythm would tend to maintain these conditions. The conditions are easily upset by the occurrence of an extrasystole and they may be re-established by other extrasystoles. I venture to suggest that a circulating excitation of this type may be responsible for some cases of paroxysmal tachycardia as observed clinically.'

G. R. Mines, *J. Physiol.* **46,** 349, 1913.

Some ten years ago, as a trainee in cardiology at the Royal Postgraduate Medical School in London, I used to spend long hours in the quiet library of the Hammersmith Hospital. One day, while thumbing through old copies of the Journal of Physiology, I came across a paper which attracted my attention because it mentioned a work of Leon Fredericq who is, deservedly, considered one of the most prominent figures in the history of my home University. At first glance, I did not like the paper very much. Quoting Leon Fredericq's views on atrioventricular transmission in auricular fibrillation, the author commented that they were 'charmingly simple'. My feelings were hurt. However, I decided to read the paper from beginning to end and soon found out that the text was one of those rare masterpieces which give its readers an intense, aesthetic pleasure. It was signed George Ralph Mines and dated 1913. Although he was not quite the very first one to do so, Mines, in this paper, laid the basis for the concept of re-entry; it is indeed amazing to remember that this text was written at a time when the dispute about the myogenic and neurogenic theories of atrioventricular transmission had just been settled.

It took some time for the concept of re-entry to attain wide acceptance, and I suspect that those who, like Pick and Langendorf, acted as pioneers in introducing the idea into clinical electrocardiography were initially considered experts in what was primarily regarded as a game of cunning and intelligence.

Nowadays, the situation has changed considerably. By using more and more sophisticated methods of investigation, electrophysiologists have been able to demonstrate that re-entry is a frequent phenomenon in cardiac patients and that its recognition may deeply influence therapeutic decisions and even lead to new approaches such as pacing or surgical techniques.

In the Fall of 1975, we felt that it might be nice to organize a meeting on Re-entrant Arrhythmias with a view to determining the present extent of our knowledge in the field. We were very lucky that most leading workers interested in re-entrant phenomena accepted the invitation to participate in this gathering. The symposium was held in late September 1976. It took place in the historical and peaceful premises of the Castle of Colonster which stands on the Campus of the University of Liege. The meeting was very friendly and the discussion most animated. It undoubtedly led to an exchange of very high level scientific information and to a most fruitful cross-fertilization of ideas. It is our sincere hope that the present book, which contains the full text of the various contributions presented at the Synposium, will be of help to all those who share an interest in the experimental and clinical aspects of cardiac arrhythmias.

H. E. Kulbertus,
Liege, December 1976

Acknowledgements

It is my pleasant duty to thank all those who, in one way or the other, have contributed to the success of the meeting.

First of all, I would like to express my grateful appreciation to the speakers who kindly agreed to participate in the Symposium and to produce their manuscripts so nicely on time. Among them, my friend H. J. J. Wellens who helped in the pre-editing and translation of some of the contributions deserves a very special acknowledgement.

The board of the University of Liege as well as the Belgian and European Societies of Cardiology sponsored the meeting; their support was most appreciated.

The Symposium was made possible by the generous financial support of Astra Chemicals, I.C.I. and Knoll, and I wish to express my deepest gratitude to the authorities of these three drug companies for their understanding of my wishes and their endeavours to meet them.

Professors A. Nizet, H. van Cauwenberge and J. Carlier acted as co-chairmen of the Symposium. Their assistance before, during and after the meeting was very efficient and is gratefully acknowledged.

Last, but not least, the secretarial work, a very heavy one indeed, was accomplished with kind dedication and meticulous competence by Mrs. B. Vervier, Miss S. Smeets and Mr. A. Vandenbroeck also worked long hours to enable the meeting to run smoothly. They surely deserve my most sincere thanks.

I would finally like to pay a tribute to Mr. Bloomer and his staff of the MTP publishers for their invaluable efforts in the production of this book.

H. E. Kulbertus

Contents

List of Contributors

Allessie, M. A.[*] Fysiologisch Laboratorium, Biomedisch Centrum
Beeldsnijdersdreef, 101
Maastricht, The Netherlands

Amat-y-Leon, J. Cardiology Section
The Abraham Lincoln School of Medicine
University of Illinois
840 South Wood Street
PO Box 6998
Chicago, Illinois 60680, U.S.A.
Division of Thoracic Surgery
Department of Surgery

Anderson, R. W. Duke University Medical Center
Durham
North Carolina, U.S.A.

Attuel, P. Clinique Cardiologique
Hôpital Lariboisière
2 rue Ambroise Paré
75475 Paris, France, Cedex 10

Bassett, A. L. University of Miami School of Medicine
PO Box 520875, Biscayne Annex
Miami, Florida 33152, U.S.A.

Boineau, J. P.[*] Cardiology Section VA Hospital
Medical College of Georgia
Augusta, Georgia 30902, U.S.A.

Bonke, F. I. M.[*] Fysiologisch Laboratorium, Biomedisch Centrum
Beeldsnijdersdreef, 101
Maastricht, The Netherlands

Cabrol, C. Service de Chirurgie Cardio-vasculaire
Hôpital de la Pitié Salpêtrière
83 Boulevard de l'Hôpital
Paris XIII, France.

Carmeliet, E.*   Laboratorium voor Fysiologie
                   Campus Gasthuisberg
                   3.000 Leuven, Belgium.

Chatelain, M. T.   Hôpital Cardiovasculaire et Pneumologique
                   28 Avenue du Doyen Lépine
                   BP Lyon Montchat
                   69394 Lyon, France

Cinca, J.   Service de Cardiologie
                   Hôpital St Eloi
                   34000 Montpellier, France

Coumel, Ph.*   Clinique Cardiologique
                   Hôpital Lariboisière
                   2 rue Ambroise Paré
                   75475 Paris, France, Cedex 10

Curry, P.*   Cardiovascular Division
                   Royal Postgraduate Medical School
                   Ducane Road
                   London W 12, England

deBakker, J. M. T. Helmholtz Institute
                   Rheinisch–Westfälischen
                   Technischen Hochschule
                   Goethestrasse 27–29
                   D-5100 Aachen, West Germany

Demoulin, J. C.*   Department of Morbid Anatomy, Institute of Pathology
                   University of Liège
                   1, rue des Bonnes Villes, 4020 Liège, Belgium

Denes, P.   Cardiology Section
                   The Abraham Lincoln School of Medicine
                   University of Illinois
                   840 South Wood Street
                   PO Box 6998
                   Chicago, Illinois 60680, U.S.A.

Dhingra, R. C.   Cardiology Section
                   The Abraham Lincoln School of Medicine
                   University of Illinois
                   840 South Wood Street
                   PO Box 6998
                   Chicago, Illinois 60680, U.S.A.

Downar, E.*   Department of Cardiology and Clinical Physiology
                   Wilhelmina Gasthuis
                   Amsterdam, The Netherlands

Elharrar, V.   Krannert Institute of Cardiology
                    Indiana University School of Medicine
                    1100 West Michigan Street
                    Indianapolis, Indiana 46202, U.S.A.

Erdin, R. A.   Cardiology Section VA Hospital
                    Medical College of Georgia
                    Augusta, Georgia 30902, U.S.A.

Facquet, J.   Service de Cardiologie
                    Hôpital de la Pitié Salpêtrière
                    83 Boulevard de l'Hôpital
                    Paris XIII, France

Fasola, A.   Eli Lilly and Co.
                    Indianapolis, Indiana 46202, U.S.A.

Fleischmann, D.*   Abteilung Innere Medizin I
                    Medizinische Fakultät
                    der Roheinisch-Westfälischen
                    Technischen Hochschule
                    Goethestrasse 27–29
                    D-5100 Aachen, West Germany

Fontaine, G.*   Service de Cardiologie
                    Hôpital de la Pitié Salpêtrière
                    83 Boulevard de l'Hôpital
                    Paris XIII, France.

Frank, R.*   Service de Cardiologie
                    Hôpital de la Pitié Salpêtrière
                    83 Boulevard de l'Hôpital
                    Paris XIII, France

Gallagher, J. J.*   Division of Cardiology
                    Department of Medicine
                    Duke University Medical Center
                    Durham
                    North Carolina 27710, U.S.A.

Gaum, W. E.   Krannert Institute of Cardiology
                    Indiana University School of Medicine
                    1100 West Michigan Street
                    Indianapolis, Indiana 46202, U.S.A.

Geer, M. R.   Duke University Medical Center
                    Durham
                    North Carolina 27710, U.S.A.

Gelband, H.   University of Miami School of Medicine
                    PO Box 520875, Biscayne Annex
                    Miami, Florida 33152, U.S.A.

Gressard, A. Hôpital Cardiovasculaire et Pneumologique
28 Avenue du Doyen Lépine
BP Lyon Montchat
69394 Lyon, France

Grolleau, R. Service de Cardiologie
Hôpital St Eloi
34000 Montpellier, France

Grosgogeat, Y. Service de Cardiologie
Hôpital de la Pitié Salpétrière
83 Boulevard de l'Hôpital
Paris XIII, France

Guiraudon, G. Service de Chirurgie Cardio-vasculaire
Hôpital de la Pitié Salpêtrière
83 Boulevard de l'Hôpital
Paris XIII, France

Harrison, L. Division of Cardiology
Department of Medicine
Duke University Medical Center
Durham
North Carolina 27710, U.S.A.

Hudson, R. D. Cardiology Section, VA Hospital
Medical College of Georgia
Augusta, Georgia 30902, U.S.A.

Hughes, D. C. Cardiology Section, VA Hospital
Medical College of Georgia
Augusta, Georgia 30902, U.S.A.

Jalife, J. Masonic Medical Research Laboratory
Utica
New York 13503, U.S.A.

Janse, M. J.* Department of Cardiology and Clinical Physiology
Wilhelmina Gasthuis
Amsterdam, The Netherlands

Kasel, J. Division of Cardiology
Department of Medicine
Duke University Medical Center
Durham
North Carolina 27710, U.S.A.

Krikler, D.* Cardiovascular Division
Royal Postgraduate Medical School
Hammersmith Hospital
Ducane Road
London W 12, England

Kulbertus, H.*   Division of Cardiology and Electrocardiology
Institute of Medicine, University of Liège
66 Bvd de la Constitution, 4020 Liège, Belgium

Lammers, J. E. P.*   Fysiologisch Laboratorium, Biomedisch
Centrum
Beeldsnijdersdreef, 101
Maastricht, The Netherlands

Miller, R. H.   Cardiology Section
The Abraham Lincoln School of Medicine
University of Illinois
840 South Wood Street
PO Box 6998
Chicago, Illinois 60680, U.S.A.

Moe, G. K.*   Masonic Medical Research Laboratory
Utica, New York 13503, U.S.A.

Mooney, C. R.   Cardiology Section VA Hospital
Medical College of Georgia
Augusta, Georgia 30902, U.S.A.

Moore, E. N.*   Department of Animal Biology and
Department of Medicine
University of Pennsylvania
3800 Spruce Street H1
Philadelphia 19174, U.S.A.

Morales, A. R.   University of Miami School of Medicine
PO Box 520875, Biscayne Annex
Miami, Florida 33152, U.S.A.

Mueller, W. J.   Bioelectronics and Computer Science Laboratory
State University of New York
Upstate Medical Center
Syracuse, N.Y., U.S.A.

Mugica, J.   Clinique Cardiologique
Hôpital Lariboisière
2 rue Ambroise Paré
75475 Paris, France

Myerburg, R. J.*   University of Miami School of Medicine
PO Box 520875, Biscayne Annex
Miami, Florida 33152, U.S.A.

Nilsson, K.   University of Miami School of Medicine
PO Box 520875, Biscayne Annex
Miami, Florida 33152, U.S.A.

Noble, R. S.   Krannert Institute of Cardiology
Indiana University School of Medicine
1100 West Michigan Street
Indianapolis, Indiana 46202, U.S.A.

Pick, A.*   Michael Reese Medical Center
29th Street and Ellis Avenue
Chicago, Illinois 60616, U.S.A.

Pop, T.   Abteilung Innere Medizin I
Medizinische Fakultät
der Roheinisch-Westfälischen Technischen Hochschule
Goethestrasse 27–29
D-5100 Aachen, West Germany

Pritchett, E. L. C.   Duke University Medical Center
Durham
North Carolina 27710, U.S.A.

Puech, P.*   Service de Cardiologie
Hôpital St Eloi
34000 Montpellier, France

Rosen, M. R.*   Departments of Pharmacology and Pediatrics
College of Physicians and Surgeons of Columbia University
630 West 168th Street
New York, NY 10032, U.S.A.

Rosen, K. M.*   Cardiology Section
The Abraham Lincoln School of Medicine
University of Illinois
840 South Wood Street
PO Box 6998
Chicago, Illinois 60680, U.S.A.

Sealy, W. C.   Division of Thoracic Surgery
Department of Surgery
Duke University Medical Center
Durham
North Carolina 27710, U.S.A.

Schlepper, M.*   Kerckhoff Klinik
Max Planck Society
Bad Nauheim, West Germany

Spear, J. F.   Department of Animal Biology and
Department of Medicine
University of Pennsylvania
3800 Spruce Street H1
Philadelphia 19174, U.S.A.

Spurrell, R. J.*   Department of Cardiology
                   St Bartholomew's Hospital, West Smithfield
                   London EC1, England

Strauss, H. C.*   Duke University Medical Center
                   Durham
                   North Carolina 27710, U.S.A.

Touboul, P.*   Hôpital Cardiovasculaire et Pneumologique
                   28 Avenue du Doyen Lépine
                   BP Lyon Montchat
                   69394 Lyon, France

Troup, P. J.   Krannert Institute of Cardiology
                   Indiana University School of Medicine
                   1100 West Michigan Street
                   Indianapolis, Indiana 46202, U.S.A.

Vedel, J.   Service de Cardiologie
                   Hôpital de la Pitié Salpêtrière
                   83 Boulevard de l'Hôpital
                   Paris XIII, France

Vexler, R. M.   Division of Cardiology
                   1650, Cedar Avenue
                   Hôpital Générale
                   Montreal H3G 1A4, Canada

Wallace, A. G.   Division of Cardiology
                   Department of Medicine
                   Duke University Medical Center
                   Durham
                   North Carolina, U.S.A.

Wellens, H. J. J.*   Department of Cardiology
                   University Hospital, Wilhelmina Gasthuis
                   Amsterdam, The Netherlands

Wit, A. L.*   College of Physicians and Surgeons of Columbia
                   University
                   630 West 168th Street
                   New York, NY 10032, U.S.A.

Wu, D.   Cardiology Section
                   The Abraham Lincoln School of Medicine
                   University of Illinois
                   840 South Wood Street
                   PO Box 6998
                   Chicago, Illinois 60680, U.S.A.

Wylds, A. C.   Cardiology Section VA Hospital
                   Medical College of Georgia
                   Augusta, Georgia 30902, U.S.A.

Wyndham, C. R.   Cardiology Section
                   The Abraham Lincoln School of Medicine
                   University of Illinois
                   840 South Wood Street
                   PO Box 6998
                   Chicago, Illinois 60680, U.S.A.

Zipes, D. P.*   Krannert Institute of Cardiology
                   Indiana University School of Medicine
                   1100 West Michigan Street
                   Indianapolis, Indiana 46202, U.S.A.

* Those contributors were active participants in the Symposium held in Liège, in September 1976.

Section I
Introductory Papers

1
Variants of Reciprocal Beating. An Exercise in Deductive Interpretation

A. PICK

Cardiovascular Institute, Department of Medicine,
Michael Reese Hospital and Medical Center, Chicago, Illinois

It was just 30 years ago that at the Michael Reese Hospital in Chicago a weird arrhythmia was observed, two bipolar chest leads (CF_1) of which are reproduced in Figure 1.1. They show an atrioventricular (AV) junctional rhythm with retrograde conduction and, in panel (b), the curious finding that the R–R intervals alternate concomitantly with the R–P intervals. The upper panel (a) obtained on another day shows diagrammatically that the lengthening of every other junctional cycle from 1.00 to 1.24 sec can be explained by antegrade re-entry of a slowed retrograde junctional impulse, completed with aberrant ventricular conduction in the middle but concealed at the beginning and the end of the record. Under each circumstance the spontaneous junctional cycle becomes reset to the same extent by 0.24 sec. A corresponding diagram explains panel (b).

There were many variants of this unusual rhythm disorder produced by digitalis and observed in numerous long records that did merit publication.[1] Yet, how little were we aware at that time, that our deductive reasoning and speculative interpretation of the various observations in this case can, and indeed have, been validated by today's advanced methods of experimental[2-7] and clinical investigation[8-13] and that such mechanisms can be applied to the explanation of a whole spectrum of common and unusual arrhythmias of supraventricular and ventricular origin[14-18]. For example Figure 1.2, three selected segments of our original observations, show that the re-entry process appeared to repeat itself, as in the first group of the lowest panel (c); and

3

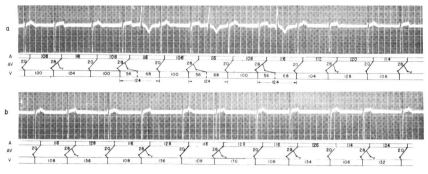

Figure 1.1 Overt and concealed AV junctional re-entry. (From Pick and Langendorf (1950) *Am. Heart J.*, **40**, 13, reproduced by permission of authors and publishers)

furthermore, antegrade as well as retrograde and repetitive re-entry processes could be considered to be partially or completely concealed within the junction, as in panels (b) and (c). We also found, as indicated diagrammatically in Figure 1.3 that a sinus P wave instead of a retrograde one was sometimes 'sandwiched' between the parent junctional beat and its ventricular echo. Measurements revealed that this occurred when the sinus P wave was inscribed at least 0.16 sec after the junctional QRS as indicated in diagrams a, b, and c. On the other hand, shorter R–P distances, or when the sinus P wave coincided with or oc-

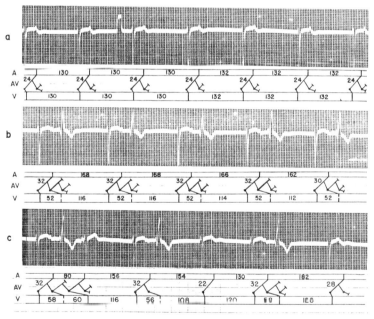

Figure 1.2 Concealed and overt repetitive re-entry in AV junctional rhythm. (From Pick and Langendorf (1950) *Am. Heart J.*, **40**, 13, reproduced by permission of authors and publishers)

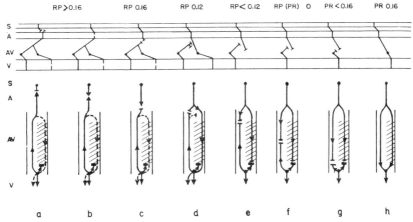

Figure 1.3 The effects of timing of a sinus impulse on the AV junctional re-entry mechanism of Figure 1.1 and 1.2. (From Pick and Langendorf (1950) *Am. Heart J.*, **40**, 13, reproduced by permission of authors and publishers)

curred shortly ahead of the junctional beat, as in diagrams d to g, echo beats failed to occur. This may be attributed to penetration of the sinus impulse into the potential re-entry loop to a progressively greater extent, thus preventing completion or the onset of the re-entry process. A sinus P wave 0.16 sec before an expected junctional impulse captured the ventricles prematurely as indicated in panel (h).

Thus, in these old observations and hypothetical diagrams, one can recognize models provided by nature in a digitalized patient of accepted conditions and postulates for initiation and maintenance of re-entry processes in general, as listed in Table 1.1.

It is remarkable that shortly after our publication Dr Peter Fleischmann reported[19] independently a strikingly similar case with an almost identical interpretation.

In the subsequent illustrations we should like to demonstrate other examples of unusual AV junctional arrhythmias we encountered in routine clinical elec-

---

TABLE 1.1   Conditions for initiation and maintenance of re-entry processes

(1) The prerequisite for a re-entry mechanism is a functional longitudinal dissociation in a part of the conduction system with unidirectional block in one and a relatively slow conduction in the other arm of a potential loop[22,28, 30−37]

(2) Delayed conduction may initiate a repetitive and sustained re-entry process and thus a paroxysmal tachycardia[2,3,8,38−41]

(3) Penetration of a critically timed independent impulse into the re-entry path may interrupt or preclude the re-entry mechanism[2,8,15,35]

(4) The specific case of AV junctional re-entry may not require inclusion of the atria into the re-entry path[2,26,27,34,35,37,42−45]

trocardiography, which, we believe, lend themselves to a reasonable deductive interpretation without the benefit of modern methods of investigation. Each will refer to one, two, or all three of the following aspects:

(1) Manifestations of concealed re-entry within the AV junction.

(2) The question of the atrial link in the reciprocating junctional tachycardias.

(3) The problem of repetitive group beating caused by simultaneous bidirectional Type I block in paroxysmal junctional tachycardias-reciprocating or focal?

In the case shown in Figure 1.4, acceleration of AV junctional impulse formation has caused incomplete AV dissociation with pairs of ventricular captures, the first of which is conducted with a P–R prolonged to 0.36 sec. Yet the distance between the consecutive capture beats of 0.98–1.00 sec is longer than

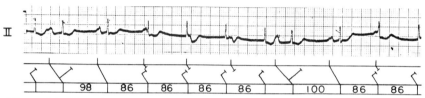

Figure 1.4 Concealed retrograde re-entry in incomplete AV dissociation. (From Pick and Langendorf (1969). *Am. Heart J.*, **76**, 553)

the junctional cycle of 0.86 sec. This can be explained by reversal of the slowly antegradely conducted sinus impulse entering a retrograde unused path in a functionally dissociated AV junction. It discharges prematurely and thus resets by about 0.12 sec, the beginning of the next spontaneous junctional cycle. Thus, the retrograde AV junctional re-entry process is concealed and revealed by its after-effect on junctional impulse formation.

Figure 1.5 shows portions of a long lead III. In the upper two panels a regular sinus rhythm is disturbed by single, and pairs, of atrial premature beats conducted to the ventricles with a prolonged P–R. In the middle of the second panel the initial atrial premature beat with the longer P–R of 0.28 sec is followed by two supraventricular premature cycles, each containing a retrograde P wave. Such sequences are characteristic of reciprocal beating of atria and ventricles. This occurs once in the upper panel and is immediately repeated in the middle panel where the mechanism is indicated by the diagram. Here this alternation of atrial and ventricular echoes comes to an end in a Wenckebach fashion in that conduction through the re-entry loop progressively slows (the R–P' lengthens). In other parts of the record atrioventricular reciprocation continued in the form of long runs of supraventricular tachycardia, the spontaneous end of which is illustrated in the panel at the bottom. At one point, indicated by the heavy arrow, the fast regular ventricular action continued although the retrograde P wave is missing. This we consider evidence

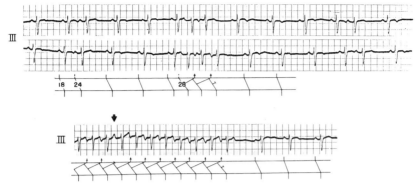

Figure 1.5 Atrial premature beats initiating repetitive AV reciprocation and re-entrant AV junctional paroxysmal tachycardia. (From Langendorf and Pick (1973). *Eur. J. Cardiol.*, **1**, 11)

that the atria are not a necessary link in the entire re-entry process. The dissociated antegrade and retrograde pathway can converge in the proximal AV junction to form a common connection with the atria. In the diagram it is indicated that the tachycardia stopped when this common path was not reached by the retrograde impulse.

Figure 1.6 demonstrates that in the middle of a Wenckebach period, at the arrow, the P–R interval after having increased from 0.28 to 0.46 sec unexpectedly shortens to 0.24 sec before its increment is resumed and the period is completed. In previous years[20] we attributed such a paradoxical P–R shortening to a supernormal phase of conduction in a depressed AV junction. In the light of recent knowledge gained in experimental and in clinical studies with intracardiac leads[21] other interpretations appear more likely and are indicated in the two diagrams. In both functional dissociation of two AV conduction pathways is postulated. In the upper diagram antegrade conduction at a critical point occurs via a path with a long refractory phase but faster conduction speed[2,22] indicated by the dashed diagonal line. The lower diagram shows the premature QRS to be unrelated to the P wave preceding it. It is attributed to a ventricular echo reflected from a concealed attempt at retrograde re-entry when the P–R interval has reached a critical length. Subsequently, another ven-

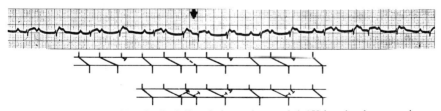

Figure 1.6 Functional longitudinal dissociation and concealed AV junctional re-entry in second degree Type I AV block. Pseudo-supernormal phase of AV conduction. (From Langendorf and Pick (1973). *Eur. J. Cardiol.*, **1**, 11)

tricular echo, after similar P–R prolongation, is prevented by penetration of the 'blocked' sinus impulse into the re-entry circuit. Again, the entire re-entry process would occur at a subatrial level of the AV junction.

In Figure 1.7 the first part shows an accelerated AV junctional rhythm, which by retrograde depolarization of the atria suppresses impulse formation in the sinus node. The retrograde conduction time progressively lengthens, until after the fifth QRS the retrograde P wave fails to appear. A ventricular pause occurs exceeding the otherwise regular junctional cycle by 0.34 sec. The returning junctional beat coincides with the P wave of an escaping sinus impulse, whereupon the regular junctional sequence with a retrograde P wave is resumed. The mechanism of the one apparently prolonged junctional cycle is explained by the diagram below the trace. The regular junctional cycle has been

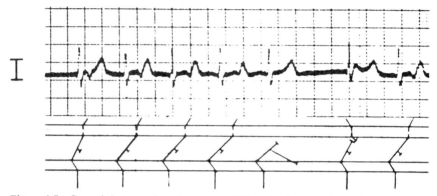

Figure 1.7   Concealed retrograde and antegrade AV junctional re-entry in accelerated AV junctional rhythm with Type 1 second degree retrograde AV block. (From Langendorf and Pick (1973). *Eur. J. Cardiol.*, **1**, 11)

reset by an attempt at a ventricular echo that failed to reach the ventricles. This antegrade re-entry was initiated by maximal delay of the retrograde impulse that proceeded to the point of re-entry but did not reach the atria – as shown by the missing of the fifth in the series of retrograde P waves. Thus, the record is interpreted as a result of two mechanisms: (a) concealed retrograde conduction causing (b) a concealed attempt at a ventricular echo.

In Figure 1.8, four different but related events are labelled (a)–(d). The basic disturbance of rhythm is seen in section (d). The P–R increases from 0.28 to 0.40 sec before the third sinus impulse is blocked. In the other sections (a)–(c), the regular sequence of sinus P waves is disturbed by premature retrograde ones, indicated by the upright arrows. These are atrial echo beats occurring after a greater and critical delay of sinus impulses in the AV junction. This reversal of impulse direction takes place regardless of whether the sinus impulse reaches the ventricles as in (c) or fails in it as in (a) and (b). Evidently, this unsuccessful concealed attempt at ventricular activation provides, in an unused

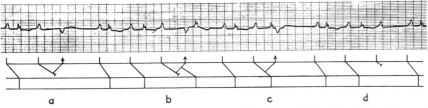

Figure 1.8 Concealed antegrade re-entry causing atrial and ventricular echoes in Type I second degree AV block. (From Pick (1973). *Am. Heart J.*, **86**, 249)

part of the AV junction, a potential avenue for reflection of impulses travelling slowly backwards and in (b), for another antegradely directed re-entry in form of a ventricular echo. This part of the record demonstrates that two successive, but oppositely directed, re-entry sweeps can take place as an after-effect of a single concealed antegrade conduction.

In Figure 1.9 the two strips of lead V_1 are continuous. Throughout the entire record, including lead II, sinus P waves can be spaced at a regular rate of 100 per min. In lead II, after a series of a constant first degree AV block, the P–R in the middle suddenly lengthens from 0.42 to 0.44 sec and subsequently ventricular bigeminy sets in, apparently due to alternation of long and shorter P–R intervals, and this, paradoxically, in that the shorter P–R follows the shorter R–P distance. Instead of postulating a supernormal phase of AV conduction, a more likely interpretation is indicated in the diagram, namely ventricular echos reflected from concealed retrograde re-entry in the AV junction, after a critical prolongation of the P–R interval to or beyond 0.44 sec (Figure 1.6).

At the start of V_1 in the middle strip, this bigeminal rhythm changes to a

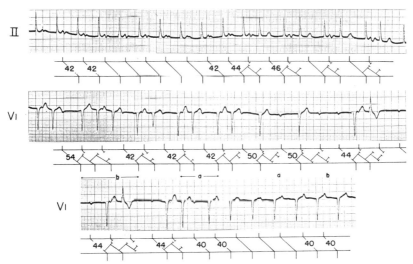

Figure 1.9 Paroxysmal (pseudo) AV block due to a repetitive bidirectional concealed re-entry mechanism in the AV junction. (From Langendorf and Pick (1973). *Eur. J. Cardiol.*, **1**, 11)

group of trigeminy that can be explained by completion of a pair of ventricular echoes induced by two consecutive unsuccessful attempts at atrial echoes. At the end of the middle strip, when the P–R of conducted sinus impulses is prolonged to 0.50 and 0.44 sec repeated attempts at both antegrade and retrograde conduction fail and remain concealed. However, evidence of their occurrence can be deduced from (1) block of single and two consecutive regular sinus P waves, (2) the observation that a long R–R interval bridging the two blocked P waves, labelled (b), is identical with that containing two consecutive echoes at the beginning of the strip, and (3), by the same token, and R–R interval labelled (a) containing one blocked P wave being equal to those containing a single ventricular echo, the cause of bigeminy of the ventricles.

The last pair of ventricular beats in the middle strip is reproduced as the first pair of the bottom strip. The right bundle branch block pattern of the second of the pair is caused by aberrant ventricular conduction due to the sequence of a short ventricular cycle after a particularly long one. This beat represents a completed ventricular echo followed by two concealed ones, the first in retrograde, the other in the antegrade direction. In the second half of this strip when P–R is again reduced to 0.40 sec reciprocation has disappeared.

The entire record, therefore, demonstrates one of the several possible mechanisms of 'paroxysmal AV block'[23–25] consisting of concealed repetitive bidirectional reciprocation, or, in other words, a temporary circulation of the cardiac impulse over functionally dissociated pathways within the AV junction without conduction to the atria and ventricles.

The last part of our presentation we should like to devote to the problem of the distinction between a focal and re-entrant origin (1.6(b)) as a particular type of supraventricular tachycardia. Of seven such cases we have observed in the course of the years, we are presenting two different examples.

Throughout lead II of Figure 1.10 atrial and ventricular complexes are arranged in repetitive groups, inverted retrograde P waves recurring in groups of three, and QRS complexes of normal shape and duration recurring in groups of four. The QRS complexes terminating each group are no longer followed by a retrograde P wave. Both P–P and R–R intervals progressively shorten. The pauses of 0.92–0.90 sec separating the atrial groups are *longer* than two successive short P–P intervals, whereas pauses between the groups of ventricular beats, measuring 0.64–0.60 sec are *shorter* than the sum of any two

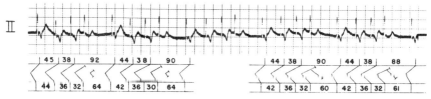

Figure 1.10 Repetitive atrial and ventricular group beating due to bidirectional second degree Type I AV block in an AV junctional tachycardia. (From Pick (1973). *Am. Heart J.*, **86**, 249)

short ventricular cycles. This repetitive atrial and ventricular arrhythmia can be explained by Wenckebach periods of forward and backward conduction of fast regular impulses arising in the AV junction and that in two ways indicated in the diagrams.

At the left, a *continuous* regular junctional tachycardia is assumed with bidirectional second degree Type I block causing a 5:4 response of the ventricles and a 5:3 response of the atria. Failure of two successive retrograde impulses to reach the atria is attributed to concealed retrograde conduction of the fourth impulse in each group. Thus, the manifest 5:3 response of the atria is an unsuccessful attempt at 5:4 response, actually occurring in the ventricles.

In the diagram at the right, the longer ventricular intervals are attributed to incomplete antegrade re-entry of junctional impulse during maximal retardation of retrograde conduction that failed to reach the atria. This re-entrant impulse also fails to reach the ventricles but resets the junctional cycle and periodically interrupts the continuity of the tachycardia (Figure 1.7).

In both diagrams a focal origin of the fast junctional impulse is assumed. Bidirectional Wenckebach periodicity as indicated in the left diagram could equally apply if the mechanism of the tachycardia were a fast regular intranodal circus motion (Figure 1.9). For the diagram at the right, two re-entry loops of different diameter may be postulated, a larger one causing the basic tachycardia and a smaller one, with a longer refractory period, which is entered only with maximal impulse retardation in the wider loop.

Another unusual variant of such a mechanism is shown in Figure 1.11, an esophageal lead. P waves, the smaller upright deflections, can be spaced throughout the tracing at a regular cycle length of 0.68 sec. The ventricular ac-

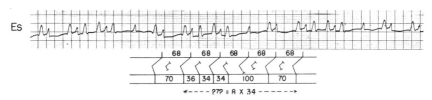

Figure 1.11   AV junctional tachycardia with 2:1 retrograde and varying second degree, Type I antegrade block. Courtesy of Dr. P. Yarvote, New York.

tion represented by the larger upright complexes is irregular but arranged in repetitive groups comprising three short R–R intervals of 0.36 and 0.34 sec and two longer ones of 1.00 and 0.70 sec. In each group the individual cycles are constant. The interpretation of one such group is presented in the diagram.

The clue to the interpretation is the finding that the sum of the ventricular cycles (272), is a multiple of one-half of the regular atrial cycle (8 × 34). This rules out an independent action of atria and ventricles and is in favour of a regular rapid junctional discharge with a cycle of 0.34 sec, corresponding to a rate of 176 per minute. The upright P waves in the esophageal lead represent retrograde conduction of the junctional impulses at a 2:1 ratio. The ventricular responses alternate between ratios of 2:1 and 6:4, the latter with a Wenckebach phenomenon. Occurrence of two consecutively blocked antegrade impulses can be attributed to concealed conduction of the first of them.

As in Figure 1.10 it is impossible to distinguish in the unipolar lead whether the rapid impulses emanate from a true ectopic focus or a circulating wave within the AV junction, presumably within the AV node representing a reciprocating or re-entrant AV junctional tachycardia. Neither of the two would exclude the possibility of a bidirectional second-degree Type I block occurring in common pathways to the atria as well as to the ventricles. Although intermittent second-degree block of antegrade *or* retrograde conduction has been demonstrated in re-entrant junctional tachycardia produced by programmed pacing[14,17,26,27] persistent repetitive bidirectional conduction disorders have, to our knowledge, no experimental counterpart.

SUMMARY

Examples are presented of unusual AV junctional arrhythmias suitable for deductive interpretation in standard leads without resorting to intracardiac records and programmed pacing. Specific aspects discussed are repetitive and concealed re-entry processes within the AV junction, the atrial participation in the re-entry path and the question of a focal or re-entrant mechanism in AV junctional tachycardias with simultaneous bidirectional exit block of Type I.

References

1. Pick, A. and Langendorf, R. (1950). A case of reciprocal beating with evidence of repetitive and blocked re-entry of the cardiac impulse. *Am. Heart J.*, **40**, 13

2. Moe, G. K. and Mendez, C. (1966). The physiologic basis of reciprocal rhythm. *Prog. Cardiovasc. Dis.*, **8**, 461

3. Han, J., Malozzi, A. M. and Moe, G. K. (1968). Sinoatrial reciprocation in the isolated rabbit heart. *Circ. Res.*, **22**, 355

4. Cranefield, P. F., Klein, H. O. and Hoffman, B. F. (1971). Conduction of the cardiac impulse I. Delay, block and one-way block in depressed Purkinje fibers. *Circ. Res.*, **28**, 220

5. Wit, A. L., Rosen, M. R. and Hoffman, B. F. (1974). Electrophysiology and pharmacology of cardiac arrhythmias. II. Relationship of normal and abnormal electrical activity of cardiac fibers to the genesis of arrhythmias. B. Re-entry Sections I and II. *Am. Heart J.*, **88**, pp. 664 and 798

6. Allessie, M. A., Bonke, F. I. M. and Schopman, J. G. (1973). Circus movement in rabbit atrial muscle as a mechanism of tachycardia. *Circ. Res.*, **33**, 54

7. Cranefield, P. F. (1975). The conduction of the cardiac impulse. Futura. Mount Kisco. New York

8. Coumel, Ph., Cabrol, C., Fabiato, R., Gourgon, R. and Slama, R. (1967) Tachycardie permanente par stimulation auriculaire et ventriculaire. *Arch. Mal. Coeur Vaiss*, **60**, 1830

9. Scherlag, B. J., Lau, S. H., Helfant, R. H., Berkowitz, W. D., Stein, E. and Damato, A. N. (1969). Catheter technique for recording His bundle activity within the AV node. *Circulation*, **39**, 13

10. Wellens, H. J. J. (1971). *Electrical Stimulation of the Heart in the Study and Treatment of Tachycardias.* (Baltimore: University Park Press)

11. Puech, P. and Grolleau, R. (1972). *L'activité du Faisceau de His. Normal et Pathologique.* (Paris: Sandoz)

12. Damato, A. N., Varghese, P. J., Lau, S. N., Gallagher, J. J. and Bobb, G. A. (1972). Manifest and concealed re-entry. A mechanism of AV nodal Wenckebach phenomenon. *Circ. Res.,* **30,** 283

13. Narula, O. S. (1975). *His Bundle Electrocardiography and Clinical Electrophysiology.* (Philadelphia: F. A. Davis Co.)

14. Janse, M. J., VanCapelle, F. J. L., Freud, G. E. and Durrer, D. (1971). Circus movement within the AV node as a basis for supraventricular tachycardia as shown by multiple microelectrode recording in the isolated rabbit heart. *Circ. Res.,* **28,** 403

15. Wellens, H. J. J. (1975). Pathophysiology of ventricular tachycardia in man. *Arch. Int. Med.,* **135,** 473

16. Zipes, D. P. (1975). Re-entry in the Ventricles: In *Recent Advances in Ventricular Conduction. Adv. Cardiol.,* **14** 51

17. Coumel, Ph., Attuel, P. and Flammang, D. (1976). The role of the conduction system in supraventricular tachycardias. In H. J. J. Wellens, K. I. Lie and M. J. Janse (eds.) *The Conduction System of the Heart. Structure, Function and Clinical Implications,* 423 (Philadelphia: Lea and Febiger)

18. Spurrell, R. A. J. (1976). Reciprocation: A mechanism for tachycardias. *Am. Heart J.,* **91,** 409

19. Fleischmann, P. (1951). The latent and manifest reciprocation mechanism. *Acta Cardiol.,* **6,** 163

20. Pick, A., Langendorf, R. and Katz, L. N. (1962). The supernormal phase of atrioventricular conduction. I. Fundamental mechanisms. *Circulation,* **31,** 398

21. Gallagher, J. J., Damato, A. N., Varghese, P. J., Caracta, A. R., Josephson, M. E. and Lau, S. H. (1973). Alternative mechanisms of apparent supernormal atrioventricular conduction. *Am. J. Cardiol.,* **31,** 361

22. Rosen, M. R., Denes, P., Wu, D. and Dhingra, R. C. (1976). Electrophysiologic diagnosis and manifestation of dual AV nodal pathways in the conduction system of the heart, In H. J. J. Wellens, K. I. Lie and M. J. Janse (eds.) *The Conduction System of the Heart. Structure, Function and Clinical Implications,* 453 (Philadelphia: Lea and Febiger)

23. Coumel, Ph., Fabiato, A., Waynberger, M., Motté, G., Slama, R. and Bouvrain, Y. (1971). Bradycardia dependent atrio-ventricular block. Report of two cases of AV block elicited by premature beats. *J. Electrocardiol.,* **4,** 168

24. Rosenbaum, M. B., Elizari, M. V., Levi, R.I. and Nau, G. I. (1973). Paroxysmal atrioventricular block related to hypolarization and spontaneous diastolic depolarization. *Chest,* **63,** 678

25. El-Sherif, N., Scherlag, B. J. and Lazzara, R. (1976). An appraisal of second degree and paroxysmal atrioventricular block. *Eur. J. Cardiol.,* **4,** 117

26. Wellens, H. J. J. (1975). Unusual examples of supraventricular re-entrant tachycardias. *Circulation,* **51,** 997

27. Wellens, H. J. J., Wesdorp, J. C., Durrer, D. R. and Lie, K. L. (1976). Second degree block during reciprocal atrioventricular nodal tachycardia. *Circulation,* **53,** 595

28. White, P. D. (1915). A study of atrioventricular rhythm following auricular flutter. *Arch. Int. Med.,* **16,** 517

29. White, P. D. (1921). The bigeminal pulse in atrioventricular rhythm. *Arch. Int. Med.,* **28,** 213

30. Scherf, D. and Shookoff, C. (1926). Experimentelle Untersuchungen über die "Umkehr-Extrasystole" (reciprocating beat). *Wien. Arch. Inn. Med.,* **12,** 501

31. Rosenblueth, A. (1958). Ventricular "echos". *Am. J. Physiol.,* **195,** 53

32. Scherf, D. and Cohen, J. (1964). *The Atrioventricular Node and Selected Arrhythmias.* p. 227–279, (New York: Grune and Stratton)

33. Korth, C. and Schrumpf, W. (1936). Über Umkehrsystolen (reciprocating rhythm). *Dtsch. Arch. Klin. Med.,* **178,** 589

34. Langendorf, R., Katz, L. N. and Simon, A. J. (1944). Reciprocal beating initiated by ventricular premature beats. *Br. Heart J.,* **6,** 13

35. Kistin, A. D. (1959). Mechanisms determining reciprocal rhythm initiated by ventricular premature systoles. *Am. J. Cardiol.,* **3,** 365

36. Mendez, C. and Moe, G. K. (1966). Demonstration of a dual AV conduction system in the isolated heart. *Circ. Res.,* **19,** 378

37. Mignone, R. J. and Wallace, A. G. (1966). Ventricular echos: Evidence for dissociation of conduction and re-entry within the AV node. *Circ. Res.,* **19,** 638

38. Samojloff, A. and Tschernoff, A. (1930). Reziproker Herz Rhythmus beim Menschen. *Z. Gesamte Exp. Med.,* **71,** 768

39. Barker, P. S., Wilson, F. N., Johnston, F. D. and Wishart, S. W. (1943). Auricular paroxysmal tachycardia with auriculo-ventricular block. *Am. Heart J.,* **25,** 765

40. Goldreyer, B. and Damato, A. N. (1971). The essential role of atrioventricular conduction delay in the initiation of paroxysmal supraventricular tachycardia. *Circulation,* **43,** 679

41. Langendorf, R. and Pick, A. (1973). Concealed re-entry in the AV junction. *Eur. J. Cardiol.,* **1,** 11

42. Schamroth, L. (1970). Case report: Reciprocal rhythm of ventricular origin during atrial fibrillation with complete AV block. *Br. Heart J.,* **32,** 564

43. Goldreyer, B. N. and Bigger, T. Jr. (1971). Site of re-entry in paroxysmal supraventricular tachycardia. *Circulation,* **43,** 15

44. Schuilenburg, R. N. and Durrer, D. (1972). Further observations on the ventricular echo phenomenon elicited in the human heart. Is the atrium part of the echo pathway? *Circulation,* **45,** 629

45. El-Sherif, N., Befeler, B., Aranda, J., Castellanos, A. and Lazarra, R. (1976). Re-entry due to manifest and concealed His bundle ectopic systoles. *Circulation,* **53,** 902

2
Possible Role of Sodium- and Calcium-Mediated Action Potentials in Re-entry

E. CARMELIET

Laboratory of Physiology, University of Leuven, Belgium

Calcium-mediated slow responses are today regarded as playing an important, if not exclusive, role in the genesis of re-entry arrhythmias. In his recent book *'The Conduction of the Cardiac Impulse'* Cranefield advances the thesis that most, and perhaps all, arrhythmias result from slow response activity, which is caused by the flow of current through a specific slow channel. This conductance channel has to be differentiated from the fast sodium channel. Under normal conditions, activation of the fast Na channel is responsible for the rapid upstroke of the action potential and propagation of the impulse through the heart. Slow channel activation on the other hand results in a slow upstroke and slow propagation of the impulse. The typical ion carrier is calcium, although sodium also permeates through the same channel to some extent[1-3].

An experimental verification of the thesis that re-entry arrhythmias are the result of slow channel activation, would have the important therapeutic implication that antagonists of the slow channel should be the anti-arrhythmic drugs of choice.

A direct demonstration of the existence of slow Ca-mediated electrical activity in the human heart and its involvement in the genesis of arrhythmia has not been reported. It is therefore of interest to look for indirect information and to find an answer to the following questions:

(1) In which way are the models, used to reproduce Ca-mediated action potentials *in vitro*, related to conditions *in vivo*?

(2) Do the characteristics of the Ca-mediated action potential fulfil the requirements for the genesis of re-entry?

15

(3) Is the Ca-mediated action potential the only type of slow response, that can result in re-entry?

MODELS FOR Ca-MEDIATED ACTION POTENTIALS

Ca-mediated action potentials have been recorded under many different experimental conditions[3].

These conditions have two characteristics in common:

(1) activation of the fast Na channel is eliminated. This is done either by omitting Na from the perfusion bath, by blocking the Na channel using a specific drug, tetrodotoxine, or by inactivating the Na channel by depolarization (high external potassium or electrical current),

(2) the flow of net inward current is favoured either by directly increasing the flow of Ca ions (catecholamines, high Ca) or by decreasing outward current (tetraethylammonium, chlorine-free medium).

Although all of these models have their specific advantages only some of them can be related to conditions *in vivo*. Increase of extracellular K together with release of catecholamines have been observed in areas of restricted perfusion (myocardial infarction). Furthermore the existence of K concentration gradients between infarcted and noninfarcted areas sets the stage for short-circuit currents, which may depolarize cells outside the ischaemic region. Such depolarization originating from K gradients has been demonstrated *in vitro*[4].

In favour of the use of these models, it must be added that the slow responses reproduce most of the characteristics of the normal action potentials in the sinoatrial node and the AV node.

REQUIREMENTS FOR RE-ENTRY

The next question to answer is whether the characteristics of Ca-mediated action potentials correspond to the conditions for re-entry. These conditions are: unidirectional block of conduction, slow conduction, and short refractory period. In connection with the latter two conditions the notion of wavelength, which is the product of conduction velocity and refractory period, is useful. The chance of inducing re-entry will be higher the shorter the wavelength of the impulse.

Unidirectional block is an extreme form of asymmetry of conduction. Some asymmetry of conduction always exists, even in normal bundles of cardiac muscle, and is due to differences in passive or active properties of the cells. Passive properties of importance in explaining propagation are membrane capacity, specific membrane resistance, specific intracellular longitudinal resistance, cell diameter and eventually resistance of the extracellular medium. Active properties include density of conductance channels, kinetics of conductance changes, and chemical gradients.

It is to be expected that asymmetry will be exaggerated in situations that depress excitability, such as high K concentration. It is also expected that the likelihood of obtaining unidirectional block will be higher the more the conduction is depressed. Ca-mediated action potentials are conducted at a speed which is only 1/10 to 1/100 of the normal conduction velocity, and unidirectional block has been observed in the presence of high external K and catecholamines[5].

The slow conduction velocity with which Ca-action potentials are propagated is responsible for the short wavelength observed for this type of electrical impulse. The long refractory period of these action potentials, however, acts in the opposite way and reduces the probability of re-entry. Long refractory periods, outlasting the repolarization of Ca-mediated action potentials, have been observed by many authors[3]. It is also known that Ca-mediated action potentials are stable only when the frequency of stimulation is low (stimulation intervals of >1 sec). At high rates of stimulation fibres seem to show a cumulative loss of excitability giving a lengthening of the refractory period instead of the expected shortening.

Taking into account the published values for conduction velocity and refractory period in different conditions one can calculate wavelengths of the order of 1–10 cm. The lowest values are about 50 times smaller than the wavelength of a typical Na-type action potential. One may thus conclude that Ca-mediated action potentials create conditions favourable for the appearance of re-entry.

ARE SLOW RESPONSES ALWAYS DUE TO ACTIVATION OF THE Ca CONDUCTANCE CHANNEL?

A critical question with respect to therapy is whether slowly conducted action potentials are always due to activation of the slow channel. The following results favour the thesis that slow responses can also be due to activation of the fast Na system.

When the external K is gradually increased in the bathing solution, the resting potential falls in proportion to the logarithm of the K concentration. Concomitant with this depolarization the upstroke velocity and the duration of the action potential decreases. Between -70 and -60 mV $(dV/dt)_{max}$ drops markedly and may become so low that propagation fails; the cells become unexcitable. The relation between $(dV/dt)_{max}$ and membrane potential is described by a sigmoidal curve and is known as the 'inactivation' curve for the fast Na conductance.

A different picture is obtained when the experiment is repeated in the presence of isoproterenol, or in Cl-free medium. Examples of results obtained in a cat papillary muscle and in a cow Purkinje fibre are shown in Figures 2.1 and 2.2. Instead of becoming unexcitable in K concentrations of $ca.$ 15 mM, the preparation continues to show action potentials characterized by a very small

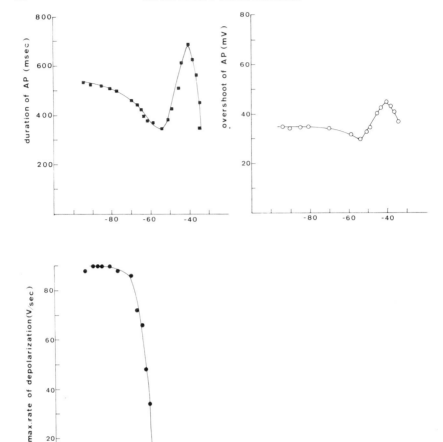

Figure 2.1   Effect of a decrease in membrane potential on the duration (■), the overshoot (○) and $(dV/dt)_{max}$ (●) of the action potential of a cat papillary muscle. The membrane potential was changed by varying the K concentration between 2.7 and 54 mM (Cl-free medium) (From Verdonck[6] by permission of the author and publishers)

upstroke velocity. In a certain potential range (−50 to −40 mV) upstroke velocity increases again before taking a second sigmoidal decline between −40 and −20 mV. This second sigmoidal relationship corresponds to the inactivation curve for slow inward current determined in voltage clamp experiments[1].

The existence of a minimum for $(dV/dt)_{max}$ at *ca.* −50 mV was unexpected and no attempt will be made here to explain the underlying mechanism. May it suffice to say that the phenomenon is not related to the K concentration but is

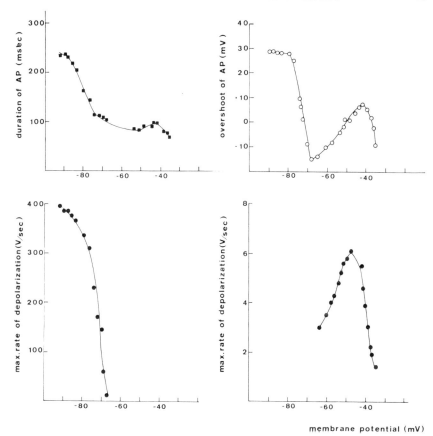

Figure 2.2   Effect of a decrease in membrane potential on the duration (■), the overshoot (○) and $(dV/dt)_{max}$ (●) of the action potential of a dog Purkinje fibre. The membrane potential was changed by varying the K concentration between 2.7 and 54 mM. Isoproterenol was added in a concentration of 2 mg/l

due to a potential dependent change in conductance. The upstroke of the action potential at this minimum is probably due to an inward movement of Ca ions because similar slow upstrokes could be obtained in the presence of tetrodotoxine (TTX)[6]. Action potentials at more negative potentials than this minimum, however, were markedly depressed in the presence of TTX and propagation was blocked. This means that action potentials with similar up-stroke velocity (on the left or right side of the minimum) but of different ionic nature can be present in cardiac cells.

It is also important to note that changes in the overshoot mirror the changes in $(dV/dt)_{max}$. The same is true for the duration of the action potential in mus-cle fibres, but less so for Purkinje fibres.

The existence of propagated slow action potentials due to Na channel activation is surprising, since the Hodgkin–Huxley equations predict that propagation fails when the Na is inactivated to less than 5% of the maximum value[7].

In cardiac muscle the situation is different because of the existence of anomalous rectification and the presence of an important Ca conductance. Even in the presence of reduced membrane potentials and partial inactivation of the Na conductance a small activation of this Na conductance may result in a depolarization sufficient to reach the threshold for a regenerative increase in Ca conductance.

Under those conditions the upstroke is seen to consist of two phases. An example obtained in a cat papillary muscle superfused with 14.8 mM K is given in Figure 2.3. The action potential consists of a 'fast' upstroke (20 V/sec) due to activation of the Na conductance followed by a second slower phase (4 V/sec) due to activation of the Ca conductance. Increasing K concentration to 22 mM resulted in a complete suppression of the first phase and inexcitability. After

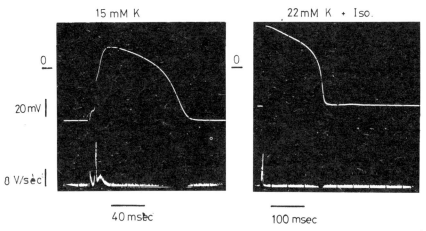

Figure 2.3   Action potentials of a cat papillary muscle in the presence of 15 mM K (left) and 22 mM K plus isoproterenol (0.2 mg/l) (right). On the left the upstroke consists of two successive phases. Note comparable $(dV/dt)_{max}$ values in both examples. Stimulation frequency 6/min

addition of isoproterenol, excitability reappeared. These facts are well known and have been documented in the literature[8–10]. It is important to note the fact that the two types of action potentials (before and after addition of isoproterenol) have a similar upstroke velocity, although they are of a different ionic nature. Both have thus the same potentiality in generating re-entry.

The two phases of the upstroke observed in the presence of an elevated K concentration are affected in different ways by local anaesthetics. Lidocaine (5 mg/l) selectively decreases the upstroke velocity of the first component while it has no effect on the rate of rise of the second component (Figure 2.4). This last observation confirms the results of previous experiments, where it was shown that local anaesthetics had no effect on Ca-mediated action potentials,

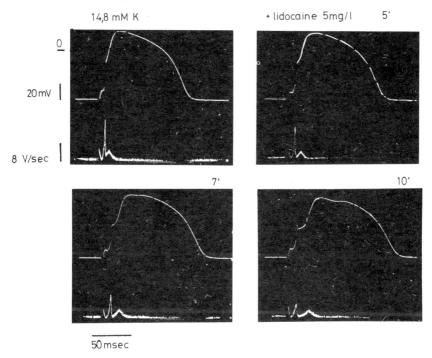

Figure 2.4   Effect of lidocaine (5 mg/l) on the action potential of a cat papillary muscle in the presence of an elevated K concentration. Lidocaine selectively depresses the amplitude and $(dV/dt)_{max}$ of the first phase of the upstroke. Stimulation frequency 6/min

while Ca antagonists (Mn, D600, verapamil) suppressed this type of activity[11]. In voltage-clamp experiments similar effects on the slow current have been described by Kohlhardt *et al.*[12].

In the preceding section it was stressed that the two types of action potentials (Na- or Ca-mediated) show a comparable upstroke velocity in the presence of elevated K. It is also important to note that the recovery kinetics of these two types of electrical activity are similar. It is known that the recovery from inactivation for the Na-type action potential is markedly slowed when the cell is depolarized by an increase in the external K concentration[13]. At −90 to −80 mV time constants are of the order of a few msec; at −60 mV they lengthen to 100 msec and more. These values are of the same order as those found for recovery of the slow inward current, determined in voltage-clamp experiments[13-15]. In Figure 2.5 examples are given for the recovery of $(dV/dt)_{max}$ of action potentials at different levels of external K. It is clear that recovery is markedly slowed when the external K is increased above 10.8 mM. At 13.5 and 14.8 mM K the upstroke of the action potentials consists of two phases corresponding to the successive activation of the fast Na and slow Ca conductance. In 14.8 mM K the first four action potentials following the test

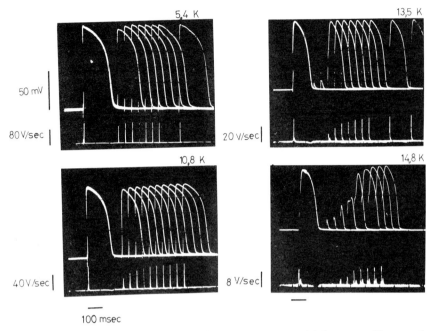

Figure 2.5   Recovery of amplitude and $(dV/dt)_{max}$ of action potentials in a cat papillary muscle superfused with solutions containing variable concentrations of K. In the presence of elevated K concentrations recovery is markedly slowed but similar for the first and second phase of the upstroke. Stimulation frequency was 60/min

stimulus were below the threshold to trigger the slow phase. For the action potentials recorded at longer time intervals, $(dV/dt)_{max}$ of both phases gradually increased with time. These observations suggest that recovery for both systems is comparable, although they are caused by different ionic mechanisms. Because changes in $(dV/dt)_{max}$ are reflected in changes in conduction velocity, they further corroborate the thesis that slow conduction can be caused by either Na- or Ca-dependent electrical activity.

References

1. Reuter, H. (1973). Divalent cations as charge carriers in excitable membranes. *Prog. Biophysics Mol. Biol.*, **26**, 3
2. Noble, D. (1975). *The Initiation of the Heart Beat.* (Oxford: Clarendon Press)
3. Cranefield, P. F. (1975). *The Conduction of the Cardiac Impulse.* (New York: Futura Publishing Co.)
4. Katzung, B. G., Hondeghem, L. M. and Grant, A. O. (1975). Cardiac ventricular automaticity induced by current of injury. *Pfluegers Arch.*, **360**, 193
5. Cranefield, P. F., Klein, H. O. and Hoffman, B. F. (1971). Conduction of the cardiac impulse. I. Delay, block and one-way block in depressed Purkinje fibers. *Circ. Res.*, **28**, 199
6. Verdonck, F. (1976). Calcium-mediated action potentials and related mechanical activity in cardiac muscle. *Thesis*, Acco, Leuven

7. Lieberman, M., Kootsey, J. M., Johnson, E. A. and Sawanobori, T. (1973). Slow conduction in cardiac muscle. A biophysical model. *Biophys. J.*, **13**, 37

8. Engstfeld, G., Antoni, H. and Fleckenstein, A. (1961). Die Restitution der Erregungsfortleitung und Kontraktionskraft des K^+-gelähmten Frosch- und Säugetiermyokards durch Adrenalin. *Pfluegers Arch.*, **273**, 145

9. Carmeliet, E. and Vereecke, J. (1969). Adrenaline and the plateau phase of the cardiac action potential. *Pfluegers Arch.*, **313**, 300

10. Pappano, A. J. (1970). Calcium-dependent action potentials produced by catecholamines in guinea-pig atrial muscle fibers depolarized by potassium. *Circ. Res.*, **24**, 379

11. Carmeliet, E. and Xhonneux, R. (1973). Electrophysiological aspects of the action of lidoflazine on the heart. *Arzneim. Forsch. Suppl.*, **26**, 16

12. Kohlhardt, M., Bauer, B., Krause, H. and Fleckenstein, A. (1972). Differentiation of the transmembrane Na and Ca channel in mammalian cardiac fibres by the use of specific inhibitors. *Pfluegers Arch.*, **335**, 309

13. Gettes, L. S. and Reuter, H. (1974). Slow recovery from inactivation of inward currents in mammalian myocardial fibres. *J. Physiol.*, **240**, 703

14. Trautwein, W., McDonald, T. F. and Tripathi, O. (1975). Calcium conductance and tension in mammalian ventricular muscle. *Pfluegers Arch.*, **354**, 55

15. Kohlhardt, M., Krause, B., Kübler, M. and Herdey, A. (1975). Kinetics of inactivation and recovery of the slow inward current in the mammalian ventricular myocardium. *Pfluegers Arch.*, **355**, 1

Section II
Sinus Node Re-entry and Atrial Arrhythmias

3
Sinoatrial Node Re-entry

H. C. STRAUSS and M. R. GEER

Duke University Medical Center, Durham, North Carolina

Iliescu and Sebastiani[1] were among the first to suggest that paroxysmal atrial tachycardia was due to re-entry within the atrium. These two authors called attention to the similarities in rate response of paroxysmal atrial tachycardia and atrial flutter to quinidine; namely in some patients receiving quinidine, the heart rate of the tachycardia decreased prior to the sudden transition to normal rhythm[1]. This mode of termination of the tachycardia lead the authors to suggest that paroxysmal atrial tachycardia might depend on a circus movement[1]. Lewis[2], on the other hand, believed that in contrast to atrial flutter, paroxysmal atrial tachycardia was due to an ectopic focus, because known values for conduction velocity in dog atria predicted a pathway for paroxysmal atrial tachycardia that was too long to be incorporated into the atrium. Ashman and Hull[3] and later Barker et al.[4] suggested that paroxysmal atrial tachycardia might be due to circus movement into and out of the sinus (SA) or atrioventricular (AV) nodes. The introduction of an element of slow conduction into the circus pathway decreased the minimal length of the pathway so that the length of the pathway was in accord with the dimensions of the atrium. In addition, Barker et al.[4] contrasted the effects of vagal stimulation on heart rate of patients in paroxysmal atrial tachycardia with those patients in atrial flutter. In the former instance, vagal stimulation sometimes decreased the rate and in the latter instance sometimes increased the rate. They argued that the increase in the rate of atrial flutter was consistent with the effects of vagal stimulation which shortened the effective refractory period of atrium and improved its conductivity, while the decrease in rate of paroxysmal atrial tachycardia was consistent with the depressant effects of vagal stimulation on AV conduction. Hence, it should be possible to differentiate between circus movement through the AV node and atrium. Further, if the effects of vagal stimulation on conduction in the SA and AV nodes were similar, then vagal stimulation should also slow the rate of a circus movement, whose pathway traversed through the SA node[4].

During the course of experiments performed on dogs, Wallace and Daggett[5] noted that during vagal stimulation reciprocal atrial beats appeared. These early atrial beats appeared to originate from the area of the SA node, suggesting that very slow intranodal conduction with block might be responsible for the generation of sinus node echoes[5,6]. Further, in 1968, Han et al.[7] argued that an atrial premature depolarization could block at one margin of the SA node while entering the SA node at another margin, propagate slowly through the SA node to reach the site of unidirectional block after sufficient delay so that it could re-emerge and re-excite the atrium. Using the isolated rabbit right atrial preparation, they demonstrated that during atrial pacing, early atrial premature depolarizations were often followed by atrial echoes. The sinus node response to the early atrial premature depolarizations was determined by recording transmembrane potentials from several locations within the sinus node and such recordings demonstrated slow intranodal conduction, incomplete excitation of the SA node, unidirectional block and electrotonic depolarizations during repolarization and diastole suggesting that nodal activation was fractionated[7]. Bonke et al.[8] demonstrated that a short atrial return cycle could also result from an early atrial premature depolarization that accelerated the sinus node pacemaker by blocking at a site outside the SA node, electrotonically depolarizing the pacemaker fibres and causing their premature discharge.

In electrophysiological studies performed in man Paulay et al.[9] observed that early atrial premature depolarizations elicited during normal sinus rhythm could cause a shortening of several subsequent atrial cycles and noted that P wave morphology and atrial activation sequences between the high and low right atrium were similar to those recorded for other sinus beats. Paulay et al.[9] also noted that the acceleration of atrial cycle length was independent of the site of stimulation, latency or current strength. In two patients, a zone in which early atrial premature depolarizations were followed by short atrial return cycles was identified, and in one patient the arrhythmia could be initiated and terminated by a single beat[9].

In acute experiments performed in dogs, Paulay et al.[10] noted that the occurrence of short atrial return cycles following early atrial premature depolarizations was more frequent during atrial pacing than during sinus rhythm, was independent of the site of stimulation and was dependent on the arrival time of the atrial premature depolarization in the region of the SA node. Such short return cycles were abolished by vagal stimulation and in those experiments in which the sinus node was crushed. In contrast, in a comparable series of dog experiments, Childers et al.[11] noted that vagal stimulation shifted the echo zone to the right. In another series of dog experiments, Ticzon et al.[12] noted that an echo zone frequently overlapped a zone of interpolation but found that once complete interpolation had occurred, short atrial return cycles could no longer be elicited by earlier atrial premature depolarizations.

These experiments have led other investigators to establish that short atrial return cycles following early atrial premature depolarizations may be demonstrated in man but that such short return cycles frequently do not generate prolonged episodes of tachycardia[9,13-16].

To further characterize the behaviour of the SA node during sinus node re-entry, we began a series of experiments in which the transmembrane potential was recorded from the SA node and an electrogram from the crista terminalis in the superfused rabbit right atrial preparation[17]. In our experiments we attempted to determine if we could predict the behaviour of the SA node by analysis of electrical activity in the atrium. Recordings of electrical activity from the surface of the crista terminalis were selected as the marker for atrial activation because activation of the crista terminalis coincides with the onset of the P wave in the body surface ECG, which would be used in the analysis of atrial cycle lengths in man. Atrial premature depolarizations were elicited during spontaneous rhythm and the atrial and SA node responses to such perturbations in rhythm were examined.

The following series of observations may in part explain why sinus node re-entry occurs relatively infrequently in man. In the isolated rabbit right atrial preparation, it has been shown that late atrial premature depolarizations (A_2) that fall within Zone I of atrial diastole are followed by compensatory atrial return (A_2A_3) cycles[12,17-21]. Atrial premature depolarizations elicited in Zone II at shorter A_1A_2 intervals are followed by less than compensatory A_2A_3 cycles. Such responses normalized by the last spontaneous sinus cycle (A_1A_1) are typically graphed in the manner that is illustrated in Figure 3.1. As the A_1A_2 interval is decreased to values that are less than 0.28 of A_1A_1 there is a sudden transition from an A_2A_3 cycle that is 1.35–1.47 of A_1A_1 to a shorter A_2A_3 cycle. Thereafter, as A_1A_2 progressively decreases, A_2A_3 decreases in value until A_2 is completely interpolated and falls on or near the interpolation line (Figure 3.1). Such interpolation responses are said to fall in Zone III of atrial diastole[12,21]. In such experiments where Zone III responses can be identified, the shortest A_1A_2 interval in Zone II has been used as a measure of the refractory period of the sinus node and/or SA junction[12,21]. However, analysis of the recordings obtained from the sinus node during such experiments revealed that A_1A_2 and corresponding sinus node intervals (SAN_1SAN_2) were not always closely correlated. In those experiments where Zone III responses were obtained, the shortest A_1A_2 intervals in Zone II were plotted as a function of the corresponding SAN_1SAN_2 interval (Figure 3.2). It can be seen that A_1A_2 responses, ranging between 125 and 135 msec, were associated with SAN_1SAN_2 intervals that ranged between 200 and 550 msec (Figure 3.2). That such a poor correlation exists between atrial and sinus node responses is not surprising and may be in part explained by referring to the ladder diagram illustrated in Figure 3.3.

We have used a traditional ladder diagram to depict the electrical activity in the sinus node, SA junction, and atrium. In addition, we have arbitrarily

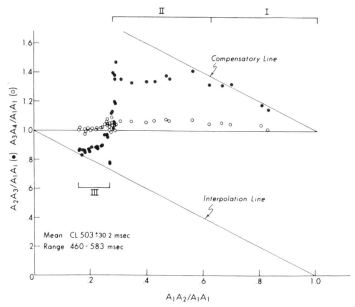

Figure 3.1   The normalized atrial return (A_2A_3/A_1A_1 ●) and post-return (A_3A_4/A_1A_1 ○) cycles are plotted as a function of the normalized atrial premature (A_1A_2/A_1A_1) cycle. The mean value ±1 SD of the A_1A_1 cycle was 503 ± 30.2 msec in this experiment, performed on a superfused isolated rabbit right atrial preparation. Late in atrial diastole atrial premature depolarizations are followed by compensatory A_2A_3 cycles that fall about the compensatory line (Zone I). As A_1A_2 is decreased A_2A_3 becomes less than compensatory (Zone II). At A_1A_2/A_1A_1 of 0.28 a discontinuity in the graph is present. Such a discontinuity suggests that different sinus node responses to A_2 are occurring. As A_1A_2 is further decreased A_2A_3 progressively decreases in value until complete interpolation occurs. Responses that are elicited at A_1A_2/A_1A_1 intervals that range between 0.16 and 0.28 are completely and incompletely interpolated (Zone III). In this experiment the long A_2A_3 cycles in Zone III coincided with large subthreshold depolarizations that depressed sinus node automaticity. As A_1A_2 decreased, the corresponding subthreshold depolarizations decreased in amplitude, presumably reflecting the shift of the site of block away from the sinus node side of the zone of perinodal fibres toward the crista terminalis side of the zone of perinodal fibres[19]. At an A_1A_2/A_1A_1 of 0.27 two short A_2A_3 cycles are noted. See text for further discussion.

designated a refractory period for the SA node that equals 250 msec. We have made three assumptions in constructing our ladder diagrams depicted in Figure 3.3: (1) SA conduction velocity is uniform throughout the sinoatrial junction; (2) antegrade and retrograde SA conduction times are equal; and (3) the effective refractory period of the SA node is independent of the SA conduction time. These three assumptions represent a gross oversimplification of the known experimental facts but the ladder diagram depicted in Figure 3.3 may still be of use in interpreting the data shown in Figure 3.2.

In Figure 3.3A where the SA conduction time equals 50 msec, A_2 elicited at an A_1A_2 interval of 130 msec encounters the effective refractory period of the SA node and is blocked. In Figure 3.3B, where the SA conduction time is 150 msec,

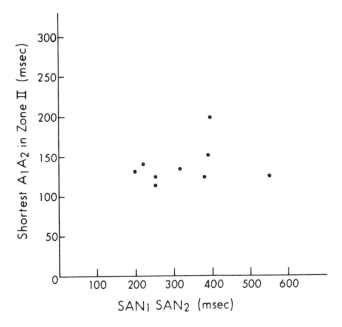

Figure 3.2 The shortest A_1A_2 cycles in Zone II (msec) are plotted against the corresponding SAN_1SAN_2 intervals (msec). These data were derived only from those experiments in which a Zone III was identified. These data show that A_1A_2 and SAN_1SAN_2 cycles do not correspond closely.

A_2 elicited at an identical coupling interval is conducted to the SA node and captures it. Hence, when A_2 is elicited during sinus rhythm the occurrence of SA entrance block will depend on the antegrade SA conduction time as well as the A_1A_2 interval, the retrograde conduction from the atrium to the SA node and the duration of the effective refractory period of the SA node and SA junction. The experimental observations depicted in Figure 3.2 would indicate that the effective refractory period of the SA node and SA junction when determined from an atrial pacing site should be determined during atrial pacing at a constant cycle length[11]. If disparity in refractoriness between the atrium and the sinus node is an important factor in the initiation of SA node re-entry, then the hypothesis depicted in the ladder diagrams in Figure 3.3 would suggest that a long sinoatrial conduction time might oppose the development of sinus node re-entry, and a short sinoatrial conduction time might favour the development of sinus node re-entry. This hypothesis would not only explain our observations illustrated in Figure 3.2 but also the observations of Paulay *et al.*[10], who demonstrated that short atrial return cycles following early atrial premature depolarizations could be more readily induced during atrial pacing than during spontaneous sinus rhythm.

We have elicited atrial extrasystoles in our isolated rabbit right atrial preparation and in many instances the pathway could not be localized with a single

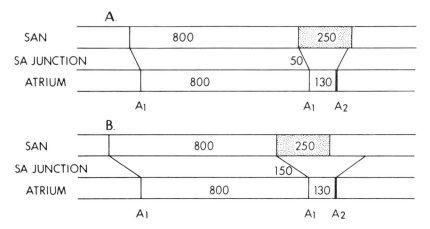

Figure 3.3 Diagrammatic representation of the effects that differences in sinoatrial conduction times might have on the ability of an atrial premature depolarization to capture and reset the SA node. It is assumed that the sinoatrial conduction time in panel A is 50 msec and in panel B 150 msec; and the refractory period of the SA node in both instances is 250 msec. The assumptions made in the ladder diagrams depicted in panels A and B are gross oversimplifications of the known experimental observations. In panel A an atrial premature depolarization elicited at an A_1A_2 interval of 130 msec fails to capture the SA node, but in panel B an A_2 at an identical A_1A_2 interval is able to conduct to the SA node and capture it. This diagrammatic representation would suggest that the antegrade sinoatrial conduction time as well as the refractory period of the SA node, retrograde conduction time between the crista terminals and SA node and A_1A_2 interval determine whether an A_2 that is elicited in normal sinus rhythm is interpolated or resets the SA node.

microelectrode. The data of the type of experiment illustrated in Figures 3.4–3.7 would most reasonably be explained by sinus node re-entrance. In the experiment depicted in Figure 3.4, atrial premature depolarizations elicited at coupling intervals between 0.985 and 0.385 of the atrial cycle A_1A_1 were followed by compensatory and less than compensatory responses as illustrated in Figure 3.1. However, at A_1A_2 intervals of <0.385 of A_1A_1 atrial premature depolarizations were followed by short A_2A_3 cycles. Two types of A_2A_3 responses were observed at short A_1A_2 intervals. A_2A_3 cycles that followed A_2 elicited at A_1A_2 intervals ranging between 0.29 and 0.38 of A_1A_1 (stippled bar) differed from the A_2A_3 cycles that followed A_2 elicited at A_1A_2 intervals that were <0.29 of A_1A_1. In the latter instance, the A_2 responses were incompletely interpolated. In the former instance, in contrast to the interpolated responses shown in Figure 3.1 as A_1A_2 decreased there was a corresponding lengthening of A_2A_3 cycles, describing a reciprocal relationship between A_2A_3 cycles. Second the A_3A_4 cycles corresponding to these A_2A_3 cycles (falling in the stippled area of the graph) are lengthened, whereas the A_3A_4 cycles corresponding to the incompletely interpolated A_2 responses are not. The short A_2A_3 cycles that fall within the stippled area of the graph are called SA node echoes or SA node re-entrant beats.

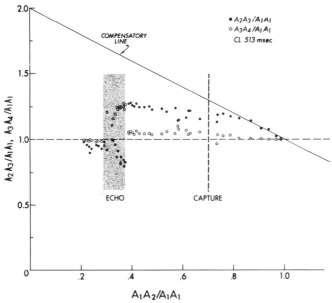

Figure 3.4   Return (A_2A_3/A_1A_1) and post-return (A_3A_4/A_1A_1) cycles are plotted as a function of the test cycle (A_1A_2/A_1A_1). As previously described[17], the transition from compensatory to less than compensatory A_2A_3 cycles occurred with late atrial premature depolarizations that failed to capture the SA node (vertical interrupted line). At A_1A_2/A_1A_1 intervals that range between 0.29 and 0.38 (stippled bar) A_2A_3 cycles are obtained that are shorter than the A_2A_3 cycles in Zone II, reciprocally related to A_1A_2, associated with prolonged A_3A_4 cycles and are interposed between the reset responses (at $A_1A_2/A_1A_1 > 0.38$) and the interpolation responses (at $A_1A_2/A_1A_1 < 0.29$). The A_2A_3 cycles that fall in the stippled area are identified as sinus node echoes.

Transmembrane potential recordings from the sinus node and electrogram recordings from the crista terminalis during a reset response, a SA node echo, and an incompletely interpolated response are illustrated in Figure 3.5. When A_2 is elicited at an A_1A_2 interval of 210 msec (panel A) it slowly conducts to the SAN recording site $(SAN_2A_2 - 135$ msec) and discharges the SA node and resets it so that A_2A_3 exceeds A_1A_1. The short SAN_2SAN_3 and SAN_3A_3 intervals suggest that a pacemaker shift has occurred. When A_2 is elicited at an A_1A_2 interval of 167 msec (panel B) the retrograde conduction time is further increased to 200 msec and now SAN_2 is followed by a short SAN_2SAN_3 cycle of 317 msec. In addition, SAN_3 and A_3 are approximately coincident in time. When A_1A_2 is decreased to 143 msec (panel C) A_2 fails to discharge the sinus node and is incompletely interpolated.

Sinus node echoes that follow atrial premature depolarizations elicited at different A_1A_2 intervals are illustrated in Figure 3.6. In panel A, an atrial premature depolarization elicited at an A_1A_2 interval of 191 msec slowly conducts to the SA node (155 msec) and is followed by SAN_3, where the SAN_2SAN_3 cycle (375 msec) is shorter than that observed following sinus node

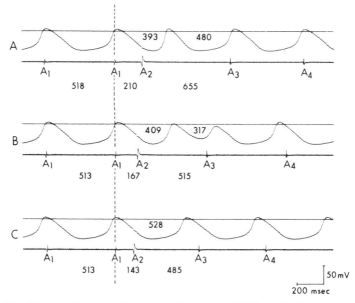

Figure 3.5 Transmembrane action potentials are recorded from the SA node and electrograms from the crista terminalis during spontaneous sinus rhythm and following A_2 elicited at three different coupling intervals. The vertical interrupted line indicates the last spontaneous atrial depolarization (A_1) that precedes A_2. In panel A, an A_2 elicited at a coupling interval of 210 msec is followed by a reset response. In panel B, an A_2 elicited at a coupling interval of 167 msec is followed by a sinus node echo. In panel C, an A_2 elicited at an interval of 143 msec is incompletely interpolated. Note that in contrast to panels A and C, the mergence between phases 4 and 0 of SAN_3 in panel B is sharp and not smooth.

reset. In addition, the sharp transition between phases 4 and 0 of SAN_3 indicates that the sinus node cell is driven and did not depolarize spontaneously. In panel A the interval between A_3 and SAN_3 is such that SAN_3 could have resulted from an A_3 that originated in the atrial appendage. As the A_1A_2 interval decreases in panels B–F of Figure 3.6 the following occurs: (1) A_2SAN_2 increases in duration; (2) SAN_2SAN_3 progressively decreases in duration, finally culminating in a fusion response (panel F); (3) coincident with the decrease in SAN_2SAN_3 interval is a progressive reduction in the diastolic membrane potential (shift toward 0 mV) between SAN_2 and SAN_3; and (4) SAN_3A_3 interval changes from a negative value in panel A to a positive value in panel E. These sequential changes between panels A and F are consistent with a premature impulse that travels behind the SA node to re-emerge and re-excite the atrium and then the SA node recording site (panel A). As A_1A_2 is decreased the pathway moves closer to the recording site in the SA node so that electrotonic interactions between the propagating impulse and the recording site occur, resulting in diastolic depolarization between SAN_2 and SAN_3 at the SA node recording site and now re-excitation of the SA node and crista terminalis coincide (panel D). A further decrease in the A_1A_2 coupling interval causes the fusion response

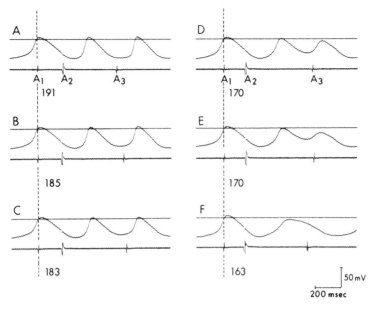

Figure 3.6 Transmembrane action potentials are recorded from the SA node and electrograms from the crista terminalis during six instances of SA reciprocation. The vertical interrupted line indicates the last spontaneous atrial depolarization (A_1) that precedes A_2. As A_1A_2 decreases from 191 msec in panel A to 163 msec in panel F there is an increase in retrograde conduction time to the SA node. A progressively more marked depolarization of the SA node occurs in the diastolic interval between SAN_2SAN_3 as the SAN_2SAN_3 interval decreases culminating in a fusion response shown in panel F. Further, the interval between SAN_3 and A_3 in panels B–F indicates that atrial re-excitation cannot account for SAN_3.

shown in panel F, as the pathway for the re-entrant SA node impulse moves even closer to the SA node recording site. The findings illustrated in Figure 3.6 would be consistent with transmembrane action potentials being recorded from the centre of a vortex of the type described by Allessie *et al.*[22] in the isolated left atrial appendage of the rabbit. If their findings can be applied to our study, one would postulate, that as A_1A_2 decreased the circuitous pathways, functionally dissociated, moved closer and closer together producing the fusion response shown in panel F. If such were the case, then the collision would have abolished the functional dissociation of the pathways and thus, the re-entrant circuit. In fact, earlier atrial premature depolarizations are blocked somewhere in the SA junction and are incompletely interpolated.

When the position of the echo zone relative to the refractory period of the SA node and SA junction is examined (Figure 3.7) one can see that refractoriness of the SA node and SA junction is quite prolonged with a marked increase in the retrograde conduction time between the crista terminalis and SA node (A_2SAN_2) occurring as the A_1A_2 interval decreases to less than 0.43 of A_1A_1. The echo zone ranged between 0.29 and 0.38 of A_1A_1 and fell in the portion of the SA node and SA

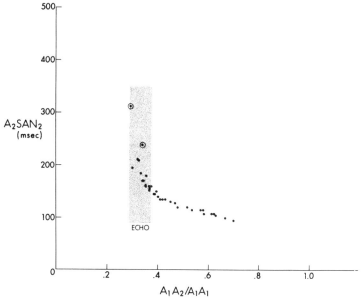

Figure 3.7 Retrograde conduction time between the crista terminalis and SA node (A_2SAN_2 msec) is plotted as a function of the normalized test cycle (A_1A_2/A_1A_1). Sinus node capture first occurs at an A_1A_2/A_1A_1 interval of 0.7. Thereafter, A_2SAN_2 increases as A_1A_2 decreases. Note that echo responses in the stippled area fall in the steep portion of the curve. The circled responses correspond to the fusion responses of the type shown in panel F of Figure 3.6.

junction relative refractory period where small decreases in A_1A_2 intervals caused large increases in A_2SAN_2 conduction times.

Exposure of the preparation of acetylcholine 1.1×10^{-6} M caused the cycle length to increase, the retrograde conduction time between the crista terminalis and the sinus node to increase, prolonged SA node and SA junction effective refractory period, widened the echo zone, shifted the echo zone to the right so that A_2 could elicit echo responses at longer A_1A_2 intervals than under control conditions and prolonged the A_2A_3 cycle of the echo. These findings would explain the results of Childers et al.[11], who showed that in the dog, vagal stimulation shifted the echo zone to the right and lengthened the A_2A_3 cycle of the echo. Presumably a greater concentration of acetylcholine would have so delayed intranodal conduction that the echoes would have been abolished. Such a sequence might explain the data of Paulay et al.[10], who observed that vagal stimulation abolished sinus node echoes. It should be pointed out that Paulay et al.[10] observed the effects of vagal stimulation in animals who had undergone excision of the stellate ganglia and the sympathetic chains.

It is apparent from these studies, that the duration of the A_2A_3 cycle of the echo is dependent on the length of the pathway, the refractory state of the tissues, and their conducting properties. In the examples shown in Figures 3.4–3.7, the A_2A_3 cycles of the echo responses were nearly equal in value to the

A_2A_3 cycles of incompletely interpolated responses. In other instances 'short' A_2A_3 cycles that fell just above the interpolation line (see A_2A_3 of 0.76 and 0.78 at A_1A_2 of 0.27 of A_1A_1 in Figure 3.1) or below the interpolation line (see Figure 3.1 of Ticzon et al.[12] and Figure 3.3 of Strauss et al.[21]) have been noted. Similar results have been observed by Paulay et al.[9] and Narula[13] who observed that the A_2A_3 cycle of sinus node re-entry may be 'short' ($A_1A_2 + A_2A_3 < A_1A_1$) or 'long' ($A_1A_2 + A_2A_3 > A_1A_1$, $A_2A_3 < A_1A_1$). Thus far we have not been able to document the pathways used by an A_2 that is followed by a 'short' A_2A_3 cycle.

Differentiation between a 'long' A_2A_3 cycle of a sinus node echo and an A_2A_3 cycle of an incomplete interpolation in man or intact animal experiments, by analysis of atrial cycles is at present uncertain. Our evidence would suggest that one should be able to demonstrate a zone of such responses that falls between a zone of reset and a zone of interpolation. In an echo zone one should be able to find a reciprocal relationship between A_2A_3 and A_1A_2, and prolonged A_3A_4 cycles. In addition vagal stimulation should shift the echo zone to the right, widen it and prolong the A_2A_3 cycle. In fact, such a reciprocal relationship between A_2A_3 and A_1A_1 has been demonstrated in one of the reported examples of 'sinus node re-entrance' with 'short' A_2A_3 cycles, i.e. the A_2A_3 cycles that fall below the interpolation line[21]. Whether such findings would indicate that such sinus node echoes associated with 'short' A_2A_3 cycles are due to similar mechanisms and utilize pathways similar to that reported in the isolated rabbit preparation is unknown. Although it is tempting to speculate on the mechanisms of such cycles reliance on P wave morphology, sequence of atrial activation between the high and low right atrium, coupled with the marked variation in spontaneous cycle length that occurs in many of these patients will make the task of establishing whether such single beats are due to SA node re-entry difficult. In those instances where multiple such beats occur, one would favour the re-entry mechanism. Further experiments are required to provide us with additional data that will then allow us to diagnose with greater certainty the arrhythmia known as sinus node re-entry in man.

Acknowledgement
This work was supported in part by US Public Health Service Grants: HL–19216, 08845, 15190, 05736, 07101, 1–K04–HL–00268 and by a Grant-In-Aid from the NC Heart Association.

References

1. Iliescu, C. C. and Sebastiani, A. (1923). Notes on the effects of quinidine upon paroxysms of tachycardia. *Heart*, **10**, 223
2. Lewis, T. (1924). *The Mechanism and Graphic Registration of the Heart Beat*, 3rd edn. (London: Shaw and Sons), pp. 240, 319
3. Ashman, R. and Hull, E. (1938). *Essentials of Electrocardiography*. 1st edn. (New York: MacMillan), p. 170

4. Barker, P. S., Wilson, F. N. and Johnston, F. D. (1943). The mechanism of auricular paroxysmal tachycardia. *Am. Heart J.*, **26**, 435

5. Wallace, A. G. and Daggett, W. M. (1964). Re-excitation of the atrium. The echo phenomenon. *Am. Heart J.*, **68**, 661

6. Hoffman, B. F. and Cranefield, P. F. (1960). *Electrophysiology of the Heart.* (New York: McGraw-Hill), p. 124

7. Han. J., Malozzi, A. M. and Moe, G. K. (1968). Sino-atrial reciprocation in the isolated rabbit heart. *Circ. Res.*, **22**, 355

8. Bonke, F. I. M., Bouman, L. N. and Schopman, F. J. G. (1971). Effect of an early atrial premature beat on activity of the sino-atrial node and atrial rhythm in the rabbit. *Circ. Res.*, **29**, 704

9. Paulay, K. L., Varghese, P. J. and Damato, A. N. (1973). Atrial rhythms in response to an early atrial premature depolarization in man. *Am. Heart J.*, **85**, 323

10. Paulay, K. L., Varghese, P. J. and Damato, A. N. (1973). Sinus node reentry. An *in vivo* demonstration in the dog. *Circ. Res.*, **32**, 455

11. Childers, R. W., Arnsdorf, M. F., de la Fuente, D. J., Gambetta, M. and Svenson, R. (1973). Sinus nodal echoes. *Am. J. Cardiol.*, **31**, 220

12. Ticzon, A. R., Strauss, H. C., Gallagher, J. J. and Wallace, A. G. (1975). Sinus nodal function in the intact dog heart evaluated by premature atrial stimulation and atrial pacing. *Am. J. Cardiol.*, **35**, 492

13. Narula, O. S. (1974). Sinus node re-entry. A mechanism for supraventricular tachycardia. *Circulation*, **50**, 1114

14. Paritzky, A., Obayaski, K. and Mandel, W. J. (1974). Atrial tachycardia secondary to sino-atrial node reentry. *Chest*, **66**, 526

15. Castellanos, A., Aranda, J., Moleiro, F., Mallon, S. M. and Befeler, B. (1976). Effects of the pacing site in sinus node re-entrant tachycardia. *J. Electrocardiol.*, **9**, 165

16. Coumel, P., Attuel, P. and Flammang, D. (1976). The role of the conduction system in supraventricular tachycardias. In: *The Conduction System of the Heart. Structure, Function and Clinical Implications.* Wellens, H. J. J., Lie, K. I. and Janse, M. J. (eds.). (Leiden: H. E. Stenfert Kroese BV), p. 424

17. Miller, H. C. and Strauss, H. C. (1974). Measurement of sinoatrial conduction time by premature atrial stimulation in the rabbit. *Circ. Res.*, **35**, 935

18. Bonke, F. I. M., Bouman, L. N. and Van Rijn, H. E. (1969). Change of cardiac rhythm in the rabbit after an atrial premature beat. *Circ. Res.*, **24**, 533

19. Strauss, H. C. and Bigger, J. T., Jr. (1972). Electrophysiological properties of the rabbit sinoatrial perinodal fibers. *Circ. Res.*, **31**, 490

20. Strauss, H. C., Saroff, A. L., Bigger, J. T., Jr. and Giardina, E. G. V. (1973). Premature atrial stimulation as a key to the understanding of sinoatrial conduction in man. *Circulation*, **47**, 86

21. Strauss, H. C., Bigger, J. T., Jr., Saroff, A. L. and Giardina, E. G. V. (1976). Electrophysiologic evaluation of sinus node function in patients with sinus node dysfunction. *Circulation*, **53**, 763

22. Allessie, M. A., Bonke, F. I. M. and Schopman, F. J. G. (1973). Circus movement in rabbit atrial muscle as a mechanism of tachycardia. *Circ. Res.*, **33**, 54

4
Paroxysmal Reciprocating Sinus Tachycardia

P. V. L. CURRY and D. M. KRIKLER

Division of Cardiovascular Medicine, The Royal Postgraduate Medical School,
Hammersmith Hospital, London

INTRODUCTION

The concept that one form of paroxysmal supraventricular tachycardia might be due to sustained impulse re-entry within the region of the sinoatrial node was proposed originally more than 30 years ago by Barker, Wilson and Johnson[1] and again, somewhat more recently, by Wallace and Daggett[2]. An analogy between the mechanisms of sinoatrial (SA) and atrioventricular (AV) nodal re-entry tachycardias arose on the basis of known similarities in the structure and electrophysiological function of these two regions, but it was only in 1968 that Han, Malozzi and Moe[3] transformed the concept into a reality by demonstrating that re-entry of an impulse in the SA node could indeed occur.

Recent studies in animals[4-7] have clarified further the features of sinoatrial reciprocation and it is from these that a more meaningful interpretation of responses observed during electrophysiological studies in man has developed[7,8]. However it should be emphasized that both our clinical and electrophysiological knowledge of this arrhythmia in man is limited especially when compared with that concerning the presentation, mechanisms, management, and prognosis of AV re-entry tachycardia. It is interesting to examine the reasons for this comparative ignorance and to see why the arrhythmia has so far been recognized more often as an interesting electrophysiological abnormality than as a significant clinical problem.

In the first instance, it is clear from the few available clinical reports that paroxysmal reciprocating sinus tachycardia (PRST)[9] produces symptoms which are usually mild and of short duration; only rarely are attacks so troublesome as to demand medical advice. This is in marked contrast to the more rapid and intense paroxysms of re-entry AV tachycardia, of which patients are less tolerant. Even where attacks of PRST are more troublesome because of repetitive occurrence, higher heart rate or association with other symptoms such as angina, the diagnosis may remain unrecognized: indeed, even where the physician has recorded the arrhythmia electrocardiographically, the appearances of sinus tachycardia at a rate which is usually between 85 and 160 beats per min, may lead him to assume that this has an 'appropriate' cause such as anxiety, and the patient is reassured about his or her 'undue awareness of the normal heart beat'. The minimum criteria for suspecting the diagnosis of PRST are a history of truly paroxysmal tachycardia associated with ECG recordings which document, on more than one occasion, the abrupt initiation and/or termination of an apparent sinus tachycardia which is *inappropriate* to the circumstances.

Only as awareness of the existence of this arrhythmia increases will some idea of its incidence be obtained; and even then, the requirements will be that the patient gives a precise account, the physician has a high index of suspicion for the disorder, and that the ECG clearly reveals the abnormality. Continuous ambulatory taped recordings of the ECG will sometimes be required.

The second diagnostic problem relates to technical difficulties which arise during the investigation of this arrhythmia using intracardiac recordings and programmed electrical stimulation. It is now realized that, while the ability to both initiate and terminate a tachycardia reproducibly by single critically timed premature beats over a specific zone strongly favours re-entry as the mechanism, more decisive evidence is provided if it can also be demonstrated that a large circuit exists (macro-re-entry): this is in contrast to impulse re-entry that occurs within a small circuit (micro-re-entry) and which may be clinically indistinguishable from focal activity. Such a demonstration entails the use of specific interventions during tachycardia with observations of their effects on regional activation times and conduction sequences in different parts of the circuit[10]. While these requirements can be met in cases of reciprocating tachycardias associated with the Wolff–Parkinson–White (WPW) syndrome, and to a lesser extent in cases of intra-AV nodal reciprocation, it is not possible when re-entry tachycardias involve the SA node. The inability to obtain recordings from within the SA node means that the locations and conduction times of both the anterograde ('α') and retrograde ('β') SA pathways and the location of their inner reflection point within the SA node remain unknown in such cases. This means that with rare exceptions[11] conclusive evidence of macro-re-entry involving the SA node in paroxysmal sinus tachycardia cannot be obtained with existing techniques.

CLINICAL FEATURES OF PAROXYSMAL RECIPROCATING SINUS TACHYCARDIA

The first clinical and electrophysiological studies of PRST were reported in 1972 by Narula[12] (two cases) and one year later by Childers *et al.*[5] (one case) and Paulay, Varghese and Damato[13] (two cases). More cases have been described since then, but to date the literature contains less than 30 such reports. The clinical features described in this chapter are based both on these reports[11,14-19] and on our own experience of eight similar cases[20], Table 4.1.

Table 4.1 Clinical details of patients with PRST

Patient	Age	Sex	Diagnosis	History	Tachycardias Incidence	Duration	Severity
1	68	F	Paroxysmal tachycardia Ischaemic HD Hypertension	6 years	frequent. up to 20 per day	1–5 min	moderate palpitations; angina provoked
2	69	F	SA node disease Brady-tachy syndrome Hypertension	1 year	variable. up to 2 per day	3–20 min	mild palpitations
3	75	F	Paroxysmal tachycardia Hypertension	2 years	variable. sometimes repetitive.	2–8 min	mild to moderate palpitations
4	51	F	Paroxysmal tachycardia WPW syndrome Type A	14 years (PRAVTS)	unknown	unknown	unknown
5	40	F	SA node disease Brady-tachy syndrome Mild hypertension	unknown (PAFibrill'n)	unknown	unknown	unknown
6	41	M	SA node disease	unknown	unknown	unknown	unknown
7	11	M	SA node disease Brady-tachy syndrome Ventricular pre-excitation Cardiomyopathy	1 year	repetitive	few beats–1 min	very mild palpitations
8	31	M	Paroxysmal tachycardia Mild hypertension	2 years	6 per week sometimes repetitive	1–2 min	mild palpitations

PRAVT = paroxysmal re-entry AV tachycardia
PAFibrill'n = paroxysmal atrial fibrillation

Age and sex
Sinus node re-entry appears to occur in all age groups although it has not yet been reported in infants. PRST was found in children in four separate studies[15,17,19,20] although the majority of reported cases occur between the ages of 30 and 70; one of the first cases reported was that of an 85-year-old male[14]. PRST appears to affect both sexes.

Association with heart disease
Some form of heart disease or hypertension (or both) is found in most patients

with PRST, but this relationship may in part reflect the selection that occurs in a situation where the specific rhythm disorder is only rarely the primary abnormality for which the patient is referred. PRST undoubtedly occurs in normal subjects: 3 of 5[19], 2 of 6[16]; 1 of 8[20]; 1 of 5[15]; or may be found in patients whose only other abnormality is a ventricular pre-excitation syndrome: 2 of 3[17]; 1 of 8[20]. What we call PRST occurred in 3 of 139 cases of WPW syndrome recently reviewed by Wellens (personal communication).

The association of PRST with SA disease is unclear: four patients in our series had suspected SA disease, as did a case reported by Coumel[11] and two of the five cases reported by Gillette[19]. In other series, resting heart rates appear to be normal although studies dealing mainly with the induction of sinus node echoes report a higher incidence of SA disease[8,12]. In contrast, sinus node echoes have been reported to occur in 11% of patients without SA disease[21].

Presentation

In our series, the mean rate of the tachycardias was 105 beats a min (range 80–142) which is similar to that reported by others[14–17]: rarely more rapid rates have been reported (187[16]; 200[19]).

Very few reports deal with the patients' description of their attacks. Mild, barely detectable or vague attacks of palpitations that were usually short-lived but which could be repetitive were the most common complaint in our series (Figure 4.1). Except for case 6, patients were aware of paroxysmal tachycardias, but in two, the documentation of tachyarrhythmias other than paroxysmal sinus tachycardia (AV re-entry tachycardias in association with the WPW syndrome, case 14; and paroxysmal atrial fibrillation, case 5) rendered the further assessment of the features of PRST from their history unreliable. In only two cases was PRST the primary reason for their referral and only in these and one other case was the diagnosis suspected before the intracardiac study; this pattern was characteristic of other series in which most cases were also diagnosed during the intracardiac study. One patient noted paroxysmal angina pectoris related more to her attacks of palpitations than to exertion.

In one series[17], all patients experienced paroxysmal tachycardias although two patients also had the WPW syndrome. Only half the patients described by Weisfogel et al.[16] had palpitations: one was asymptomatic while two others had either dyspnea or vague dizziness. We would like to stress that PRST in association with symptomatic bradycardia constitutes one form of the bradycardia–tachycardia syndrome.

Narula[14] recently reported 20 patients whose ages ranged from 49 to 85 years in whom it was possible to induce sinus node echoes; however in only two of these was the PRST sustained (in one after the administration of atropine) While only one patient in this group had unexplained palpitations, six had atrial tachyarrhythmias including atrial fibrillation and atrial flutter, and many had dizziness or syncope. Eight had underlying coronary heart disease, while

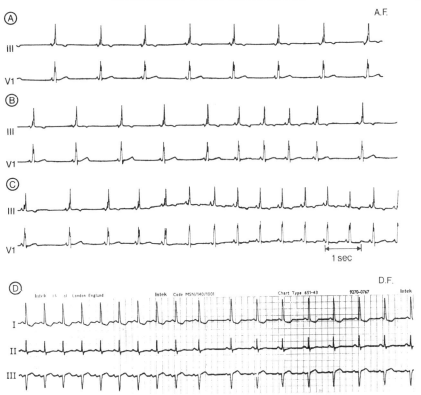

Figure 4.1   The three panels A, B and C show non-continuous ECG recordings of standard lead 1 simultaneously with lead V₁ in case 7. Upper panel A shows the basic sinus bradycardia (rate 50–60 b.p.m.) while in the central panel B, the spontaneous initiation and termination of a brief paroxysm of sinus node tachycardia and in the lower panel C, the spontaneous initiation of a sustained attack of PRST without an antecedent atrial extrasystole can be seen. The heart rate during sinus node tachycardia is *ca.* 90 b.p.m. (panel C)

In panel D (Case 3), simultaneous ECG recordings of standard leads I, II and III show the characteristically abrupt termination of PRST following a slight prolongation of the last cycle of the tachycardia. The P wave configuration during PRST is similar to that during the basic sinus rhythm

five had valvular, pulmonary vascular or myopathic heart diease. Four had average heart rates of less than 60 beats per min during sinus rhythm; but only two had significant prolongation of the sinus node recovery time.

INTRACARDIAC STUDIES IN PATIENTS WITH PRST

Methods

As indicated earlier, most cases of PRST are only recognized incidentally at the time of an electrophysiological study undertaken to investigate other specific abnormalities of rhythm. Occasionally, PRST is noted only during the detailed analysis following the intracardiac study. As a consequence, few investigators have undertaken detailed mapping of the SA node region during attacks of PRST, or have performed tests to confirm the presence or absence of macro-re-entry during the (usually brief) attacks. The minimum number of recording sites in the right atrium required for the study of PRST is two: the high right atrium (HRA), and the His bundle electrogram (HBE) which includes the low right atrium (LRA)[22]. In our series at least one other right or left atrial (coronary sinus, CSE) electrode was in position in each case. Four surface electrocardiograms (Leads I, III, V1 and V6) were recorded simultaneously with the regional endocardial bipolar electrograms; any changes that occurred in the P wave configuration during the induction of PRST[20,23] were more obvious this way. Filtering and amplification of all atrial electrograms (frequency response range as for HBE; 50–500 Hz) permitted more detailed observations of changes which occurred in their individual configurations during induced changes in rhythm, and was particularly valuable in the case of HRA recordings.

Sinus node function was studied using two standard pacing programmes (Devices stimulator 4279): the right atrial extrastimulus test during sinus or regularly paced rhythm in which the cardiac cycle was scanned by introducing single premature depolarizations at progressively shorter coupling intervals down to the atrial effective refractory period[3,24]; and continuous atrial pacing[25,26] at different rates (90, 120, 150 beats per min) for different periods (30, 60, 180 sec). Where sustained tachycardias were initiated by either one or both of these techniques, the tachycardia cycle was scanned by triggered premature depolarizations to define the nature and location of the mechanism[10,27]. Similarly, the effects of carotid–sinus massage (CSM) on the tachycardia were examined where possible. In five patients, these tests were repeated following the intravenous administration of verapamil; atropine was given in two other cases.

Definition of terms

(1) Electrograms

A1   the atrial electrogram of either a sinus or paced beat of the spontaneous or regularly driven basic rhythm respectively.

A2   the atrial electrogram of a premature depolarization induced at a specified site in the atria.

A_3, A_4, A_5 (etc.)   the atrial electrograms of the first, second, third, (etc.) spontaneous return beats following A_2 due variously to sinus node escape beats, sinus node echoes or atrial repetitive firing.

(2) Intervals and conduction times (measured in msec)

A_1–A_1 the duration of spontaneous or regularly paced cycles of the basic rhythm prior to induction of the premature atrial beat A_2.

A_1–A_2 duration of the shortened test cycle.

A_2–A_3 (A_3–A_4, etc.) duration of the first (second, etc.) atrial return cycle following the induced premature atrial beat A_2.

Sinus node recovery time

the longest sinus node escape time following sinus node suppression by over-drive atrial pacing[25,26].

Sinoatrial conduction time

the sum of the anterograde and retrograde conduction times of the sinoatrial node calculated by subtracting the cycle length of sinus rhythm (A_1–A_1) from the first post-extrasystolic return cycle (A_2–A_3) when values for the latter inter-val have become virtually constant and indicate reproducible invasion and reset of sinus node pacemaker cells by the atrial premature beats introduced during the latter half of a spontaneous sinus cycle. The value and limitations of this test have recently been reviewed[24].

A review of the electrophysiological criteria used to diagnose sinus node re-entry during the studies is given later.

Illustrative cases

Figure 4.1 shows examples of paroxysmal reciprocating sinus node tachycardia (PRST) documented electrocardiographically prior to intracardiac elec-trophysiological studies in cases 7 (panels A–C) and 3 (panel D). Note the similarity in P wave configuration between beats of the spontaneous sinus rhythm and those of the PRST. Both the termination and the initiation of PRSTs in Figure 4.1 occur spontaneously following a minor change in cycle length but without being due to an extrasystole. In neither case was there an 'appropriate' reason for such a sudden change in heart rate during the routine recording of their ECG. The termination in Figure 1(D) is very similar to that in a recent report[18].

Table 4.2 shows the variation in heart rate of the basic sinus rhythm for each

Table 4.2   Studies in Sinus Rhythm

Case	Sinus rate (b.p.m.)	PA (msec)	AH (msec)	HV (msec)	Sinoatrial conduction time (msec)	Sinus node recovery time (msec)	Presence of V to A conduction	ERPA (msec)
1	64–77	50	70	50	330	800–1120	0	260
2	55–76	40	100	30	280	1300 1600	0	300
3	65–75	60	70	45	200	950–1350	0	280
4	85–102	35	95	30	220	800–940	+	220
5	55–66	50	80	30	211	800–1050	0	340
6	44–52	50	115	30	200	1300–1500	+	310
7	50–60	30	70	20	280	1100–1600	0	220
8	68–82	45	100	35	230	800–900	0	200

ERPA = effective refractory period of the atria

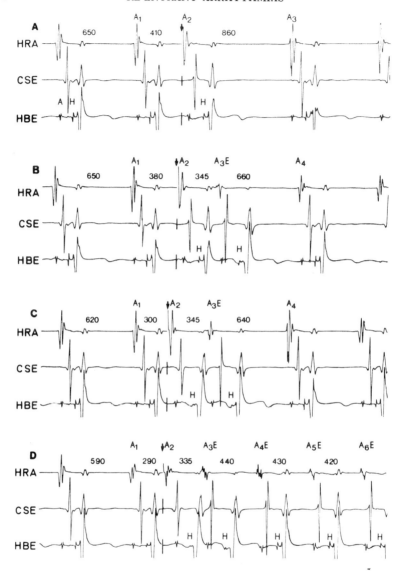

Figure 4.2 Case 4: Panels A to D show the responses obtained from an atrial extrastimulus test during sinus rhythm (BCL 590–650 msec). Each panel shows recordings from three intracardiac leads: the high right atrium, HRA; the coronary sinus, CSE; and the His bundle, HBE. In the upper panel A, a high right atrial extrastimulus with an A_1–A_2 coupling interval of 410 msec produces the first reset of the SA node (A_1–A_3 = 860 + 4; P = *1270* msec; which is slightly less than twice the sinus cycle, *1300* msec) giving an estimated SA conduction time of 210 msec $[(A_2$–$A_3)$–$(A$–$A_1)]$. In panels B and C, premature atrial extrastimuli (A2) induce sinus node echoes (A3E) over a wide A_1–A_2 coupling zone (300–380 msec). In panel D a slightly earlier extrastimulus (A_1–A_2 290 msec) initiates sinus node re-entry tachycardia whose cycle length is 420–440 msec

of the eight patients with PRST; four cases (2, 5, 6 and 7) had heart rates that were frequently lower than 60 beats per min between attacks. The intracardiac conduction intervals for intra-AV nodal conduction (AH), His bundle to ventricle conduction (HV) and for inter-nodal intra-atrial conduction (PA), were normal in all patients during sinus rhythm with the exception of case 3 in whom the PA time was slightly prolonged at 60 msec, and case 7 who had ventricular pre-excitation and consequently a shortened HV interval of 20 ms. Case 4, who had intermittent WPW syndrome, only rarely showed evidence of ventricular pre-excitation and consequently a shortened HV interval of 20 msec. Case 4, who patients exceeded a value of 215 msec; a value found in 38% of patients with symptomatic SA disease in a recent study by Strauss et al.[8]. Three patients had atrial effective refractory periods (ERPA, defined as the longest A1–A2 interval at which the extrastimulus A2 just fails to activate the atrium during an extrastimulus test) with values of greater than 300 msec although all three also had sinus bradycardia during their extrastimulus tests. Three patients (cases 2, 6 and 7) had sinus node recovery times exceeding 1500 msec[8,26]. Only two patients showed intact ventriculo-atrial conduction during ventricular pacing (cases 4 and 6).

Table 4.3 presents the collected data on sinus node re-entrant phenomena induced during the electrophysiological studies in the eight patients. In all patients there was a 'zone' over which coupled extrastimuli introduced at different specified sites evoked sinus node echoes and initiated reciprocating sinus node tachycardia (PRST). In five patients (cases 1, 2, 5, 7 and 8) sinus node re-entry was initiated by extrastimuli more reproducibly, and over a wider A_1–A_2 coupling zone, during a regularly paced rhythm than during spontaneous sinus rhythm. In the two patients with intact ventriculo-atrial conduction, ventricular pacing also initiated sinus node re-entry (cases 4 and 6). The zone over which coupled premature atrial extrastimuli induced sinus node re-entrant responses was independent of the stimulation site during regular pacing. Weisfogel et al.[16] showed that a slightly wider and later zone for PRST initiation (250–470 msec) was obtained when extrastimuli were given from the HRA when compared with that obtained by stimulating the coronary sinus (CS; 280–420 msec) during sinus rhythm in one of their patients.

PRST was initiated with extrastimuli during sinus rhythm in seven patients; however, in one of these (case 5) two consecutive extrastimuli were needed (Figure 4.4). In seven patients who also had extrastimuli introduced during regular paced rhythms, PRST could be initiated by single premature beats alone. In only two patients did sinus node echoes occur in a zone of responses which included completely and incompletely interpolated A_2 extrastimuli (cases 5 and 8); the distinction between these two types of response was sometimes impossible unless two consecutive echoes or PRSTs were initiated at the same A_1–A_2 coupling interval. In both of these cases the 'gap' phenomenon in retrograde conduction into the SA node was seen during the atrial extrastimulus test[28,29].

Table 4.3 Paroxysmal Reciprocating Sinus Tachycardia (PRST)

Case	Initiation of sinus node re-entry by:				Paroxysmal re-entry sinus tachycardia (PRST)					Termination of PRST		
	Atrial extrastimulus tests			Atrial pacing; lowest atrial rate which starts PRST (b.p.m.)	BCL in msec (rate, b.p.m.)	Duration (maximum)	P wave on ECG	PA interval (msec)	HRA electrogram	Pacing site for termination by single APB	Spontaneous terminations	Effect of CSM
	Pacing site	BCL of basic rhythm (msec)	PRST initiation 'zone' (A₁–A₂: msec)									
1	HRA HRA	800 SR 670 AP	620 325–390	not initiated	420–490 (143) (122)	sustained	slight change	40	changed	HRA	+	slows and stops
	LA	670 AP	360–380							LA		
2	HRA HRA	900 SR 650 AP	— 330–370	150	450–470 (133) (128)	sustained	slight	30	changed	HRA	+	slows
3	MRA	800 SR	390–480	90	670–720 (90) (83)	sustained	as for SB	50	changed	MRA	+	slows and stops
4	HRA RV	630 SR 600 VP	280–300 335	160	420–500 (143) (120)	26 beats	slight change	35	changed	—	+	not tried

5	HRA	930 SR (only double extra-stimuli) 350–640 400	165	500–660 (120)(91)	10 beats	as for SB	50	sl. changed	—	+	not tried
	HRA	780 AP								
6	HRA RV	1100 SR 695 VP 700 655	not initiated	670–750 (90)(80)	20 beats	as for SB	50	as for SB	—	+	slows and stops
7	HRA	1100 SR 400	120	590–670 (120) (90)	30 beats	as for SB	30	as for SB	HRA	+	not tried
	HRA	620 AP 320								
8	HRA	750 SR 270	150	540–600 (111) (100)	18 beats	as for SB	45	as for SB	—	+	slows and stops
	HRA	600 AP 260–270								

SR = sinus rhythm; AP = atrial pacing; VP = ventricular pacing; SB = sinus beats; CSM = carotid sinus massage; APB = atr al premature beat; BCL = basic cycle length; PA = intra-atrial conduction time between sinus and AV node; LA = Left atrium; RV = Right ventricle; HRA = High right atrium

Figure 4.2 shows the induction of sinus node echoes and the initiation of PRST during an atrial extrastimulus test in case 4. The sinus node echo zone is wide, but PRST is only initiated during a specific part of this zone. The fixed sinus node echo cycle (A_2-A_{3E}) and constant second return cycle of the first sinus node escape beat $(A_{3E}-A_4)$ are best explained by assuming an induced delay in retrograde (atrio-sinus) conduction time caused by the premature atrial stimulus A_2 which also resets the sinus node. The sequence of atrial activation both in sinus node echo beats and during PRST is similar to that of sinus beats; the high right atrial electrogram (HRA) however changes during sinus node re-entrant responses.

Figure 4.3 shows both the initiation (upper panel A) and termination of PRST (lower panel B) by a critically-timed atrial premature beat (case 3). The sequences of atrial activation for both sinus and sinus node re-entrant beats are identical, but the high right atrial electrogram is again altered during PRST. The P waves of sinus beats and of PRST beats are similar in leads I, III, V_1 and V_6. The phenomenon of 'polarization of conduction' is shown in this figure in the two spontaneous sinus node escape beats following termination of the tachycardia in the lower panel B. The mechanism of this phenomenon is discussed later (Figure 4.13).

Figure 4.4 shows the initiation of PRST in case 5 by two atrial extrastimuli (upper panel A) and at the same time demonstrates the independence of the PRST mechanism from AV nodal behaviour. The second atrial extrastimulus initiates PRST at a time when the AV node is refractory. In the lower panel B, AV nodal conduction is restored at a slightly longer A_1-A_2 interval, but even with optimal intra-AV nodal delay, PRST fails to start.

Figure 4.5 shows the wide A_1-A_2 coupling interval which starts PRST (lower panel B) in case 7, and that the PRST mechanism is not only independent of induced AV nodal conduction delays but also of intra-atrial delays which occur in the atrial relative refractory period (upper panel A).

In six cases, PRST could be initiated by continuous atrial pacing such as is used to measure the sinus node recovery time. All spontaneously initiated attacks of PRST which were documented electrocardiographically appeared to start following gradual shortening of the spontaneous sinus cycle length, a mechanism which may be related to that whereby PRST is initiated during continuous atrial pacing (Figure 4.6).

Intra-atrial conduction times were slightly altered in three patients (cases 1–3) during PRST compared with values recorded in sinus rhythm. The sequence of atrial activation was otherwise similar before and during PRST in all cases. P wave configurations altered slightly in four patients while HRA configurations changed in five patients during PRST and in sinus node echo beats when compared with those recorded in sinus rhythm. 'Polarization' of sinus node exit pathways affected the configurations of the HRA electrograms of the first one or more sinus node escape beats following termination of PRST in cases 2 and 3.

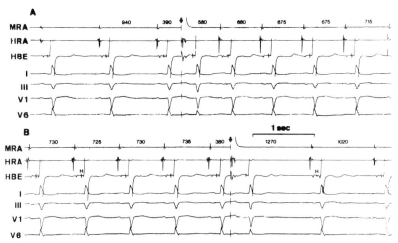

Figure 4.3 Case 3: In the upper panel A, an atrial premature depolarization (arrowed) introduced in the mid right atrium (MRA) with an A_1–A_2 coupling interval of 390 msec initiates PRST whose cycle length varies betwen 675 and 735 msec. The sequences of atrial activation and intra-atrial conduction times during PRST remain similar to those seen in sinus rhythm, however the configuration of the high right atrial electrogram (HRA) has changed. P wave configurations in the simultaneously recorded ECG leads I, III, V_1 and V_6 are similar in both of the spontaneous and re-entrant sinus node rhythms. In the lower panel B, a critically timed atrial extrastimulus with an A_1–A_2 coupling interval of 380 msec terminates the tachycardia.

Note that the HRA electrogram of the first sinus node escape beat after the termination of PRST has a configuration similar to that seen during the tachycardia while that of the second spontaneous sinus beat resembles that seen in sinus rhythm prior to the initiation of the tachycardia (for an explanation of this phenomenon see text and Figure 3.11)

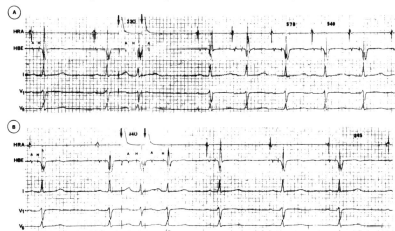

Figure 4.4 Case 5: The upper panel A shows the initiation of reciprocating sinus node tachycardia by double premature atrial extrastimuli (arrowed) introduced at the high right atrium (HRA) during sinus rhythm. The second stimulus activates the atrium but fails to be conducted through to the His bundle being blocked in the AV node (A, but no H on the HBE); it is therefore highly unlikely that the mechanism of the tachycardia involves the AV node. The lower panel B is included for comparison, showing failure of the paired atrial premature beats to initiate sinus node re-entry tachycardia when the second extra stimulus is only 10 msec later than in the upper panel A; despite conduction through the AV node being restored providing long intra-AV nodal delays

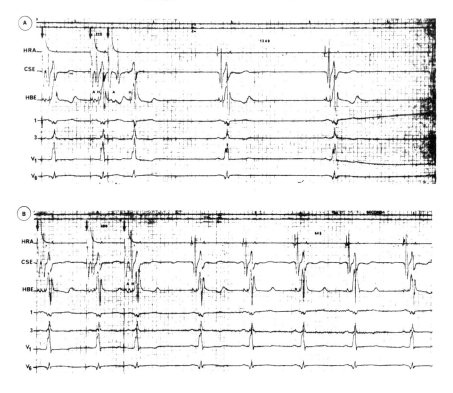

Figure 4.5 Case 7: A shows an interpolated atrial premature beat introduced in the high right atrium (HRA) with an A_1-A_2 coupling interval of 225 msec after the eighth beat of a regularly paced atrial rhythm (BCL 620 msec). The sinus node escape time which is calculated from the last beat of the basic driven rhythm to the first sinus node escape beat is 1600 msec. In the lower panel, B, an atrial premature beat at an A_1-A_2 coupling interval of 480 msec, initiates a reciprocating sinus node tachycardia which has a cycle length of 645 msec. Initiation of the tachycardia is clearly not dependent on critical changes in AV nodal conduction time (AH) induced by premature atrial beats

The cycle length of PRST ranged from 420 to 750 msec (mean = 570 msec). The maximum cycle length variation was 160 msec (case 5) although some variation was seen in all cases. In only four cases were attacks of PRST sustained for long enough periods to permit the study of the effects of triggered extrastimuli on the tachycardia mechanism from one or more different sites. Figure 4.7 shows the initiation of PRST in case 1 (upper panel A) and compares the efficacy of single premature beats, triggered to interrupt the tachycardia from two different sites: the mid right atrium (MRA) in panel B and the left atrium (LA) in panel C respectively. The MRA extrastimulus given nearer to the PRST circuit terminates the tachycardia (panel B) despite its having been given later in the tachycardia cycle than the LA extrastimulus which fails to

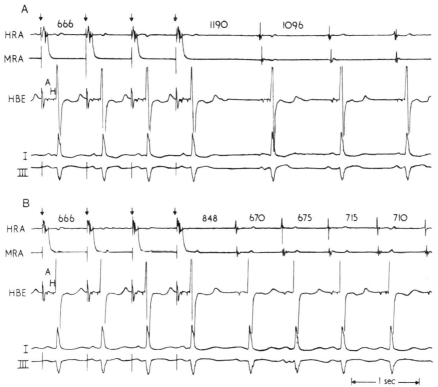

Figure 4.6 Case 3: Upper panel A. The sinus node recovery time after atrial pacing for 30 sec at a BCL of 666 msec (90 b.p.m.) is 1190 msec. In the lower panel B, atrial pacing at the same BCL is continued for 60 sec which results in the initiation of paroxysmal reciprocating sinus node tachycardia (PRST) with a cycle length of 670 and 715 msec

terminate PRST due to loss of 'effective' prematurity in traversing the much greater intra-atrial distance between its site of introduction and the SA node.

Attacks of PRST could terminate spontaneously in all patients; sometimes abruptly (Figure 4.8), at other times after a variable period of slowing. Figure 4.9 shows the initiation of PRST in case 4 by a suitably timed HRA extrastimulus (upper panel A) and the subsequent gradual slowing and spontaneous termination of the tachycardia with restoration of sinus rhythm (lower panel B).

All five patients in whom the effects of carotid sinus massage on PRST were assessed showed slowing of the tachycardia; four had attacks terminated by this method (Figure 4.10).

Verapamil was given intravenously (10 mg) during sustained PRSTs in two patients and in both terminated the tachycardia within one minute. Attempts to reinitiate PRST after verapamil in five patients were unsuccessful; even sinus node echoes were suppressed. Atropine (0.6 mg) favoured the initiation and maintenance of PRST in two patients.

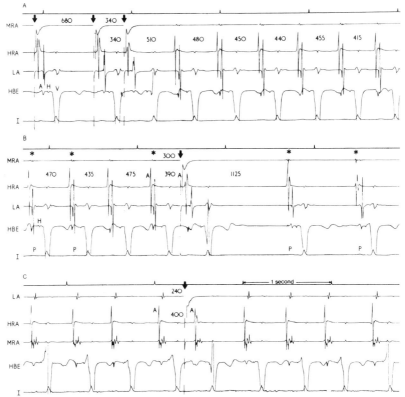

Figure 4.7 Case 1: Upper panel A shows the initiation of PRST by an atrial premature depolarization with an A_1–A_2 coupling interval of 340 msec during a regularly driven atrial rhythm (BCL 680 msec). The cycle length of the tachycardia varies between 415 and 480 msec. The centre panel B, shows termination of the tachycardia by a premature atrial beat with an A_1–A_2 coupling interval of 300 msec at mid right atrium (MRA) but whose 'effective' coupling interval at the high right atrium (HRA) is 390 msec. Limited by an atrial effective refractory period (ERPA) of 230 msec (not shown), the earliest atrial depolarization which can be introduced into the tachycardia cycle from the left atrium (LA) has an A_1–A_2 coupling interval of 240 msec (lower panel C). This gives an 'effective' HRA_1–HRA_2 coupling interval of 400 msec which fails to terminate the tachycardia. The left atrial electrode is obviously further away from the re-entry circuit than the mid right atrial electrode

Criteria for diagnosing paroxysmal sinus node tachycardia (PRST) in man during electrophysiological studies

Localization to region of sinoatrial node

The sequence of atrial activation and intraatrial conduction times of sinus node echoes and during PRST must be similar to that of sinus beats, i.e. high to low and right to left. Ideally, many different intraatrial recording sites should be used simultaneously for mapping of activation sequences; only in this way can the re-entrant circuit and its behaviour be more clearly defined.

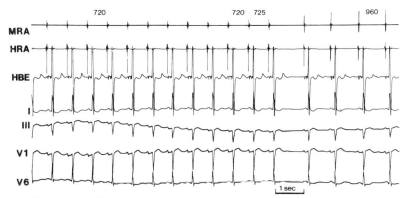

Figure 4.8 Case 3: Shows the abrupt spontaneous termination of paroxysmal reciprocating sinus node tachycardia recorded simultaneously on three intracardiac leads (MRA – mid right atrium; HRA – high right atrium and HBE – the His bundle electrogram) and on four surface ECG leads (I, III, V_1 and V_6). The basic cycle length of the tachycardia (BCL) is 720 msec compared with a BCL of 960 msec in sinus rhythm. The post-tachycardia sinus node recovery time is 1255 msec.

Note the similarity in the sequence of atrial activation and in the P wave configuration between both the spontaneous and the re-entrant sinus node rhythms

The P wave configuration on the surface electrocardiogram representing atrial depolarization by sinus node re-entrant beats must be similar to that of sinus beats although minor differences both in the P wave and in the high right atrial electrogram (HRA) would not be unexpected as parts of the sinoatrial node normally used anterogradely in sinus rhythm may instead be used retrogradely during PRST thereby disturbing the sequence of local atrial activation near the re-entrant pathway[3]. (See Figures 4.3, 4.9 and 4.11.)

The sinus node re-entry mechanism must be shown to be independent from the AV node which may also demonstrate functional changes in its refractoriness and conducting properties that can clearly parallel those which occur in the sinus node during atrial extrastimulus tests and atrial pacing procedures (Figures 4.4 and 4.5). Usually, the varying conduction delays induced in the AV node do not relate to the critical coupling zone over which atrial depolarizations reproducibly induce sinus node echoes, indeed the AV node may be refractory at a coupling interval which is suitable for the initiation of sinus node re-entry. The absence of retrograde conduction through the AV node also argues against its involvement in this re-entry circuit mechanism[14,16]. The development of fixed or varying second degree AV block at AV nodal level during PRST, perhaps following carotid sinus massage, is an additional indication that the persisting atrial tachyarrhythmia is independent of the AV node.

Additional localizing criteria and the tachycardia mechanism
It should be possible *reproducibly* to initiate sinus node echoes and PRST by premature beats over a zone dependent on the 'effective' A_1–A_2 coupling inter-

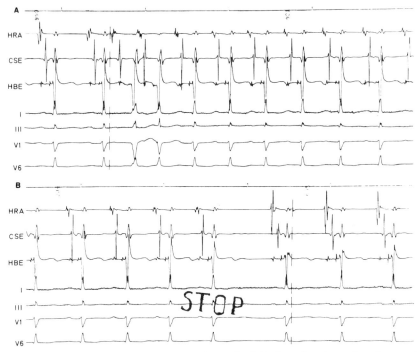

Figure 4.9 Case 5: The upper panel A shows the initiation of reciprocating sinus node tachycardia (PRST) by a single critically timed atrial extrastimulus given at the high right atrium (HRA). The cycle length of the tachycardia which is at first 430 msec, gradually increases over the subsequent 30 cycles (not shown, non-continuous recordings) until finally the tachycardia stops spontaneously (lower panel B). Note the sequence of atrial activation which is similar during both the spontaneous and the re-entrant sinus node rhythms. In contrast, the configurations of the HRA electrogram and P wave in PRST differ slightly from those in sinus rhythm.

The word 'STOP' (lower panel B) occurs coincidentally but characteristically on this page (p. 995) of the recording paper (Elema Schönander, Sweden).

vals obtaining at the HRA during sinus rhythm, but which is independent of the pacing site during regularly driven rhythms (Figure 4.13A and B). This 'initiation zone' during sinus rhythm may be found with an extrastimulus test either before or after entrance pathways into the SA node have become refractory, i.e. before or during the zone of interpolation. In the latter case it might be assumed that the re-entry mechanism involves only the outer parts of the sinus node; perhaps only the SA junction and not the central pacemaker region. Alternatively, the mechanism may be similar to that whereby sinus node re-entries can be initiated by premature beats over a zone which is quite *late* in the spontaneous sinus cycle (cases 1 and 6). The factor common to these two situations is that the re-entry mechanism may be started by an escaping spontaneous sinus beat re-entering after an invading extrastimulus has caused uni-

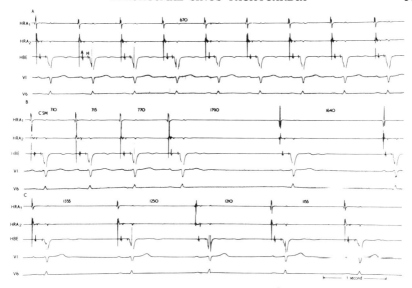

Figure 4.10 Case 6: The three panels A, B and C (which are not continuous) each show simultaneous recordings from electrodes positioned near the sinus node (HRA1 and HRA2), and the His bundle (HBE), as well as from two surface ECG leads: V_1 and V_6. The upper panel (A) shows the sustained sinus node re-entry tachycardia (BCL 670 msec). The centre panel (B) shows the last three cycles of the tachycardia which is slowed and finally terminated by carotid sinus massage (CSM, onset of application not shown). The lower panel (C) shows the basic sinus rhythm after the effects of CSM have worn off. The atrial activation sequence and P wave configuration of both tachycardia and sinus beats are similar

directional exit block and delay for the escaping beat by concealed retrograde conduction into the sinus node. In this way PRST may be initiated in both the zones of non-reset and of interpolation during sinus rhythm (Figure 4.12). The mechanism whereby PRST is initiated by a single extrastimulus during regular paced ('overdriving') rhythm probably differs from that which follows an extrastimulus during spontaneous ('escaping') sinus rhythm and resembles more closely the initiation mechanism for re-entry AV tachycardias.

PRST is rarely very fast; in this and in other series the range of heart rates is from *ca.* 85–160 beats per min although rarely more rapid attacks have been reported[16,19]. If heart rates are <90 beats per min in PRST, the basic spontaneous rhythm is sinus bradycardia (Table 4.2).

Spontaneous initiation of PRST by a sudden antecedent shortening of the sinus cycle in sinus rhythm is common in such cases and is comparable to a mechanism previously described for re-entrant AV tachycardias[25]. PRST can frequently be initiated by continuous atrial pacing at only moderate rates; these attacks are to be distinguished from the brief runs of sinus tachycardia which very frequently follow other rapid spontaneous or induced arrhythmias that produce hypotension.

Attacks of PRST are poorly sustained and are sensitive to changes in vagal tone as might be expected from the slow rate, the variability in cycle length and the location of the circuit within a region richly supplied with autonomic nerve fibres. Cycle length 'alternation' during PRST may support the assumption that the mechanism is re-entrant[30].

Sustained PRST can be terminated by critically timed beats over a definite coupling zone which is dependent on the 'effective' coupling interval obtaining usually at the HRA (Figure 4.13C and D); however, where the circuit is large and includes significant parts of the right atrium in addition to the sinus node, the 'effective' coupling zone may relate to those A_1–A_2 coupling intervals obtaining at MRA[11].

HRA electrograms that had changed at the onset of PRST in two patients, failed at the end of an attack to return immediately to the configuration seen in sinus rhythm before initiation of the tachycardia, but did so gradually over the next two or three beats (Figure 4.11). A similar phenomenon is sometimes seen after a paroxysm of orthodromic AV re-entry tachycardia in the WPW syn-

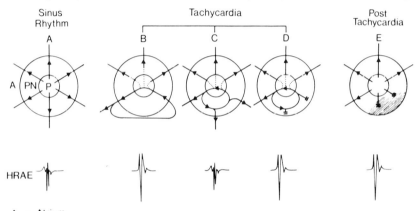

A = Atrium
PN = Peri-Nodal
P = 'P' cell area

Figure 4.11 Diagrammatic representation of the different sequences of activation within and surrounding the SA node; and the resultant configurations of the high right atrial electrograms (HRAE) during: A – sinus rhythm (radial excitation originating from the centre of the SA node); B to D sinus node re-entry tachycardias (PRST); and E – the first few escape beats of sinus rhythm immediately after the termination of PRST. The re-entry tachycardia circuit may include the atrium, the peri-nodal cells and the central pacemaker region of the sinus node (B) in which case the local sequence of atrial activation during PRST may differ from that in sinus rhythm (A) resulting in an altered HRAE and possibly also an altered P wave on the surface ECG, since some of the exit pathways used in sinus rhythm are now used retrogradely as re-entrant pathways. Alternatively, the circuit may be entirely within the SA node when the sequence of atrial activation during PRST (C) may be identical to that in sinus rhythm unless rate dependent aberration is induced in some of the exit pathways (D). 'Polarisation' of sinus node exit pathways used retrogradely in PRST may occur particularly following prolonged attacks, leaving these pathways relatively refractory for a varying period which may extend over one to four cycles of the subsequent sinus rhythm. In this case the HRAE in the few cycles of sinus rhythm will retain a configuration similar to that seen during PRST (E)

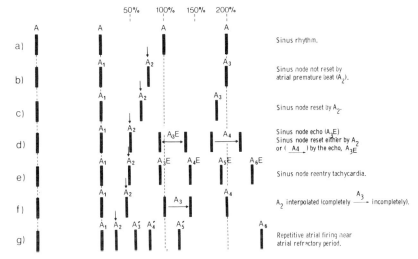

Figure 4.12 Diagram of the responses which may be obtained in the course of a single atrial extrastimulus test during sinus rhythm.

Both A and A_1 represent high right atrial electrograms of the basic sinus rhythm. A_2 is the induced atrial extrastimulus while A_3 to A_6 are return beats following the introduction of A_2. The letter 'E' after a response indicates sinus node re-entry (echoes or tachycardia). Abnormal sequences of intra-atrial depolarization are indicated as in $A_3'' - A_5''$

drome when the pattern of ventricular pre-excitation, previously always apparent in sinus rhythm, fails to return immediately in the first two or more sinus beats. We have used the term 'polarization of conduction' here to indicate an orientation of conduction pathways used unidirectionally and linked 'in series' during a re-entry mechanism that only gradually alters to permit conduction 'in parallel' after re-entry has finished.

Response to anti-arrhythmic agents and atropine
Very little is known about the value of anti-arrhythmic drugs in PRST in man, though there have been studies on the effects of digoxin[31] and quinidine[32] on sinus node re-entry in dogs. In our series verapamil suppressed both PRST and sinus node echoes in five cases; two patients who have subsequently received verapamil prophylactically have reported a marked reduction in the number of attacks of PRST (cases 1 and 3; follow-up longer than 1 year). The responses to either quinidine-like agents on the one hand and verapamil-like agents on the other during studies on PRST may indicate the relative dependency of the re-entry circuit on atrial (sodium activated) and intranodal (calcium-activated) cells respectively.

Acknowledgement
We thank the British Heart Foundation who supported this work and Miss Jean Powell for the preparation of the Figures.

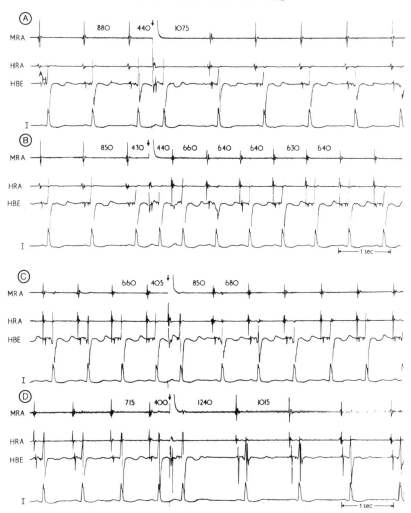

Figure 4.13   Case 3: An atrial premature beat introduced from the mid right atrium (MRA) with an A_1–A_2 coupling interval of 440 msec (arrowed in panel A) resets the sinus node while one introduced at a slightly shorter coupling interval during the basic sinus rhythm (A_1–A_2 – 430 msec, panel B) initiates a reciprocating sinus node tachycardia whose cycle length (630–660 msec) is only 200 to 250 msec shorter than that of sinus rhythm (850–880 ms).

In panel C, a single suitably-timed atrial premature beat (A_1–A_2 coupling interval, 405 msec) introduced from the mid right atrium (MRA) during a sustained sinus node re-entry tachycardia captures and advances the tachycardia by 85 msec. A slightly earlier atrial premature beat with an A_1–A_2 coupling interval of 400 msec terminates the tachycardia (panel D). Note the changing configuration of the high right atrial electrogram (HRA) in the four cycles following the termination of the tachycardia; the configuration gradually returns to that seen in sinus rhythm before the tachycardia.

HRA – high right atrial electrogram; HBE – His bundle electrogram; I – standard lead I of surface ECG

References

1. Barker, P. S., Wilson, F. N. and Johnson, F. D. (1943). The mechanism of auricular paroxysmal tachycardia. *Am. Heart J.*, **26**, 435

2. Wallace, A. G. and Daggett, W. M. (1964). Re-excitation of the atrium. The echo phenomenon. *Am. Heart J.*, **68**, 661

3. Han, J., Malozzi, A. M. and Moe, G. K. (1968). Sinoatrial reciprocation in the isolated rabbit heart. *Circ. Res.*, **22**, 355

4. Bonke, F. I. M., Bouman, L. N. and Schopman, F. J. G. (1971). Effect of an early premature beat on activity of the sinoatrial node and atrial rhythm in the rabbit. *Circ. Res.*, **29**, 704

5. Childers, R., Arnsdorf, M., De La Fuente, D., Gambetta, M. and Svenson, R. (1973). Sinus nodal echoes: clinical case report and canine studies. *Am. J. Cardiol.*, **31**, 220

6. Paulay, K. L., Varghese, P. J. and Damato, A. N. (1973). Sinus node re-entry: an *in vivo* demonstration in the dog. *Circ. Res.*, **32**, 455

7. Ticzon, A. R., Strauss, H. C., Gallagher, J. J. and Wallace, A. G. (1975). Sinus nodal function in the intact dog heart evaluated by premature atrial stimulation and atrial pacing. *Am. J. Cardiol.*, **35**, 492

8. Strauss, H. C., Bigger, J. T., Saroff, A. L. and Giardina, E-G. V. (1976). Electrophysiological evaluation of sinus node function in patients with sinus node dysfunction. *Circulation*, **53**, 763

9. Curry, P. V. L., Gallowhill, E. A. and Krikler, D. M. (1976). Paroxysmal reciprocating sinus tachycardia. *Br. Heart J.*, **38**, 311

10. Coumel, Ph. (1975). Supraventricular Tachycardias. In Krikler and Goodwin. *Cardiac Arrhythmias: the modern electrophysiological approach.*, 1st edn. (London: W. B. Saunders), p. 116

11. Coumel, Ph., Attuel, P. and Flammang, D. (1976). The role of the conduction system in supraventricular tachycardias. In Wellens, Lie, Janse (eds.). *The Conduction System of the Heart: Structure, Function and Clinical Implications.* 1st edn. (Leiden: H. E. Stenfert Kroese), p. 424

12. Narula, O. S. (1972). Sinus node re-entry: mechanism of supraventricular tachycardia (SVT) in man. *Circulation*, **46**, (II), 11

13. Paulay, K. L., Varghese, P. J. and Damato, A. N. (1973). Atrial rhythms in response to an early atrial premature depolarization in man. *Am. Heart J.*, **85**, 323

14. Narula, O. S. (1974). Sinus node re-entry: a mechanism for supraventricular tachycardia. *Circulation*, **50**, 1114

15. Pahlajani, D. B., Miller, R. A. and Serratto, M. (1975). Sinus node re-entry and sinus node tachycardia. *Am. Heart J.*, **90**, 305

16. Weisfogel, G. M., Batsford, W. P., Paulay, K. L., Josephson, M. E., Ogunkelu, J. B., Akhtar, M., Seides, S. F. and Damato, A. N. (1975). Sinus node re-entrant tachycardia in man. *Am. Heart J.*, **90**, 295

17. Wu, D., Amat-y-Leon, F., Denes, P., Dhingra, R. C., Pietras, R. J. and Rosen, K. M. (1975). Demonstration of sustained sinus and atrial re-entry as a mechanism of paroxysmal supraventricular tachycardia. *Circulation*, **51**, 234

18. Childers, R. W. (1976). Classification of cardiac arrhythmias. *Med. Clin. North Am.*, **60**, 3

19. Gillette, P. C. (1976). The mechanisms of supraventricular tachycardia in children. *Circulation*, **54**, 133

20. Curry, P. V. L., Evans, T. R. and Krikler, D. M. (1977). Paroxysmal reciprocating sinus tachycardia. *Eur. J. Cardiol.*, in the press

21. Dhingra, R. C., Wyndham, C., Amat-Y-Leon, F., Denes, P., Wu, D. and Rosen, K. M. (1975). Sinus nodal responses to atrial extrastimuli in patients without apparent sinus node disease. *Am. J. Cardiol.*, **36**, 445

22. Scherlag, B. J., Lau, S. H., Helfant, R. H., Berkowitz, W. D., Stein, C. and Damato, A. N. (1969). Catheter technique for recording His bundle activity in man. *Circulation*, **39**, 13

23. Curry, P. V. L. (1975). Fundamentals of arrhythmias: Modern methods of investigation. In: Krikler and Goodwin (eds.) *Cardiac Arrhythmias; the modern electrophysiological approach,* (London: W. B. Saunders Co.). p. 39

24. Narula, O. S., Samet, P. J. and Javier, R. P. (1972). Significance of the sinus node recovery time. *Circulation,* **45,** 140

25. Krikler, D. M., Curry, P. V. L., Attuel, P. and Coumel, Ph. (1976). Incessant tachycardias in Wolff–Parkinson–White syndrome. 1: Initiation without antecedent extrasystoles or PR lengthening, with reference to reciprocation after shortening of cycle length. *Br. Heart J.,* **38,** 885

26. Mandel, W., Hayakawa, H., Danzig, R. and Marcus, H. S. (1971). Evaluation of sinoatrial node function in man by overdrive suppression. *Circulation,* **44,** 59

27. Wellens, H. J. J. (1971). *Electrical Stimulation of the Heart in the Study and Treatment of Tachycardias,* 1st edn. (Leiden: H. E. Stenfert Kroese)

28. Wit, A. L., Damato, A. N., Weiss, M. B. and Steiner, C. (1970). Phenomenon of the gap in atrio-ventricular conduction in the human heart. *Circ. Res.,* **27,** 679

29. Curry, P. V. L. and Krikler, D. M. (1977). The 'gap' phenomenon in retrograde sinoatrial conduction (in preparation)

30. Curry, P. V. L. and Krikler, D. M. (1976). Significance of cycle length alternation during drug treatment of supraventricular tachycardia. *Br. Heart J.,* **38,** 882

31. Paulay, K. L. and Damato, A. N. (1975). Effect of digoxin on sinus node re-entry in the dog. *Am. J. Cardiol.,* **35,** 370

32. Paulay, K. L., Weisfogel, G. M. and Damato, A. N. (1974). Sinus nodal re-entry. Effect of quinidine. *Am. J. Cardiol.,* **33,** 617

5

The Effects of Carbamylcholine, Adrenaline, Ouabain, Quinidine and Verapamil on Circus Movement Tachycardia in Isolated Segments of Rabbit Atrial Myocardium

M. A. ALLESSIE, F. I. M. BONKE and
W. J. E. P. LAMMERS

Department of Physiology, Biomedical Centre, University of Limburg, The Netherlands

Since 1887[1] it has been known that atrial flutter can be induced by strong faradic stimulation. Some years later Mines[2] and de Boer[3] established that also a single stimulus can initiate fibrillation or produce a series of extrasystoles, provided that the stimulus is applied very early after the recovery of excitability. West and Landa[4] reported that a minimal mass of more than 30 mg is required to start tachycardias in segments of rabbit atrial muscle. Although this is suggestive of a re-entrant mechanism[5] the true nature of these atrial tachycardias remained unknown. Some years ago we started a series of investigations to analyze the underlying mechanism of these tachycardias[6]. Segments of left atrial muscle, measuring about 15 × 15 mm, were isolated and put in a tissue bath. Under normal conditions these preparations did not show spontaneous activity and therefore they were paced at a regular rhythm (basic length 500 msec). After every 20th basic stimulus one early test stimulus of four times diastolic threshold was delivered via the same electrodes through which the basic stimuli were applied. In most preparations one or more areas could be found where a properly timed premature beat repeatedly initiated a period of rapid repetitive activity. By extensive mapping of the excitation sequence during the initiation of these paroxysms of tachycardia with multiple exploring leads, we could directly demonstrate that circus movement of the impulse through a relative small part of the myocardium was responsible for the tachycardia. The impulse was trapped in a circuitous route if (1) the premature impulse was conducted in one direction while it was blocked in another direction and (2) the area where propagation of the premature impulse failed was activated with such delay that the fibres proximal to the block were allowed to restore their excitability again. In a later study[7], the occurrence of local block, which sets the stage for circus movement, was related to the spatial dispersion in refractory periods of the atrium. Comparison of the spread of activation of the premature beat with the naturally existing non-uniformity in recovery of excitability, made clear that local conduction block of the premature impulse was associated with areas of retarded restoration of excitability. In separate experiments in which differences in refractory periods were induced artificially by regional application of carbamylcholine, it could be established that a disparity in refractory periods of about 14 msec between adjacent areas was already sufficient to cause conduction block.

To get more detailed information about the exact nature of the present type of circus movement we further made multiple intracellular recordings during the tachycardia. This resulted in the observation that the local responses exhibited by the fibres in the area where the premature impulse was blocked, served as a temporary barrier of refractoriness for the impulse on its first roundtrip, thus preventing an early lateral invasion of the blocked area. This may explain that despite the absence of an anatomical obstacle, the premature impulse was forced to travel all around the region of local block, giving the fibres proximal to the block the opportunity to restore their excitability sufficiently to be re-entered by the turning impulse.

Finally in the third part of the study[8], we focused our attention on the centre of the circus movement. Since in the isolated segments of the atrium there was no gross anatomical obstacle, it seemed essential to be informed of what was going on in the centre of this type of circulating excitation. During long lasting stable tachycardias with a constant coupling interval, the activation of about 100 individual fibres was recorded with the multiple microelectrode technique[9], and the spread of the activation, including that in the centre, could be reconstructed accurately. It turned out that the centre of the circuit was invaded by multiple centripetal wavelets arising from the main circulating wave front. In the very centre of the circuit these centripetal wavelets collided, thus preventing each other from cutting off part of the circuit. Thus in case of circulating excitation without the involvement of an anatomical obstacle, the circulating impulse creates its own functional obstacle consisting of a number of converging centripetal wavelets.

THE LEADING CIRCLE HYPOTHESIS

From the observations summarized above, we have come to the following concept of circulating excitation in the absence of an anatomical obstacle.

(1) Since the circuit with the smallest dimensions can be expected to have the shortest revolution time, the rate of the tachycardia will be determined by the smallest possible circuit in which the impulse can continue to circulate. In such a 'leading circuit' the efficacy of the circulating wave front as a stimulus is just enough to excite the tissue ahead which is still in its relative refractory phase. Because of this tight fit between the crest and the tail of the leading circulating impulse, there is no gap of full excitability in the circuit.

(2) The dimensions of the leading circuit are determined by electrophysiological properties such as refractory period, conduction velocity and stimulating efficacy of the activation wave. Neither the position nor the dimensions of the leading circuit are fixed, but may change with variations in electrophysiological conditions. So prolongation of the refractory period will increase the minimal length of the re-entrant pathway; an increase in the conduction velocity will have the same effect.

(3) The revolution time of the circulating impulse is determined by the time course of recovery of excitability of the tissue and the efficacy of the circulating wave front as a stimulus. It equals the time which the fibres in the leading circuit need to restore their excitability just sufficiently to be excited again by the circulating impulse.

THE EFFECT OF CARBAMYLCHOLINE ON THE LEADING CIRCLE TACHYCARDIA

To test the validity of the leading circle model and to study the behaviour of the related tachycardia under different conditions, we studied the effect of some arrhythmogenic and anti-arrhythmic drugs. In Figure 5.1 the effects of carbamylcholine are shown, both on the dimensions and on the revolution time of the leading circle. In panel A the spread of activation is shown as reconstructed from more than 100 electrograms recorded during a single long lasting tachycardia. The cycle length of the tachycardia was constant and amounted to 90 msec. As can be seen from panel A the impulse was circulating in a clockwise direction. Analysis of the electrograms taken from the centre of the circuit revealed that the centripetal wavelets emerging from the leading circuit were blocked along a longdrawn area in the centre. Block of the centripetal wavelets is indicated by double bars, while in the scheme beneath the map the dimensions of the leading circuit are given. In this case the length of the circuit can be estimated to be $ca.$ 30 mm. During the course of the tachycardia carbamylcholine was added to the tissue bath in a concentration of 10^{-6} g/ml. This resulted in a gradual increase in the rate of the tachycardia, the cycle length being shortened from 90 to 60 msec. After the coupling interval of the

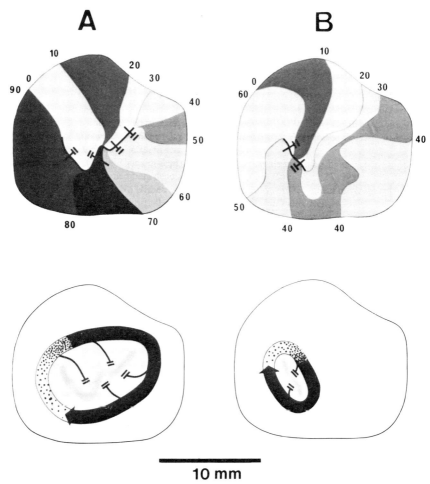

10 mm

Figure 5.1 The effect of carbamylcholine on circus movement tachycardia in isolated left atrium of the rabbit. Panel A shows the map and a schematic drawing of the spread of activation during a long lasting tachycardia under normal conditions (interval 90 msec). Panel B shows the same tachycardia after addition of carbamylcholine (10^{-6} g/ml) to the tissue bath. Under the influence of the drug the revolution time of the circulating impulse has been diminished to 60 msec. This increase in the rate of the tachycardia is caused by a narrowing of the circuitous pathways. Obviously the shortening of the refractory period caused by carbamylcholine enabled the circulating impulse to cut off a part of the circuit

tachycardia had become constant again, the mapping procedure was repeated. Panel B shows the result. The impulse is still travelling in a clockwise direction; however, it is now circulating in a much smaller circuit. The shortening of the refractory period, brought about by the administration of carbamylcholine, obviously enabled the circulating excitation to cut off a part of the circuit. The observed acceleration of the tachycardia under the influence of carbamylcholine thus must be attributed directly to a reduction in size of the circuitous pathway. This reduction of the minimal mass required for circus movement may also explain why acetylcholine and its derivatives, or vagal stimulation, highly favour the initiation of tachycardia[10] and why under these circumstances tachycardia frequently passes into fibrillation[11].

ADRENALINE

In Figure 5.2 the effect of adrenaline (10^{-6} g/ml) on tachycardia in an isolated segment of atrial muscle is shown. As a control the response of a spontaneously beating isolated right atrium, put in the same tissue bath, is given too. Before the administration of adrenaline the interval of sinus rhythm was 940 msec. This slow discharge of the sinus node was caused by the fact that carbamylcholine (10^{-7} g/ml) was present in the perfusion fluid to facilitate the in-

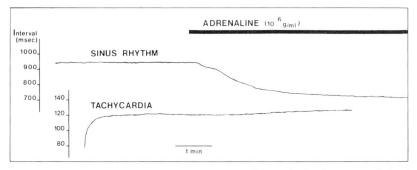

Figure 5.2 The effect of adrenaline on the frequency of sinus rhythm (spontaneously beating isolated right atrium of the rabbit) and on circus movement tachycardia induced in the isolated left atrium of the rabbit. Both preparations were in the same tissue bath. During the whole course of the experiment carbamylcholine (10^{-7} g/ml) was present in the perfusion fluid. Whereas sinus rhythm was markedly accelerated under the influence of adrenaline, the interval of the tachycardia was hardly affected

duction and to favour the perpetuation of tachycardias. During the first minute after the induction of tachycardia with the single stimulus method, the interval of the tachycardia gradually increased from <80–120 msec. This initial lengthening of the beat to beat interval is very characteristic for the present type of circus movement[6]. After the rate of the tachycardia had become constant adrenaline was added. The effect of adrenaline on both rhythms was markedly different. While sinus rate, as expected, accelerated considerably, the effect on the interval of the tachycardia was negligible. At best there was a slight prolongation of the cycle length. This remarkable failure of adrenaline to influence the rate of this reciprocating rhythm is not so surprising as it may seem. Although adrenaline has a strong effect on pacemaker tissues and impulse conduction mediated by slow channels, it has little effect on the electrical activity of atrial muscle. Most investigators have reported no significant alterations in either the resting potential, the velocity of depolarization or the amplitude of the action potential, while the action potential duration is affected only slightly[12].

OUABAIN

It is well known that many cases of atrial flutter or paroxysmal tachycardia can be treated successfully with digitalis. However, there is still much uncertainty about the mechanism behind this success. One possible explanation is that, if the tachycardia is associated with congestive heart failure, the positive ino-tropic effect on the ventricles may diminish the concomitant dilatation of the atria. Removal of the stretch of the walls of the atria then may be sufficient to terminate the paroxysm of tachycardia. Another possibility is that the effect is mediated by reflex vagal stimulation. However, besides these indirect effects, ouabain may exert its anti-arrhythmic action by a direct influence on the elec-trophysiological properties of the atria. In Figure 5.3 such a direct effect of ouabain on circus movement tachycardia is demonstrated. During the first phase

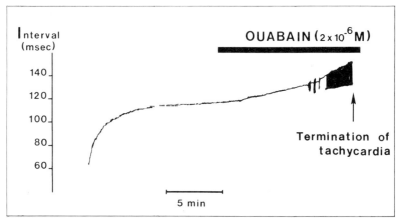

Figure 5.3   The effect of ouabain on atrial tachycardia. The drug first causes a slowing of the tachycardia. After a period of alternating beats the tachycardia then is suddenly terminated

of its development the interval of the tachycardia gradually increased from 60 to 115 msec. After the rate of the tachycardia had become constant, ouabain (2 × 10⁻⁶ M) was added to the tissue bath. This initially resulted in a further lengthening of the coupling interval; after a while, however, the tachycardia became irregular, exhlbiting alternating responses. In other cases, not shown here, a sudden jump in cycle length was observed, presumably caused by a sudden change in the pathway of the circulating impulse. Frequently the tachycardia was abruptly terminated by the effects of ouabain, in this case as soon as the revolution time had increased to 150 msec. This direct anti-arrhythmic action of ouabain on tachycardias based on circulating excitation in atrial myocardium, probably must be attributed to the decrease in amplitude and rate of rise of the action potential and the delay in recovery of excitability of atrial muscle fibres brought about by the drug.

QUINIDINE

Together with ouabain, quinidine is one of the most useful drugs to control tachycardia and fibrillation of the atria. It is known to prolong the effective refractory period in isolated rabbit atria and isolated ventricular muscle and Purkinje fibres; excitability and conduction velocity are depressed[13,14]. In addition quinidine has an anticholinergic effect. Figure 5.4 shows the effect of quinidine on circulating rhythm in a piece of rabbit atrial muscle under the in-

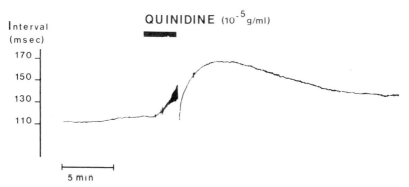

Figure 5.4 The effect of quinidine on the revolution time of circus movement tachycardia in the atrium. The beat to beat interval of the arrhythmia is markedly prolonged by the drug. (See text for further discussion.)

fluence of carbamylcholine (10^{-7} g/ml). The effect closely resembles the effect of ouabain. The interval of the tachycardia is prolonged while alternation in cycle length supervenes. During this period of alternation the tachycardia is suddenly interrupted. Rapid restarting of the tachycardia reveals a further increase in cycle length up to 170 msec. During the wash-out of quinidine, the tachycardia accelerates again, showing that the effect of the drug is reversible. The observed graded slowing of the frequency of the circus movement tachycardia by quinidine can be understood in terms of the actions on atrial muscle fibres described above. Refractory period is increased, directly as well as indirectly, due to the anticholinergic action of the drug. Such delay in the process of recovery of excitability, together with a decrease of amplitude and rate of rise of the action potential, will lengthen the shortest possible interval between successive beats. Since in the leading circle model a tight fit between the crest and the tail of the circulating impulse is assumed, this will lead to an increase in the revolution time of the impulse.

VERAPAMIL

Recently, clinical reports have appeared that some cases of supraventricular tachycardia can be terminated by the administration of verapamil[15,16]. It is argued that in these cases a re-entrant mechanism involving the SA or AV node is responsible for the tachycardia. Experimental evidence has been gathered that verapamil depresses electrical activity in the nodes and may abolish experimentally induced nodal re-entrant tachycardia[17]. In Figure 5.5 the effect of verapamil on circus movement tachycardia in atrial muscle is shown. It is

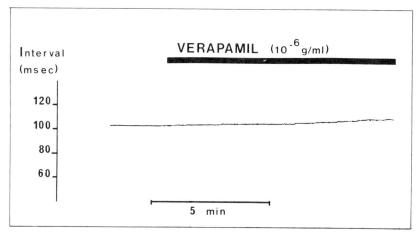

Figure 5.5　Administration of verapamil during a long lasting regular tachycardia in a segment of the left atrium of the rabbit. There is almost no effect. At most there is an increase of the interval of 10 msec

quite clear that verapamil does not have much effect on this type of tachycardia. Only a very slight increase in cycle length was recorded. This observation seems to strengthen the idea that, if verapamil is effective against a supraventricular tachycardia, the sinoatrial or atrioventricular regions are involved in the origin of the arrhythmia.

References

1. McWilliam, J. A. (1887). Fibrillar contraction of the heart. *J. Physiol.*, **8**, 296
2. Mines, G. R. (1914). On circulating excitations in heart muscle and their possible relation to tachycardia and fibrillation. *Trans. R. Soc. Can.*, **4**, 43
3. de Boer, S. (1921). On recurring extrasystoles and their relation to fibrillation. *J. Physiol.*, **54**, 410

4. West, Th. C. and Landa, J. F. (1962). Minimal mass required for induction of a sustained arrhythmia in isolated atrial segments. *Am. J. Physiol.*, **202**, 232

5. Garrey, W. E. (1914). The nature of fibrillary contraction of the heart – its relation to tissue mass and form. *Am. J. Physiol.*, **33**, 397

6. Allessie, M. A., Bonke, F. I. M. and Schopman, F. J. G. (1973). Circus movement in rabbit atrial muscle as a mechanism of tachycardia. *Circ. Res.*, **33**, 54

7. Allessie, M. A., Bonke, F. I. M. and Schopman, F. J. G. (1976). Circus movement in rabbit atrial muscle as a mechanism of tachycardia. II. The role of nonuniform recovery of excitability in the occurrence of unidirectional block, as studied with multiple microelectrodes. *Circ. Res.*, **39**, 168

8. Allessie, M. A., Bonke, F. I. M. and Schopman, F. J. G. (1977). Circus movement in rabbit atrial muscle as a mechanism of tachycardia. III. The 'leading circle' concept: a new model of circus movement in cardiac tissue without the involvement of an anatomical obstacle. *Circ. Res.*, **40**

9. Schreurs, A. W., Selij, A. P. L., Allessie, M. A. and Bonke, F. I. M. (1974). A concentrically and radially adjustable holder for ten microelectrodes. *Pfluegers Arch.*, **346**, 167

10. Winterberg, H. (1907). Studien über Herzflimmern. I. Mitteilung. Über die Wirkung des N. vagus und accelerans auf das Flimmern des Herzens. *Pfluegers Arch.*, **117**, 223

11. Lewis, T., Drury, A. N. and Bulger, H. A. (1921). Observations upon flutter and fibrillation. Part VII. The effects of vagal stimulation. *Heart*, **8**, 141

12. Hoffman, B. F. and Cranefield, P. F. (1960). *Electrophysiology of the Heart.* (New York: McGraw-Hill)

13. Hoffman, B. F. (1958). The action of quinidine and procainamide on single fibers of dog ventricle and specialized conducting system. *An. Acad. Bras. Cien.*, **29**, 365

14. West, T. C. and Amory, D. W. (1960). Single fiber recording of the effect of quinidine at atrial pacemaker sites in the isolated right atrium of the rabbit. *J. Pharmacol. Exp. Ther.*, **130**, 183

15. Schamroth, L., Krikler, D. M. and Garret, G. (1972). Immediate effects of intravenous verapamil in cardiac arrhythmias. *Br. Med. J.*, **1**, 660

16. Härtel, G. and Hartikainen, M. (1976). Comparison of verapamil and practolol in paroxysmal supraventricular tachycardia. *Eur. J. Cardiol.*, **4**, 87

17. Wit, A. L. and Cranefield, P. F. (1974). Effect of verapamil on the sinoatrial and atrioventricular nodes of the rabbit and the mechanism by which it arrests re-entrant atrioventricular nodal tachycardia. *Circ. Res.*, **35**, 413

6

Observations on Re-entrant Excitation Pathways and Refractory Period Distributions in Spontaneous and Experimental Atrial Flutter in the Dog

J. P. BOINEAU, C. R. MOONEY, R. D. HUDSON,

D. G. HUGHES, R. A. ERDIN, JR. and A. C. WYLDS

Section of Cardiology, Veterans Administration Hospital, Department of Medicine, Medical College, Augusta, Georgia

INTRODUCTION

The object of this paper is to report two sets of observations in atrial flutter. The first set of observations led to the second, and together they demonstrate the process and the mechanism of this atrial arrhythmia. Both sets of data were obtained in the intact canine heart. The first deals with certain totally unique observations on spontaneous atrial flutter in a dog. The data obtained in this dog demonstrated that an abnormality in conduction due to a structural defect in the right atrium was the primary basis for the arrhythmia. However, the structural defect alone could not account for the initiation of the event. Therefore, an experimental study was begun to define the factors which initiated the atrial flutter.

After completion of the first phase of the investigation, we read the work of Allessie et al.[1,2]. It is now obvious that our two groups approached the problem from opposite directions, and that each group defined one variable and identified a second absent factor needed to complete the picture. Interestingly, each group focused on the other's missing factor. The two components fit together and provide a new and more comprehensive explanation of atrial flutter.

Briefly, the two factors are: (1) A fixed structural component identified as a relative discontinuity in the right atrial conduction pathway which slows the normal rapid and preferential conduction; and (2) A dynamic functional component represented by the changing non-uniform distribution of the atrial refractory period. The two interacting factors represent, at any moment, the intrinsic capacity (or threshold) of the atria to flutter. The actual occurrence of atrial flutter depends on the interaction with a third factor, the premature atrial beat.

METHODS

Twenty mongrel dogs weighing 40–60 lb were anaesthetized with α-chloralose 100 mg/kg and morphine sulphate 3 mg/kg. The heart was exposed through a median sternotomy and cradled in the pericardium.

Electrodes

After careful dissection of the posterior atrial and mediastinal structures, 24 individual bipolar electrodes (IE) were affixed to the atrium (Figure 6.1A). These low-inertia electrodes were spaced uniformly over the right and left atria and anterior interatrial band (Bachmann).

In addition to the 24 individual electrodes (IE), a macro-patch containing 24 bipolar electrode pairs was placed over the mid-right atrium (Figure 6.1A). This 20 × 25 mm rectangular array contained four rows of six electrode pairs. Each pair of electrodes was separated by 1 mm and 5 mm along the short and long axes respectively. The patch was moved to different atrial regions during the study to obtain greater spatial resolution in the activation of critical regions.

Atrial stimulation and extra stimulus method

Spontaneous sinus rhythm (SR) and driven (S_1) atrial beats were recorded. The atrial driving stimulus was delivered near the sinus node at the electrode site recording earliest atrial activity during sinus rhythm. A digital pulse generator (Figure 6.1B) was used to drive an isolated stimulator which delivered a 2 msec pulse 1.1 × diastolic threshold.

A series of 12 stimuli (S_1) at a constant cycle length of 375 msec (rate 160) was delivered to individual electrode locations or to the patch electrode positions. The 12th driving stimulus (S_1) was followed by a premature atrial stimulus (S_2). The $S_1 S_2$ interval was initially set at 60 msec and gradually lengthened until the S_2 elicited either a propagated premature atrial contraction (R_2) or a run of repetitive activity, i.e. $R_2 R_3 R_4 \ldots R_n$. In this way the refractory period was scanned and the effective refractory period (ERP) was deter-

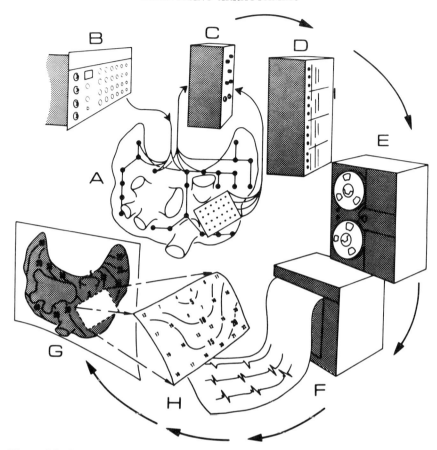

Figure 6.1 Methods for mapping the atrial activation sequence. In A the 24 individual atrial bipolar electrodes and the 24 point macroelectrode array are shown. B indicates the digital pulse generator used to drive the atrium and deliver atrial premature stimuli at any of the electrode locations. C indicates the input-selector box containing the input amplifiers and switching for recording between different sets of 24 bipolar electrodes. D indicates the 28 channel system for amplifying and filtering the bipolar electrogram. E indicates the 28 channel analogue tape recorder. F indicates the 28 channel strip chart recorder. G is the global map of atrial activation and H represents a detailed map of a small atrial region from the patch electrode

mined. The ERP was the longest S_1S_2 interval which did not result in a propagated R_2.

Activation recordings

The 24 atrial activation signals were fed through an input-selector box containing FET amplifiers of 10^{11} Ω input impedance (Figure 6.1C). The signals were amplified and filtered at a bandwidth of 40–2000 Hz (Figure 6.1D). Thus, the various combinations of electrodes were used to obtain 24 simultaneous bipolar atrial electrograms, a constant reference atrial electrogram, a lead II surface ECG, a time code, and a voice comment.

All data were recorded on a 28 track analogue magnetic tape recorder at a speed of $7\frac{1}{2}$ IPS (Figure 6.1E). The tape recorded data were displayed on a 28 channel strip chart recorder for monitoring, editing, and data analysis (Figure 6.1F).

Activation maps

Global atrial activation sequence maps (Figure 6.1G) and regional activation maps (Figure 6.1H) were constructed from the electrograms recorded with the 24 individual electrodes and the patch electrodes. Activation times were determined by computing the time difference between peaks or fastest deflections of each electrogram. The reference electrogram was used to relate (time align) sets of data recorded at different times.

Reproducible periods of repetitive atrial flutter were produced in 12 of 20 dogs. In addition, in the dog with spontaneous flutter, numerous runs of repetitive activity were recorded. In all other animals, the extra stimulus technique was used to initiate identical or closely similar runs of flutter allowing mapping of up to 96 points during an event (i.e. 24 IE and three patch positions).

Using these methods, activation sequence maps were made for normal sinus conduction, driven atrial conduction (S_1), and atrial repetitive activity (RA). In addition, maps of the ERP distribution were constructed from the individual determinations made using the extra stimulus method.

Atrial transillumination

A new method was used for visualizing the distribution of the right atrial myocardium. After completion of the electrophysiological studies, the dogs were sacrificed, and the atria fixed in 10% formalin solution. Subsequent to fixation, the atria were positioned, first endocardium down, later reversed on a plastic translucent platform and illuminated by a 12 V high intensity light source suspended in a box below the platform. f stops and shutter speeds (exposure values) were determined for each atrial exposure. Thus, comparisons between different atria could be made by making prints from all negatives with the same exposure value for each heart. All processing and printing of comparative atria were performed identically.

RESULTS

Atrial anatomy

Figure 6.2 illustrates a posterior (left) and anterior (right) transilluminated view of a normal dog right atrium. Underneath these are schematic drawings

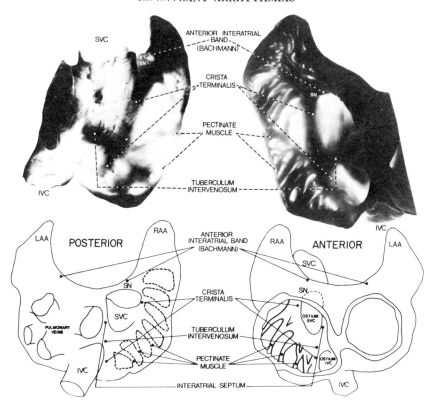

Figure 6.2 Transilluminated anatomy and organization of the atrial muscle. On the left is a transillumination of the right atrium viewed posteriorly (above) and the schematic diagram of the entire atrium viewed posteriorly. On the right is an anterior view with the light source positioned posteriorly. Note that the atrial myocardium is organized into dense bundles of compact tissue and adjacent thin, transparent regions of less concentrated muscle. These regions have been defined and related to the schematic atrial diagrams below. Atrial activation sequence maps to follow will be displayed on a schematic outline of the posterior atrium (lower figure, left panel). To relate activation map details to the distribution of atrial muscle compare this figure with those to follow

demonstrating the locations of important structures also identified in the trans-illuminated photographs above. Note the dense concentrations of myocardium organized into bands. These bands have been identified according to several anatomic sources[3-5]. The anterior interatrial band, crista terminalis, and the tuberculum intervenosum, are the locations indicated by James[6] for his anterior, posterior and middle internodal tracts. Note also the position of the sinus node (SN) which was estimated from the earliest area of epicardial atrial activity in this heart. Note that this region (SN) occupies a position central to the trifurcation of atrial muscle bundles. Also, observe that the regions adjacent to the chief muscle masses or bundles are quite transparent and contain myocardium which is obviously less dense.

Note that the pectinate muscles run perpendicular to the superior–inferior axis of the atrium, and that the confluence of pectinate muscles at the right lateral margin of the right atrium forms another region of superior–inferior continuity at the atrial ring.

By relating the actual transilluminated anatomy to the schematic figures below, it is possible to relate the activation sequence maps with the important atrial structures.

Normal sinus activation

Figure 6.3 demonstrates the epicardial atrial activation sequence in four dogs. A represents the activation sequence in the dog with spontaneous atrial flutter, and B, C and D demonstrate atrial activation in three normal dogs for com-

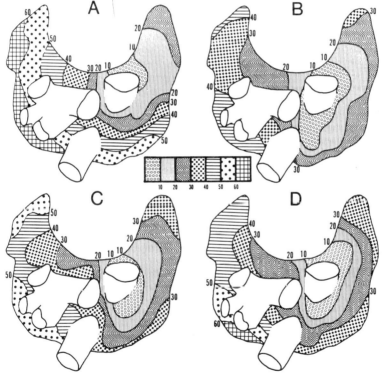

Figure 6.3 Comparison of abnormal and normal atrial activation during sinus rhythm. Isochronous or isotemporal maps are used to display the sequence of atrial activation. The time key indicates the activation time gradient encompassed by each pattern. The lines between patterns indicate the position of the activation wavefront for each 10 msec instant during atrial depolarization. Map A illustrates the activation sequence during sinus rhythm in the dog with atrial flutter and should be compared with Maps B through D which show normal sino-atrial activation. Note the absence of normal, preferential conduction inferiorly over the crista terminalis and superiorly over the anterior interatrial band in Map A

parison. In the latter three dogs, note the normal preferential atrial activation pattern with rapid spread from sinus node region to inferior vena cava along the pathway of the crista terminalis. This non-uniform spread of atrial activation is consistent with observations reported by other investigators[7-10]. In addition, note the more rapid spread from sinus node into the left atrium over the anterior interatrial band. Particular attention should be directed toward the isochronous lines at 10, 20 and 30 msec in comparing Map A with B, C and D. In the dog with flutter (Map A), during sinus activation, there is no evidence of normal preferential atrial activation, either inferiorly along the crista terminalis or superiorly and leftward over the anterior interatrial band. Also note the persistent slowing as represented by the closely adjacent isochronous lines between 20 and 50 msec beginning just below the superior vena cava and extending laterally to the right atrial margin. The latest inferior right atrial activation time in this dog is 56 msec and this point is located adjacent to the inferior vena cava at the bottom of the right atrium. Note, in addition, that the total atrial activation time is >60 msec and the latest time to be activated is in the inferior left atrium adjacent to the left pulmonary veins at 67 msec.

Thus, the dog with atrial flutter demonstrates an abnormality in normal sinus activation characterized by the absence of normal preferential atrial conduction.

Spontaneous atrial flutter
Activation potentials
In Figure 6.4 note the 24 simultaneous atrial electrograms recorded during two different types of spontaneous atrial flutter in this dog. This is the same animal which exhibited abnormal atrial activation during sinus rhythm in Figure 6.3A. Type 1 atrial flutter is demonstrated in A and Type 2 atrial flutter is demonstrated in B. In A, note that the electrocardiogram recorded in lead II demonstrates a pattern frequently observed in atrial flutter in human subjects. The flutter waves are characterized by continuous undulation with maximum positive convexity and a brief nadir of intervening negativity. Also note the presence of characteristic 2:1 AV block. By contrast, note the electrocardiogram in Type 2 atrial flutter demonstrated in B. Note that between each QRS complex, a positive or upright flutter wave is present, (F wave or P wave in surface ECG) and a second F wave is hidden by the superimposed QRS complex.

Inspection of the time relationships in the electrograms of adjacent points reveals that the activation sequences in the two types of flutter are quite different. For example, notice the relationship in the time of the peaks of the electrogram at points 17 and 18. In A (Type 1 flutter) 18 precedes 17, and this sequence is reversed in B (Type 2 flutter) Also note that electrograms at certain locations exhibit marked alternation in bipolar potential amplitude. The locations exhibiting most marked alternation do so in both types of atrial flutter; for example, positions 2, 9, 20 and 24.

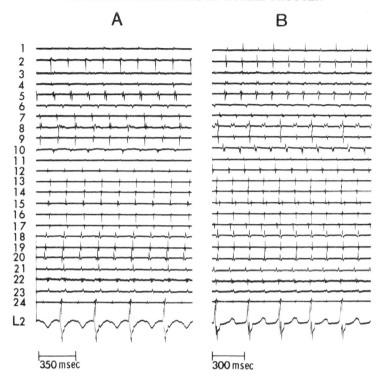

Figure 6.4 Atrial potentials during two types of spontaneous atrial flutter. Twenty-four individual bipolar electrograms are shown together with a lead II surface electrocardiogram. These potentials during flutter were recorded from the dog whose map during sinus rhythm is shown in Figure 6.3A. Note the differences in the electrocardiogram in A and B. In both cases atrial flutter with 2:1 AV block is present. In B only every other P wave is visible. Alternate P waves are masked by superimposed QRS. Note that the electrocardiogram in A is characteristic of human flutter. See text for further discussion

These two forms of atrial flutter were the only types of repetitive activity observed in this dog. Neither type spontaneously reverted to the other; for Type 2 to succeed Type 1 flutter, Type 1 first had to be terminated. Note that in Type 2 flutter (Figure 6.4B) the electrocardiogram exhibits what appears to be a flat baseline between the F wave peaks.

Atrial activation sequence – Type 1 flutter
A map of the sequence of atrial excitation during Type 1 atrial flutter is illustrated in Figure 6.5. The pathway of the wavefront during this form of atrial flutter is depicted in two ways in this figure. To the left, each 10 msec time zone is indicated by a different colour, and the colour key below indicates the activation times as the flutter wave passed different atrial electrode positions. Additionally, the time key is correlated with a single flutter cycle and a solitary

flutter wave. The figure to the right schematically represents the direction of the wavefront and its instant by instant direction is indicated by the arrows.

Figure 6.5 shows that one complete cycle lasted 175 msec and that the earliest evidence of atrial activity was located between the two venae cava to the right on the right main pulmonary vein spreading superiorly and bilaterally. The left wave blocked and rightward excitation spread inferiorly both above and below the superior vena cava at a very slow velocity as indicated by the

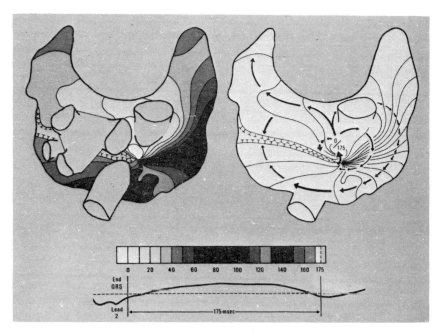

Figure 6.5 Map of atrial activation sequence during Type 1 flutter. To the left the position of the wavefront at each 10 msec instant of atrial activation is indicated by different colours. The colour key below indicates the time period between each 10 msec instant. To the right is a schematic representation demonstrating the direction and relative velocity of the activation wavefront for one flutter cycle. The activation times are correlated with the beginning and end of one flutter wave below. Note that the cycle length of one cycle is 175 msec. The T symbols indicate a region of block for both clockwise and anticlockwise moving waveforms

closeness of the isotemporal lines. Note that a vortex effect is created by considerably slower velocity near the origin of the wave with more rapid propagation away from the centre.

Also, note that propagation of the wave is slowest to the right and inferior of the superior vena cava between 20 and 120 msec. Because of the unique spatio–temporal relationships between late excitation waves and the location of earliest activation and recovery, re-entry from latest to earliest area occurred. This pattern was repeated with each successive cycle. Thus this complex form of intra-atrial re-entry resembles the theoretical models of circus rhythm and satisfies the conditions of one-way block and opposite one-way conduction. This recurring activity occurred in the absence of artificial barriers to conduction. Additionally, the superior vena cava orifice was not an essential part of the re-entrant pathway. The critical pathway was that portion located between the two venae cava in the region of the tuberculum intervenosum.

Correlation between the activation pattern and the surface F wave of the ECG in Type 1 flutter

Epicardial atrial activity was continuously present at locations adjacent to the vortex throughout the entire cycle. Note that from 0 to ca. 20 msec the activation wavefront spreading superiorly formed a closed surface interrupted only by the discontinuity of the superior vena cava. Because of maximum cancellation, closed surfaces of activation produce extremely small or no detectable changes in surface ECG. Upon reaching the superior aspect of the atrium, two wavefronts resulted: one spreading clockwise, rightward and subsequently inferiorly, and the other spreading leftward, counterclockwise and superior to the pulmonary veins, and then inferiorly. Thus, for most of excitation after 20 msec, wavefronts were directed laterally and predominantly inferiorly. This was associated with a predominantly positive F wave from 20 to 140 msec. At 140 msec, the wavefront spreading clockwise in the inferior right atrium propagated across the inferior vena cava and moved superiorly in the left atrium adjacent to the pulmonary veins. This latter period of superiorly directed left atrial activation was associated with a decreasing and finally negative potential in the undulating ECG waveform. The dotted line in Figure 6.5 associated with the surface ECG represents the position of the baseline.

Atrial activation sequence – Type 2 flutter

The sequence of atrial activation in spontaneous Type 2 atrial flutter is illustrated in Figure 6.6. The format is the same as that of Figure 6.5, and the time key similarly indicates the times of local excitation during a single cycle of atrial flutter for different locations of both right and left atrium.

In contrast to Type 1 flutter, the region of earliest activity began near the right atrial margin at the junction between the right atrial appendage and body of the right atrium. From this point, the wavefront propagated slowly in all directions, but most slowly in the right to left axis. The result was an elongated, nearly closed surface of electrical activity with two pseudopods of clockwise, extending superior and counterclockwise inferior activity. This highly cancelling surface of slow atrial excitation continued for 80 msec. At this point, the inferior pseudopod of excitation blocked inferiorly and to the right of the superior vena cava. Coincident with the block of the inferiorly travelling wavefront, excitation moved across the superior vena cava, into the sinus node area and leftward into the anterior interatrial band. At this point the propaga-

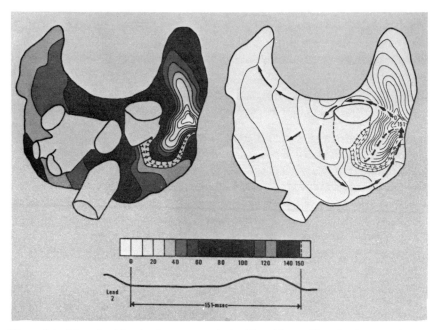

Figure 6.6 Map of atrial activation sequence during Type 2 flutter. Note that in comparison to the Type 1 flutter, Type 2 begins at the right atrial margin and progresses slowly superiorly and inferiorly in two pseudopods of activity. Also note that until *ca.* 80 msec the wavefront forms a nearly closed surface of electrical activity with a small opening at the lateral AV margin. The inferior portion of the wavefront blocks at 80 msec whereas the superior portion continues into the anterior interatrial band and inferiorly around the SVC. Once again due to the spatial apposition between early and late regions of activation, re-entry occurs

tion velocity increased as the wave spread around the superior vena cava and inferiorly into the region of the posterior atrial septum between the right pulmonary veins and superior vena cava. The wavefront continued at a near normal propagation velocity laterally and inferiorly in the left atrium. Note that in contrast to the pattern of Type 1 flutter in Figure 6.5, the unblocked portion of electrical activity progressed in a counterclockwise sequence around the superior vena cava, finally arriving in the inferior right atrium at 110 msec. The inferior wavefront at this point blocked on refractory tissue initially depolarized by the earlier blocked, inferiorly directed pseudopod of activation. However, the unblocked portion of the wavefront continued through a narrow pathway of undepolarized myocardium, resulting in close spatial apposition of late wavefronts and the initially activated region now undergoing recovery. Thus the wave re-entered the point of origin and the process was repeated with each subsequent cycle. Note that in Type 2 flutter (Figure 6.6), the cycle length was only 151 msec. Thus Type 2 flutter was associated with a faster atrial rate and a greater tendency to higher degrees of AV block than Type 1 flutter.

Correlation between the activation pattern and the surface F wave of the ECG in Type 2 flutter

Correlation of the activation pattern with the body surface ECG in Type 2 flutter revealed that, because of the nearly closed loop of excitation from 0 to 80 msec, very little change was generated in the surface ECG due to the effect of maximum cancellation of opposing wavefronts. At 80 msec due to block and disappearance of the inferior pseudopod and superior wavefront in the right atrial appendage, the unopposed wavefronts propagating inferiorly and leftward resulted in an increasing positive deflection in the body surface ECG. Note the notch in the F wave between 110–130 msec. As indicated by the activation sequence map, the second F wave peak coincides with the period of left atrial excitation. Between 130 and 140 msec the remaining wavefronts in the low left atrium and midlateral region of the right atrium had diminished markedly in area (size). Also, the direction of opposing wavefronts resulted in greater cancellation. This resulted in decreasing positivity of the F wave in the surface ECG.

Thus, the differences in the electrocardiographic manifestations of these two forms of atrial flutter reflect the marked differences in the patterns of activation. There is a tendency to oversimplify the process and distinguish between clockwise and anticlockwise right atrial flutter by the form of the electrocardiographic F wave. A more accurate analysis should consider that, in both types of flutter, there is predominant leftward and inferior unopposed electrical activity resulting in positive F waves. Also, that in Type 2 flutter, the presence of an apparent baseline does not indicate an absence of activation wavefronts, but a slowly propagating, almost closed surface of electrical activity resulting in cancellation of the ECG field for 80 msec even though activity is present the entire time.

The anatomy of atrial flutter

Figure 6.7 illustrates a posterior transillumination of four atria viewed from the anterior aspect looking through the tricuspid valve and viewing the endocardium of the posterior right atrial wall. By referring to Figure 6.2, the structures can be identified. As all of these atria were photographed and processed under identical conditions comparisons between the size and length of atrial conduction pathways, and the relative continuity of each atrial pathway can be made. The atrium in Figure 6.7A is that of the dog with spontaneous atrial flutter. The arrow indicates the region of slow sinus rhythm conduction between 10 and 20 msec illustrated in Figure 6.3A. B, C and D are normal atria of the dogs for which activation patterns were shown in Figure 6.3B, C and D.

Observe that in all four atria, the crista terminalis laterally, and the septum medially, and the crossing bridges of the anterior interatrial band superiorly and the tuberculum intervenosum centrally form a flat top A or a figure of 8. Also note the geometric differences in each of the dogs B, C and D. Although

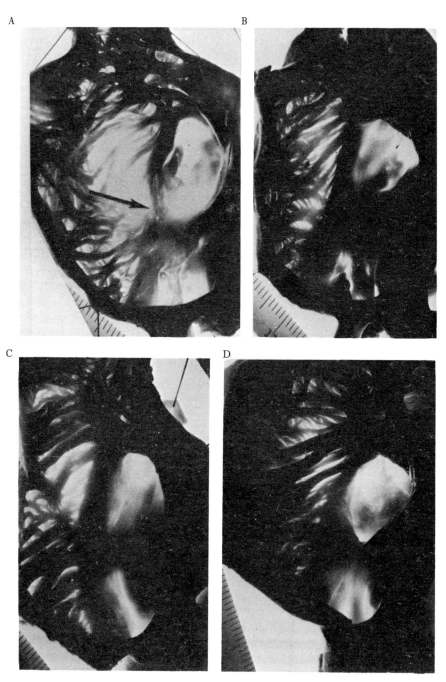

Figure 6.7 The anatomy of atrial flutter. Four transilluminated right atrial specimens are compared. The light source is posterior and the view is of the anterior right atrial endocardium. By referring to Figure 6.2 the components of the atrial myocardium can be identified. A shows the transilluminated right atrium of the dog with spontaneous atrial flutter to be compared with the right atria of three normal dogs. Note the generalized hypoplasia of the atrial muscle and in A specifically note the relative discontinuity between the superior portion of the crista terminalis and the tuberculum intervenosum (arrow). Also note the relative hypoplasia of the pectinate muscles particularly in the superior right atrium lateral to the crista terminalis

normal, each dog atria can be identified by the minor differences, shapes, sizes and densities of the structures forming the A or figure of 8. These variations were reflected in the minor differences in the atrial activation sequence during normal sinus conduction in these animals.

In contrast to the normal dogs, the dog with spontaneous atrial flutter (Figure 6.7A) demonstrated a generalized hypoplasia of the right atrial myocardium. This was characterized by more narrow bands of atrial muscle composing the crista terminalis, anterior interatrial band and tuberculum intervenosum. Additionally, the crista terminalis appeared to taper markedly in its superior aspect and as it approached the tuberculum intervenosum it became almost discontinuous. Also, the pectinate muscles in the region between the crista terminalis and the right atrial margin appeared atrophic with a decrease in the bridging pectinate bundles connecting the crista with the lateral margin of atrial ring myocardium.

Production of flutter by crista ligation

With the exception of the dog with spontaneous flutter, atrial repetitive activity with cycle lengths in excess of 140 msec and electrocardiographic manifestations resembling human atrial flutter were not encountered in any other dogs studied. The studies on the experimental stimulation of flutter-like repetitive activity will be presented later.

In a normal dog, an attempt was made to produce conditions favourable to atrial flutter by focal suture ligation of the crista terminalis at the level of the tuberculum intervenosum. This intervention was suggested by the observations on the anatomy and electrophysiology of the dog with the spontaneous atrial flutter. Thus, a 5 mm width of atrial myocardium at the junction of the crista terminalis and tuberculum intervenosum was ligated by placing a suture around the crista terminalis at this location. Figure 6.8 demonstrates the results. In the left panel, the global excitation sequence of the atria during normal sinus activation (A) and during atrial flutter (B) is demonstrated. To the right are enlarged maps of the activation sequence constructed by the rectangular dotted lines on the atrial maps to the left. The location and width of the atrial suture is indicated by the sawtooth within the rectangle.

The atrial activation time from sinus node to the inferior right atrium was prolonged after suture ligation of the crista terminalis. Also, the activation sequence resembles that in Figure 6.3A of the dog with spontaneous atrial flutter. Thus, normal sinus activation was modified resulting in slowing of conduction in the crista terminalis and altering the normal pattern of preferential conduction. The detailed map for the patch during normal sinus activation (Figure 6.8) demonstrates slowing of activation spreading from superior to inferior atrium characterized by the closeness of isotemporal lines between 15 and 50 msec.

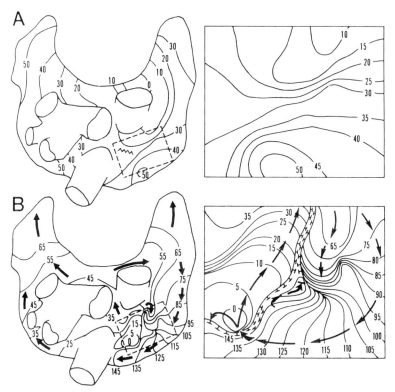

Figure 6.8 Production of flutter by ligation of the crista terminalis. In this normal dog flutter could not be stimulated until a 5 mm suture was placed around the crista terminalis at its approximate junction with the tuberculum intervenosum (sawtooth line in A, on left). Maps of the global atrial excitation sequence during sinus rhythm and during flutter are shown on the left. Detailed maps produced from the electrodes on the macro-patch are shown on the right. The position of the macro-patch during the recording is shown by the dotted rectangular area on the atrial maps

Figure 6.8B shows the sequence of activation and the complex re-entrant pathway during atrial flutter induced by premature atrial stimulation from the patch. Note that the initial area of excitation begins at the lower left corner of the patch which represents the site of premature stimulation and moves slowly superiorly, blocking along a boundary indicated by the T-shaped symbols. The wavefront moves to the top of the patch and pivots just below the superior vena cava in the tuberculum intervenosum. It subsequently propagates inferiorly with an exceedingly slow velocity in a non-uniform manner.

The conduction velocity at the periphery is considerably more rapid than that at the centre of the patch, resembling the vortex in the dog with spontaneous flutter. The inferiorly moving vortical wavefront also blocks on the boundary running from the top to the bottom left side of the patch. Thus, the sequence of activation is characterized by block of the wavefront moving inferiorly and to the right along a 15 mm boundary running from top to bottom of the patch. The return wavefront blocked on the refractory boundary of the initial wavefront at the same location. Terminal activation waves were located in the left inferior corner of the patch, and a pseudopod of late activity at the centre of the patch. Because of early recovery of the region of initial excitation and the apposition of the late wave in relationship to this area, re-entry occurred at the bottom left corner of the patch. The late area at the centre of the patch blocked and terminated in a cul-de-sac of tissue still in the refractory state.

This experimental production of flutter by focal interruption of the crista terminalis further emphasizes the importance of this critical discontinuity in atrial conduction in the genesis of atrial flutter.

Experimental atrial flutter
Some form of atrial repetitive activity was produced in 12 of 20 dogs using the extra stimulus method. In eight of these 12 dogs, reproducible short runs of repetitive activity resembling atrial flutter were mapped by the methods previously outlined. Compared to the animal with spontaneous atrial flutter, however, cycle lengths were considerably less regular and of shorter duration. An example of such an arrhythmia is illustrated in Figure 6.9. In this dog, 22 electrograms were recorded from the epicardial surfaces of the left and right atrium along with the reference atrial electrogram and a lead II ECG. Note the constant sequence of activation of the last four cycles, A3 through A6.

Figure 6.10 shows the response in one of these dogs to a progressive decrease in the premature beat (S_1S_2) interval. At an S_1S_2 interval of 129 msec, only one spontaneous re-entrant response (R_3) was noted. Two re-entrant responses were noted with a decrease in the S_1S_2 interval to 124 msec, and three responses were noted to an S_1S_2 interval of 123 msec. Finally, when the S_1S_2 interval was shortened to 100 msec, a long run of atrial repetitive activity of rapid rate, short cycle length, and irregular interval was noted.

Figure 6.11 shows two cycles from a run of atrial repetitive activity in response to a premature atrial stimulus delivered to the left atrium. Note that the re-entrant pathway is located in the left atrium and related to the site of premature atrial stimulation. Note that the cycle length of this arrhythmia barely exceeds 100 msec. Although there is a similar recurring overall pattern of atrial activation with each cycle, there are cycle to cycle differences between A and B (and subsequent cycles) due to the presence of dissociated wavelets. These dissociated wavelets are inconsistent in location and timing. Note in A the independent or dissociated wavelet beginning at 50 msec at the right atrial margin and in B note the independent wavelet rising in the inferior right atrium immediately to the right of the inferior vena cava at 170 msec. Observe the non-uniform spread of activation pseudopods with block of the impulse propagating inferiorly in the left atrium and propagation of activity superiorly

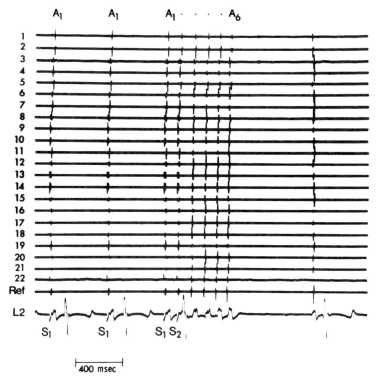

Figure 6.9 Induced repetitive activity in normal dogs. The extra stimulus method was used to induce runs of atrial repetitive activity in dogs with normal atrial anatomy. Note that 22 individual bipolar electrograms are recorded with a reference atrial bipolar electrogram and a lead II electrocardiogram. S_1 indicates the basic driving stimulus to the atrium, S_2 the premature stimulus, A_1 the response to S_1, A_6 the last of a series of six repeating cycles of re-entrant atrial activation induced by the S_2. See text for discussion

toward the left atrial appendage, then left to right in the anterior interatrial band, and subsequently a clockwise return to the point of origin. Also note the pseudopod of activation at 91 msec in A which does not re-enter and dies out in a cul-de-sac. This is repeated again in B 101 msec later. Thus, as in the dog with spontaneous flutter, the actual occurrence of re-entry depends upon some spatiotemporal continuity between late wavefronts and initially excited regions recovering their excitability in time to be restimulated or re-entered.

Correlation between atrial potentials, non-uniform atrial refractory period distribution, asymmetric atrial conduction, block and re-entry

To investigate the mechanism for the event initiating atrial repetitive activity and re-entrant excitation, correlations were made between the non-uniform activation present during the re-entrant cycles and the non-uniform distribution

S₁S₂ (msec)

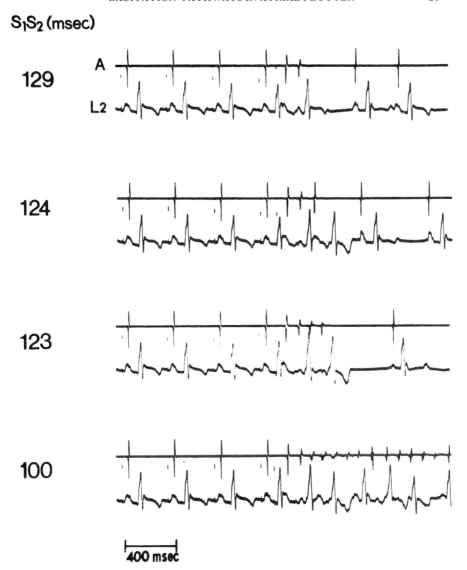

Figure 6.10 Pattern 2 – repetitive response. Note that in this dog successive decreases in the premature beat (S₁–S₂) interval resulted in increasingly longer runs of repetitive activity. This response which has been noted in the isolated atrium is less frequent in the intact heart

of the atrial ERP. Figure 6.12 indicates this relationship in a dog with experimental atrial repetitive activity. To the left in this figure, bipolar electrograms recorded from 21 of 24 epicardial locations are illustrated together with a reference bipolar electrogram and a lead II ECG. S₁A₁ indicates the stimulus and response of the last of a series of 12 driven stimuli delivered to

A   B

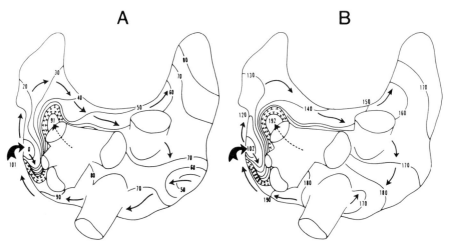

Figure 6.11 Repetitive activity due to left atrial premature stimulation. A represents one cycle from the middle of a run of atrial repetitive activity. B represents the cycle following A. Successive cycles resembled A and B. Note that the repeating cycle is only 101 msec

location 12. S_2A_2 represents the premature stimulus, which was delivered 126 msec after S_1, and the response, and A_3 represents a single re-entrant response as a result of premature stimulation. W_1 and W_2 represent the dissociation of the response to S_2 into two complexes. This fragmentation is seen best in rows 2, 3, 5, 6 and 7. These two widely separated components represent electrodes responding to an early and later wavefront.

The two waves are shown in the A_2 map to the right. The key to this map is indicated below. Each bipolar electrode pair is indicated by the large centre dot in the key. The distance between each of the bipolar electrode pairs is indicated above and to the right. The numbered position of each bipolar electrode pair and the corresponding atrial electrogram to the left is indicated by the number in the upper left hand quadrant. The upper case number in the upper right quadrant represents the ERP of that location, corrected for the activation time of the preceding S_1. The numbers in the two lower quadrants represent the arrival time of the wavefronts. Wavefront 1 (W_1) is indicated by the diagonal line pattern and wavefront 2 (W_2) is indicated by the small circle pattern. The premature stimulus (S_2) was delivered at an S_1S_2 interval of 126 msec at point 12. The wavefront propagated downward and was unimpeded. The wavefront propagating upward and leftward blocked. By correlating the activation times of wave 1 (W_1) with the corrected ERP, the mechanism for the block along this boundary is indicated. If W_1 arrived at an electrode location before the end of the refractory period (i.e. W_1 activation time was less than the corrected ERP time), then the wave blocked at that point. Because of block at that location, the tissue distal to this region was not excited and was thus responsive to a returning wave (W_2) which blocked on the same boundary which was again

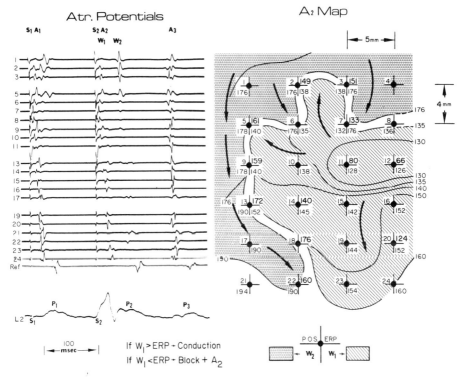

Figure 6.12 Correlation between refractory period distribution, one-way block-propagation, and repetitive response. On the left are the atrial potentials and stimulus artifacts recorded from 21 of the 24 point electrode patch. S_1 is the last of the series of basic driving stimuli, A_1 is the last response to the series of S_1. S_2 is a premature atrial stimulus and A_2 is the atrial response. W_1 and W_2 represent the fragmentation of A_2 into two components. A_3 represents a spontaneous re-entry response. Potentials are recorded together with a reference bipolar atrial electrogram and a lead II electrocardiogram. In the ECG, P_1 P_2 and P_3 represent the P waves associated with the three atrial cycles. To the right is a map of the premature stimulus (S_2) response (A_2). The map was constructed from the activation times determined from the bipolar electrograms. In the potentials recorded on the left note that several rows demonstrate two bipolar complexes whereas others demonstrate only one. This fragmentation is the result of these locations recording two wavefronts. The code below the map on the right indicates the meaning of each of the numbers associated with the 24 electrode positions. The black dot represents the location of the bipolar pair of electrodes. The number in the upper left hand corner indicates the numbered electrode position. The upper case number in the upper right hand corner represents the effective refractory period of that location corrected for S_1 activation time. The two numbers in the two lower quadrants represent the activation times of wave 1 and the later wave 2

refractory due to the earlier blocked wave (W_1) that had activated the tissue up to this point. Note at electrode location 3, the ERP is 151 msec and W_1 arrives before recovery at 138 msec and blocks. At 176 msec W_2 arrives at this same point.

In regions where the wavefront occurred after the refractory period of the tissue, it propagated without impediment. At position 14 the activation wave arrived at 145 msec which was 5 msec later than the refractory period. Similar correlations demonstrating the effect of the non-uniform distribution of the atrial refractory period on atrial conduction were observed in other dogs. However, because of the moment to moment changes in refractory period durations, this correlation was not conclusive in all dogs.

DISCUSSION

Re-entry concept

The fundamental basis for understanding atrial flutter is the result of early work by Mayer[11,12], Garrey[13], Mines[14,15] and Lewis and his co-workers[16,17]. These investigators demonstrated a theoretical basis for non-uniform or asymmetrical conduction referred to as re-entry. This concept proposes, for simple geometries such as those associated with major discontinuities, uni-directional block of a prematurely initiated impulse with slow circular propagation of the impulse in the opposite direction, returning to the site of initial activation. Re-entry and circus motion persist with one-way conduction around the loop if the excitation wave arrives at the site of initial stimulation after it has recovered its excitability.

An alternate hypothesis for atrial flutter is based on the microelectrode observations demonstrating enhanced automaticity in atrial fibres[18-20]. Although there is a large mass of data accumulated from microelectrode studies to implicate this latter mechanism, there is no conclusive electrophysiological data in the intact heart which definitely establishes automaticity as a basis for atrial flutter. In this regard, the cinematographic studies of Prinzmetal[21] demonstrating repeating wave motion from a central origin could be explained on the basis of focal microdissociation with re-entry into the surrounding tissue.

Studies by Rosenblueth and Garcia-Ramos[22] and also by Kimura et al.[23] on the experimental creation of flutter in the intact animal heart support the concept of circus rhythm and re-entry as the mechanism of atrial flutter. The major drawback to these previous studies, however, is the conditions under which the flutter was created, namely the production of barriers to conduction which essentially reduce the evidence for re-entry to another theoretical model. Thus, although flutter can be produced by creating barriers with compression and incision, the fact that it occurs naturally in the absence of these lesions leaves the question of actual mechanism unanswered.

The normal discontinuities of the human atrium, such as the superior and inferior vena cava and pulmonary veins have been invoked as the natural discontinuities about which the flutter wave moves[24].

Non-uniform recovery and excitation

The studies of Moe and his associates[25,26] are essential to the problem of flutter. They have shown that a premature beat encountering myocardial tissue with asymmetric or non-uniform recovery of excitability will result in non-uniform conduction, characterized by block in some areas and conduction in other areas.

Allessie and his co-workers[1] have recently demonstrated, in the isolated rabbit left atrium, complex forms of re-entrant circus rhythm which they mapped with multiple simultaneous electrodes. The re-entrant pathways demonstrated by this group resemble vortex motion with slow activation at the centre adjacent to the site of premature stimulation, and more rapid activation at the periphery of the atrial tissue. It follows that their premature beats encountered an inhomogeneous distribution of refractory atrial tissue producing this unique moulding of the wavefront associated with one-way block and one-way conduction. A subsequent study by their group[2] confirms this thesis, and demonstrates correlations between block locations and conduction and the gradient of the refractory period. Their studies were confined to isolated tissue of small dimensions. Also, the cycle lengths they observed were quite short and do not approach the cycle lengths (or lower heart rates) observed in spontaneous human atrial flutter. Thus, they recognized the importance of a missing factor, namely slowing of the unblocked return wave.

Speculations on the role of slow conduction

In the absence of an excessively long pathway over which the unblocked returning wave propagates, slowing of this wave in some part of its circuit must take place so that enough time elapses for the tissue to be re-entered to recover from its previous excitation. Atrial flutter in human subjects commonly exhibits cycle lengths between 180 and 215 msec. If spontaneous human flutter is due to intra-atrial re-entry as suggested by the studies of Allessie et al.[1,2], what then accounts for the longer cycle lengths? A certain degree of slowing is inherent as the premature wavefront encounters partially refractory tissue. However, this alone is not sufficient to explain the longer cycle lengths. Thus, there is some other factor needed for maintaining the re-entrant wave and allowing the receiving tissue to recover evenly and propagate the return wavefront smoothly.

There are numerous observations in single cardiac cells using microelectrode techniques which attempt to relate the action potential upstroke velocity to slow propagation or block in a system or matrix of cells. These studies do not and cannot define the larger problem which is the effect of a system of simultaneously activating cells on downstream conduction. Propagation in such a system of fibres depends on the spatio-temporal field associated with the wavefront of synchronously firing fibres. This synchrony determines the stimulus strength or stimulating efficacy at any moment and interacts with the overall excitability of downstream fibres and their particular geometry to determine the propagation velocity in the very next segment of the conduction pathway. Thus, a model consisting of: (1) Stimulus strength or efficacy; (2) Excitability of downstream cells; and (3) The specific geometry of the downstream cellular matrix is essential to any rational concept of conduction. These three interacting factors may also explain the effect of a system of exciting cells on the response of single cells. In addition, the interaction of these variables could account for the different effects of particular geometries on conduction, a factor essential to understanding differential or segmental variation in conduction velocity, block and arrhythmias. Recent studies in which extracellular bipolar activation potentials have been used to demonstrate dissociation of the activation wave[27,28] emphasize that simple dissociation or complex desynchronization accompanies the slowing. Although at present there are no established models relating precise geometries to conduction velocity and block, there is strong circumstantial evidence that in addition to individual fibre diameter, fibre direction and anisotropy, fibre packing density and the overall dimensions of a group of fibres exert a significant influence on conduction velocity.

Thus, if stimulating efficacy is related to the spatial current density of synchronously firing fibres, then a loose packing density or large gaps in conducting matrices will produce a decrease in the current density of the instantaneous field and reduce the stimulating efficacy of the wavefront and result in decremental slow conduction or block downstream.

Mechanism of slow conduction in atrial flutter
Figures 6.3, 6.5 and 6.6 in the dog with spontaneous atrial flutter, all demonstrate the greatest degree of slowing during sinus rhythm and atrial flutter in the same region. That region is to the right of the superior vena cava. Figure 6.7A demonstrates that this is the area of greatest abnormality in the atrial myocardial distribution of that dog. Note that in the area of the arrow, the crista terminalis decreases in density and becomes nearly discontinuous; and that lateral to this, the pectinate muscles are hypoplastic and the atrium in this region becomes almost transparent. Although the evidence obtained in single animals is not final proof of mechanism, the combination of observations lead us to conclude that the hypoplasia of right atrial myocardium and relative discontinuity of the crista terminalis are the basic substrates for atrial flutter in this dog.

The importance of atrial myocardial organization
Data obtained in this study indicate that the atrial myocardium rather than containing specialized tracts is *specially organized* to propagate rapidly the sinus node impulse. Whereas Purkinje fibres are insulated from surrounding

ventricular septal muscle, the areas of major atrial conduction are not. However, most recent studies show that atrial activation is definitely preferential, most rapid down the crista terminalis, and over the anterior interatrial band, and depends on the impulse being initiated in, or very near, the sinus node. The transillumination studies show why the site of the impulse initiation is so critical to the pattern of preferential conduction. Its location is at the junction or trifurcation of the major muscle bundles of the right atrium.

The present study suggests that situations where there is absence of preferential conduction may also be associated with atrial flutter. This is in contrast to the concepts that the 'specialized atrial tracts' are the site of the re-entrant circuits or automatic firing of special cell types located in these regions.

Initiation of repetitive activity – Role of non-uniform recovery

Our studies on experimental flutter confirm those of Allessie et al.[2] that the particular distribution of the refractory period interacting with the specific location and timing of an atrial premature beat, are the key variables which determine the initiation of a re-entrant cycle characterized by one-way block and one-way return conduction. Figure 6.13 indicates that it is the non-uniform refractory state of the atrium which moulds the premature wavefront giving rise to areas of block and other areas of conduction that eventually return to the site of initiation of the impulse.

The short re-entrant cycle lengths in our studies in dogs were similar to those reported by Allessie et al.[1,2] in their studies in the isolated left atrium of the rabbit. In inducing repetitive activity in dogs, we frequently noted cycle lengths of <100 msec. However, these cycle lengths in the intact dog heart were noted to be quite irregular when comparing different cycles. Rates as high as those observed by Allessie in isolated rabbit atrium and also by our group in the intact dog atria cannot be sustained in a regular pattern of flutter in larger atrial masses. Because of the larger mass of cells and the greater overall difference of refractory durations, as well as the distances and dimensions away from the principle re-entrant circuit, the process will be irregular, i.e. flutter–fibrillation. Thus in the studies by Allessie, a very localized event is described, which in a larger intact heart would have been similar to ours, i.e. flutter–fibrillation or fibrillation.

Relationship between atrial flutter and fibrillation

In the studies on experimentally induced repetitive activity, re-entrant vortices were frequently encountered. They were often associated with various degrees of dissociated activity in the form of secondary waves at varying distances from the primary, central pathway of the repeating wave. Also, these dissociated waves were observed to interrupt the repeating event which had initiated the repetitive activity. In any case the greater the degree of dissociation, the more irregular were the atrial cycle lengths. Thus, the repetitive action noted in the extrastimulus studies in normal dogs, without a mechanism for slowing the return wave, was an impure form of flutter and in reality, flutter–fibrillation.

Thus the definition of flutter which has evolved in these studies is a stable, repeating, spatio-temporal continuity of wave activity without dissociation or the presence of discontinuous activity. Thus fibrillation is defined as the presence of any degree of dissociation. Even though dissociated, because there is a repeating cycle of activity with predominant spatio-temporal continuity, the surface ECG and many individual electrograms can resemble those of flutter. This could also be called flutter–fibrillation. It seems obvious now that any degree of dissociation could be present and that previous observations describing both flutter and fibrillation simultaneously in the same heart are relevant to these current findings.

Components of atrial flutter

This study suggests that the following interacting variables are responsible for atrial flutter: (1) Structural discontinuity or disorganization of atrial myocardium, specifically, the crista terminalis, and secondly, the pectinate muscle hypoplasia. The pectinate muscles represent an alternate path of less direct conduction. Also their confluence at the lateral margin of the right atrium forms another potential pathway. (2) Non-uniform refractory period distribution or gradient. (3) Premature atrial beat — its precise location and timing.

The combination of factors (1) and (2) determines the intrinsic state of vulnerability or threshold to flutter. This state is constantly being altered by the changing individual refractory periods and the overall refractory period distribution. For flutter to occur, there must be optimum coincidence between factors (1), (2) and (3). The potential for flutter resides in the existence of factor (1), which may be congenital or acquired. The paroxysmal nature of atrial flutter and its presence, absence, frequency and duration are related to the changing nature of factors (2) and (3), which are extremely labile and influenced by multiple secondary or tertiary effects. These peripheral factors, which are commonly associated with the occurrence of flutter, produce their effects through the final common pathway of the autonomic nervous system, and primarily affect the refractory period distribution of the atrial myocardium.

The concept of a three-factor basis for atrial flutter has implications beyond this specific arrhythmia. Modified by the special conditions of each unique myocardial region, it can be used as an intermediate working model in unravelling specific mechanisms of other cardiac arrhythmias. However, each arrhythmia will have to be approached as a separate and unique problem, using techniques for recording multiple simultaneous extracellular potentials, determining multiple refractory period durations, and correlating these measurements with abnormalities of the cardiac geometry.

Acknowledgement

We are exceedingly grateful to the efforts of Wanda Rice and Linda Lantz for preparing the manuscript and to the Division of Medical Illustration of the Medical College of Georgia for their efforts in preparation of the illustrations. This work was supported by NHI grant No. HL–18398 and VA grant No. 1013.

References

1. Allessie, M. A., Bonke, F. I. M. and Schopman, F. J. G. (1973). Circus movement in rabbit atrial muscle as a mechanism of tachycardia. *Circ. Res.*, **33**, 54

2. Allessie, M. A., Bonke, F. I. M. and Schopman, F. J. G. (1976). Circus movement in rabbit atrial muscle as a mechanism of tachycardia. II. The role of non-uniform recovery of excitability in the occurrence of unidirectional block, as studied with multiple microelectrodes. *Circ. Res.*, **39**, 168

3. Licata, R. H. (1961). Anatomy of the heart. In: *Development and Structure of the Cardiovascular System*, A. A. Luisada (ed.). American College of Cardiology Monograph. (New York: McGraw-Hill Book Co.) pp. 1–35

4. Netter, F. H. (1969). *The Ciba Collection of Medical Illustrations*, Vol. 5, Heart, Sec 1, Plate 7. Ciba Pharmaceutical Company, p. 8

5. James, T. N. (1962). Anatomy of the sinus node of the dog. *Anat. Rec.*, **143**, 251

6. James, T. N. (1963). The connecting pathways between the sinus node and the A-V node and between the right and the left atrium in the human heart. *Am. Heart J.*, **66**, 498

7. Goodman, D., van der Steen, A. B. M. and van Dam, R. T. (1971). Endocardial and epicardial activation pathways of the canine right atrium. *Am. J. Physiol.*, **220**, 1

8. Spach, M. S., Lieberman, M., Scott, J. G., Barr, R. C., Johnson, E. A. and Kootsey, J. M. (1971). Excitation sequences of the atrial septum and the AV node in isolated hearts of the dog and rabbit. *Circ. Res.*, **29**, 156

9. Sano, T. and Yamagishi, S. (1965). Spread of excitation from the sinus node. *Circ. Res.*, **16**, 423

10. Holsinger, J. W., Jr., Wallace, A. G. and Sealy, W. C. (1968). Identification and surgical significance of the atrial internodal conduction tracts. *Ann. Surg.*, **168**, 447

11. Mayer, A. G. (1906). Rhythmical pulsation in scyphomedusae. *Carnegie Institution Publication No. 47*, 1

12. Mayer, A. G. (1905). Rhythmical pulsation in scyphomedusae. II. *Carnegie Institution Publication No. 102*, **1**, 115

13. Garrey, W. E. (1914). The nature of fibrillary contraction of the heart – Its relation to tissue mass and form. *Am. J. Physiol.*, **33**, 397

14. Mines, G. R. (1914). On circulating excitations in heart muscles and their possible relation to tachycardia and fibrillation. *Trans. R. Soc. Can. (Biol.)*, **8**, 43

15. Mines, G. R. (1913). On dynamic equilibrium in the heart. *J. Physiol. (London)*, **46**, 349

16. Lewis, T., Feil, H. S. and Stroud, W. D. (1920). Observations upon flutter and fibrillation. Part II – The nature of auricular flutter. *Heart*, **7**, 191

17. Lewis, T., Drury, A. N. and Iliescu, C. C. (1921). A demonstration of circus movement in clinical flutter of the auricles. *Heart*, **8**, 341

18. Hoffman, B. F. and Cranefield, P. F. (1960). *The Electrophysiology of the Heart*. (New York: McGraw-Hill Book Co.)

19. Singer, D. H., Ten Eick, R. E. and DeBoer, A. A. (1973). Electrophysiologic correlates of human atrial tachyarrhythmias. In: *Cardiac Arrhythmias*, L. S. Dreifus and W. Likoff (eds.). (New York: Grune and Stratton) pp. 97–111

20. Hogan, P. M. and Davis, L. D. (1968). Evidence for specialized fibers in the canine right atrium. *Circ. Res.*, **23,** 387

21. Prinzmetal, M., Corday, E., Brill, I. C., Oblath, R. W. and Kruger, H. E. (1952). *The Auricular Arrhythmias.* (Springfield Ill.: Charles C. Thomas)

22. Rosenblueth, A. and Garcia Ramos, J. (1947). Studies on flutter and fibrillation. II. The influence of artificial obstacles on experimental auricular flutter. *Am. Heart J.*, **3,** 677

23. Kimura, E., Kato, K., Murao, S., Ajisaka, H., Koyama, S. and Omiya, Z. (1954). Experimental studies on the mechanism of the auricular flutter. *Tohoku J. Exp. Med.*, **60,** 197

24. Wiener, N. and Rosenblueth, A. (1946). The mathematical formulation of the problem of conduction of impulses in a network of connected excitable elements, specifically in cardiac muscle. *Arch. Inst. Cardiol. Mex.*, **16,** 205

25. Moe, G. K., Rheinboldt, W. C. and Abildskov, J. A. (1964). A computer model of atrial fibrillation. *Am. Heart J.*, **67,** 200

26. Moe, G. K. (1975). Evidence for re-entry as a mechanism of cardiac arrhythmias. *Rev. Physiol. Biochem. Pharmacol.*, **72,** 55

27. Boineau, J. P. and Cox, J. L. (1973). Slow ventricular activation in acute myocardial infarction. *Circulation*, **48,** 702

28. Walston, A., II, Boineau, J. P., Alexander, J. A. and Sealy, W. C. (1976). Dissociation and delayed conduction in the canine right bundle branch. *Circulation*, **53,** 605

7
Pathological Correlates of Atrial Arrhythmias

J. C. DEMOULIN and H. E. KULBERTUS

Division of Cardiology and Electrocardiology, Institute of Medicine, University of Liège

INTRODUCTION

By elegant experimental procedures, or complex clinical techniques of investigation, the electrophysiologists have furthered considerably our understanding of the mechanisms of cardiac arrhythmias. Our knowledge of the pathological correlates of rhythm disturbances has in the meantime, unfortunately, remained relatively poor.

About two years ago, a programme was started in this institution to compare pathological data gathered from a series of patients with overt cardiac disease, but normal sinus rhythm, with data obtained from subjects with chronic atrial dysrhythmias, or evidence of sino-atrial disease. The purpose of this paper is to report on the preliminary results of this investigation.

MATERIAL AND METHODS

Studies were made of 26 hearts obtained from subjects who could be subdivided into three subgroups. Details regarding the clinical features can be found in Table 7.1.

The first subgroup consisted of 14 patients with overt cardiac disease, but normal sinus rhythm. There were ten male and four female ranging in age from 47 to 90 years. Nine subjects had a history of myocardial infarction, five a complete heart block, two a bacterial endocarditis and one a mitral insufficiency.

The second subgroup was made up of six cases with atrial fibrillation (five) or recurrent paroxysmal atrial tachycardia (one). There were four male and two female ranging in age from 48 to 69 years. They presented with coronary heart

Table 7.1 (a)   Patients with Overt Heart Disease, but Normal Sinus Rhythm

Case No	Sex	Age	Clinical features	Coronary arteries	Pathological findings of the SA region
1	M	69	Recent myocardial infarction	LAD: obst. Cx: st Recent thrombosis of RCA	Moderate fibrosis of SA node. Medial hypertrophy of SA node artery. Diffuse, severe fibrosis of atrial myocardium with leucocytic infiltrations (Type II)
2	M	73	Septicaemia Heart failure	LAD, Cx and RCA: st.	Mild fibrosis of SA node. Severe alterations of intrinsic ganglia. Severe fibrosis of atrial myocardium with large scars and inflammatory infiltration (Type III). Fibrotic pericarditis. Thrombosis of additus ad antrum
3	M	58	Inferior myocardial infarction	LAD, Cx and RCA st.	Necrotic areas within atrial myocardium. (Type III)
4	F	70	Bacterial endocarditis (aortic valve). Complete heart block	Within N. L.	Severe alterations of the ganglionated plexus. Haemorrhagic infiltration of nerves. Haemorrhagic and inflammatory infiltration of pericardium
5	F	87	Diabetes mellitus Mitral insufficiency. Complete heart block	Diffuse atheroma without significant narrowing	Diffuse fibrosis of atrial myocardium with scars and amyloid deposits (Type III)
6	M	58	Anthracosilicosis Anterolateral myocardial infarction	LAD: obst. RCA; Cx: st	Mild fibrosis of SA node and nodoatrial connections. Medial hypertrophy of SA node artery. Focal areas of pericardial thickening
7	M	85	Inferolateral myocardial infarction	RCA: st. Cx: obst.	Severe fibrosis of SA node. Disruption of nodoatrial connections. Severe, diffuse fibrosis of atrial wall (Type II). Lymphocytic infiltration of pericardium. Thrombosis of additus ad antrum

8	F	75	Complete heart block	Within N. L.	Mild fibrosis with small necrotic patches in SA node. Medial hypertrophy of SA node artery. Diseased ganglia and inflammatory infiltration of nerves. Conspicuous, diffuse fibrosis of atrial myocardium (Type II)
9	M	72	Anterolateral myocardial infarction	LAD: obst.	Diffuse and severe fibrosis of atrial wall (Type II). Pericardial leucocytic infiltration
10	M	90	Complete heart block	RCA; LAD and Cx: st.	Severe fibrosis of SA node. Thickening of the wall of the SA node artery. Fibrinous pericarditis. Thrombosis of additus ad antrum.
11	F	65	Old inferior and recent septal infarction	RCA: obst.	Severe fibrosis of SA node. Disruption of nodoatrial connections. Diseased nervous ganglia. Severe diffuse fibrosis of atrial wall with scars and amyloid deposits (Type III)
12	M	65	Old apical infarct Complete heart block	Cx: obst.	Mild SA node fibrosis. Severe fibrosis of atrial wall with scars (Type III). Inflammatory pericarditis
13	M	47	Old anterior infarct VF during an anginal attack	LMCA: st. LAD and Cx: ost. RCA: st.	Thickened wall of SA node artery
14	M	63	Old inferior infarct Recent anterior myocardial infarction. Pericardial effusion	Cx: obst. RCA and LAD: st.	Haemorrhagic effusion in pericardium

Table 7.1 (b) Patients with Atrial Tachyarrhythmias

Case No	Sex	Age	Clinical features	Coronary arteries	Pathological findings of the SA region
15	F	48	Mitral stenosis Chronic bronchitis Pulmonary emboli. Atrial fibrillation	Within N. L.	Marked fibrosis of SA node and nodoatrial connections. Diseased SA ganglionated plexus. Inflammatory infiltration of nerves, myocardium (Type II), and pericardium. Pericardial thickening
16	M	48	Corrected transposition of great arteries. Atrial fibrillation	Within N. L.	Severe fibrosis of SA node
17	F	62	Mitral valve disease Uremia; scleroderma. Atrial fibrillation	Within N. L.	Severe fibrosis of SA node with recent haemorrhagic and inflammatory infiltration. Lymphocytic infiltration of nerves. Medial hypertrophy of SA node artery. Severe, diffuse fibrosis of atrial myocardium (Type II). Inflammatory infiltration of pericardium
18	M	61	Recent anterior infarct. Atrial fibrillation	LAD: obst. RCA, Cx: st.	Conspicuous fibrosis of SA node and nodoatrial connections. Inflammatory infiltration of nerves. Severe, diffuse fibrosis of atrial myocardium (Type II). Thrombosis of additus ad antrum
19	M	69	Old inferior infarction. Atrial fibrillation	RCA: obst.	Mild fibrosis of SA node and nodoatrial connections. Moderate, diffuse fibrosis of atrial wall (Type II). Diseased SA node ganglionated plexus. Pericarditis
20	M	67	Aortic valve disease. Recent septal infarction. Pericarditis. Recurrent paroxysmal atrial tachycardia	LAD: st.	Fibrosis of nodoatrial connections with haemorrhagic infiltrations. Thickened wall of SA node artery. Diseased ganglia. Fibrosis and focal areas of coagulation necrosis in atrial myocardium (Type III). Inflammatory infiltration in pericardium

Table 7.1 (c) Patients with Sinoatrial Disease

Case No	Sex	Age	Clinical features	Coronary arteries	Pathological findings of the SA region
21	M	63	Old inferolateral myocardial infarction. Recent anterolateral infarction. Brady-tachycardia syndrome	RCA, Cx: obst. LAD: st	SA connections destroyed by fibrosis and haemorrhagic infiltration. Thickened wall of SA node artery. Type III involvement of atrial myocardium. Altered ganglia. Pericardial inflammatory infiltration
22	M	20	Diphteric myocarditis Bradytachycardia syndrome	Within N. L.	Severe fibrosis of SA node and nodoatrial connections. Leucocytic infiltration of nodoatrial junctions. Pericardial thickening. Thrombosis of additus ad antrum
23	M	72	Old apical and inferior myocardial infarct. Bradytachy-cardia syndrome	LAD: obst. Cx, RCA: st.	Severe fibrosis of SA node. Type III fibrosis of atrial myocardium with lymphocytic infiltration. Altered ganglia. Thrombosis of additus ad antrum
24	M	67	Cardiac failure. Syncopal attacks. Bradytachycarcia syndrome	Within N. L.	Amyloid deposits and severe fibrosis of SA node, nodo-atrial connections and nerves. Amyloid deposits and thickening of the wall of SA node artery. Severe fibrosis with amyloid deposits in atrial myocardium. (Type III)
25	F	75	Atrial septal defect. (Ostium primum). Sinus bradycardia; sinus arrest or sino-atrial block	Within N. L.	Severe fibrosis and haemorrhagic infiltration of SA node and nodoatrial connections. Altered ganglia and haemor-rhagic infiltration of nerves. Severe fibrosis (with scars) of atrial myocardium (Type III) with amyloid deposits. Thrombosis of additus ad antrum
26	F	66	Inferolateral myo-cardial infarction. Sinus arrest or sinoatrial block	RCA: obst.	Severe fibrosis, coagulation necrosis and inflammatory infiltration of SA node and nodoatrial connections Severe fibrosis of atrial wall with scars and necrotic patches (Type III). Pericardial thickening

disease (three cases), aortic valve disease (one case), mitral valve disease (two cases), or corrected transposition of the great arteries (one case).

The third group consisted of six patients with documented sino-atrial disease, manifesting itself either by a tachycardia–bradycardia syndrome (four cases), or by sustained sinus bradycardia with episodes of SA block or sinus arrest and slow escape junctional rhythm (two cases). There were four male and two female, ranging in age from 28 to 75 years. Three had a history of myocardial infarction, one had a diphteritic myocarditis, one suffered from amyloidosis and the last one had an atrial septal defect of the ostium primum type.

In each heart, the region of the SA node was obtained in the following manner (Figure 7.1). A first cut was made from the orifice of the inferior vena cava to the upper part of the right atrial appendage. The second cut passed

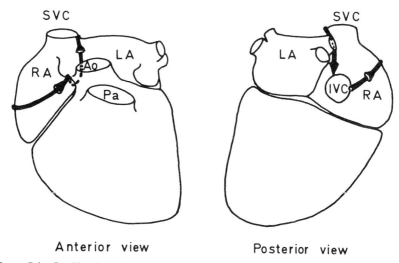

Anterior view   Posterior view

Figure 7.1 On this schematic representation of the anterior and posterior aspects of the heart, the dark line indicates how the cut was made to obtain the fragment containing the sinus node and the adjacent structures (see text for description). RA: right atrium; LA: left atrium; Pa: pulmonary artery; Ao: aorta; SVC: superior vena cava; IVC: inferior vena cava

posterior to the right atrial appendage and was directed towards the orifice of the superior vena cava. Finally, the last cut went from the superior to the inferior vena cava thus separating a block which was fixed in formalin and embedded in paraffin. Sections 10μm thick perpendicular to the axis of the superior vena cava, were prepared. Each 20th section was stained by haematoxylin–eosin, Azan–Heidenhain's solution, or Masson's Trichrome. Furthermore, in each case, 20–40 sections were stained by orcein or Congo Red with a view to studying the pathological changes of elastic fibres and to searching for amyloid deposits. The nervous structures were observed by using Bodian's staining.

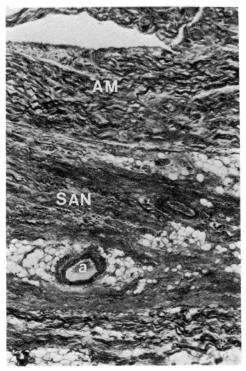

Figure 7.2 Section through a SA node centred by its artery (a) which is directly surrounded by a small area of lipomatosis. The node (SAN) contains nodal cells and fibrotic tissue in approximately equal amounts. This can hardly be judged on a white and black photograph whereas it is quite easy, at microscopic examination, since nodal cells and collagen tissue then appear in different colours. The node is surrounded by normal atrial myocardium (AM). Azan–Heidenhain × 48

This paper will only describe the pathological alterations of the SA node, nodoatrial junctions, atrial myocardium, sinus node artery and nervous structures.

The following morphological criteria and descriptions were used:

(1) *SA node*: severe fibrosis of the node was diagnosed when only a few scattered nodal fibres were left embedded in a mass of collagen tissue. (Figures 7.2 and 7.3). Haemorragic or inflammatory infiltrations were also carefully looked for.

(2) *Nodeatrial junctions*: we have always been unable to clearly demonstrate the presence of specialized atrial internodal pathways in the human heart. It remains however that areas of nodoatrial continuity are consistently seen along the margins of the compact sinus node (Figure 7.4). Such areas of blending of nodal and atrial muscle cells are notably found[1] in the regions presumed to be the origin of the bundles described by Bachmann[2], Wenckebach[3] and Thorel[4]. These areas of nodoatrial continuity most probably

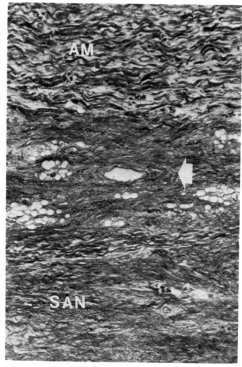

Figure 7.3 Severe fibrosis of the sinoatrial node (SAN) in which only very few nodal cells could still be found. The node was totally isolated from the atrial myocardium (AM) by a thick shell of fibrotic tissue which interrupted all areas of nodoatrial continuity. This is evidenced on this picture by the presence of a thick fibrous band indicated by an arrow. Azan–Heidenhain × 48

represent important structural bridges between the node and the atrial myocardium and were, therefore, carefully studied. Severe fibrosis of these structures was said to be present when they were all, largely or totally, replaced by intranodal or perinodal fibrosis (Figure 7.3).

(3) *Atrial myocardium*: the pathological changes in the atrial myocardium were graded according to Bailey's classification[5]. In grade I, (Figure 7.5) the atrial myocardium only shows minimal changes and is, in fact, grossly normal. Grade II specimens show moderate to severe fibrosis with preservation of muscle mass and architecture (Figure 7.6). Grade III specimens are characterized by extensive fibrosis, with loss of muscle and architecture (Figure 7.7).

(4) *Sinus node artery*: the pathological changes of the sinus node artery were noted: they consisted of intimal thickening or medial hypertrophy.

(5) *Ganglia and nerves*: the alterations of the nerves ganglia and fibres were diagnosed according to the descriptions made by Rossi[6]. The ganglia were thought to be abnormal when their cells showed vacuolar degenerescence or atrophy or when alterations in the pericellular processes and capsular cells were

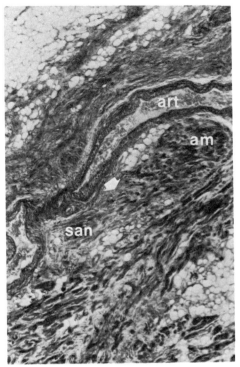

Figure 7.4 In the vicinity of the artery (art), this picture shows (arrow) an area of blending of rather pale nodal cells (san) with darker atrial muscle cells (am). Azan–Heidenhain × 48

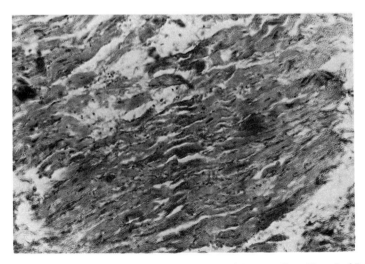

Figure 7.5 Section through an area of rather normal atrial myocardium (Type I of Bailey's classification)[5]. Hematoxylin–eosin × 100

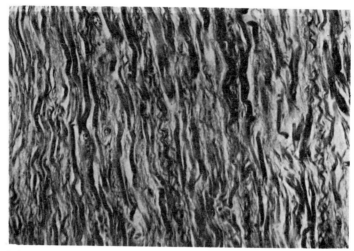

Figure 7.6 Atrial myocardium with severe, but diffuse fibrosis (Type II of Bailey's classification)[5]. Azan–Heidenhain × 100

present (Figure 7.8). Haemorrhagic and inflammatory infiltrations of the nervous fibres were also carefully searched for (Figure 7.9).

RESULTS

A detailed description of the observed findings is given in Table 7.1.

In the group of patients with *sinus rhythm,* three showed extensive fibrosis of the SA node accompanied twice by disruption of all nodoatrial connections.

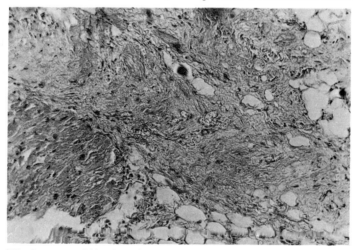

Figure 7.7 Presence, within the atrial myocardium, of a large fibrous scar surrounded by adipose cells. Such areas of loss of tissue may of course constitute definite localized anatomical obstacles. This is an example of Type III of Bailey's classification[5]. Hematoxylin–eosin × 100

Five further hearts were found to have some fibrotic or necrotic changes within the node, but these alterations were considered trivial or moderate. Rather severe fibrosis of the atrial myocardium was far from being uncommon. It was found in nine out of 14 cases and was graded as type II in four instances, and as type III in the remaining five. Amyloid deposits were also depicted in two cases and inflammatory infiltrations of the atrial wall in three. Five subjects had a diseased nodal artery and the nervous structures showed significant pathological changes in another five.

Among the six subjects with *atrial dysrhythmias,* four were discovered to have a sinus node which was nearly totally destroyed by a fibrotic process which also interrupted the nodoatrial connections in two instances. One patient only had a moderate loss of nodal fibres and in the last, inflammatory infiltrations were seen within the node. Atrial wall lesions were present and graded II in four patients and III in one. Arterial changes were observed in only one heart, but the nervous structures were clearly abnormal in five.

In five of the six patients, *with SA disease,* the node was almost totally replaced by connective tissue and only very few scattered nodal cells could still be seen embedded in a sea of collagen fibres. In four of these, the nodoatrial junctions were disrupted by fibrosis or by haemorrhagic or inflammatory infiltrations, a feature which was also present in the only instance where the node was not entirely destroyed. Grade III lesions were found in the atrial wall of five of these patients who also had severe pathological changes of the studied nervous structures. In only one subject was the nodal artery abnormal.

Discussion

Analysis of the histological findings in the sinus node area of normal subjects indicate that with advancing age, there is a gradual increase in the amount of connective tissue and a gradual reduction in the number of nodal muscle fibres[7,8]. Lev[7] considers that by the age of 40 years, the muscle and interstitial elements are present in about equal amounts. No further changes would take place after 60 years. As mentioned by Truex[1], when disease is superimposed on these ageing processes, it is often difficult to demonstrate more than a few nodal cells lost in a dense area of connective tissue. Sometimes, the node is so badly damaged that only its central artery can be identified with certainty. It may seem puzzling that three of our subjects with normal sinus rhythm did show extremely severe lesions of the sinus node accompanied in two cases by disruption of nodoatrial connections. Such a situation is however not exceptional and others have previously drawn attention to similar observations[8,9]. Considering that the extensive distribution of pacemaker type cells in the SA region usually covers a much larger zone than that occupied by the node itself, it seems possible that a proper impulse can still be generated in the SA region, for example closer to the crista terminalis even when most of the node has been destroyed[10]. Furthermore, the minimum number of living nodal cells which is needed to ensure a satisfactory pacemaking function remains unknown and probably depends on several factors, both anatomical and physiological.

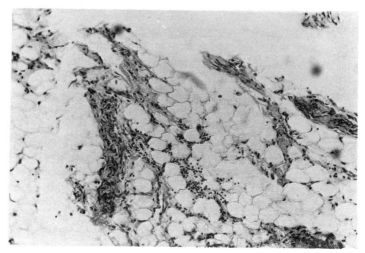

Figure 7.8 This picture shows a section through a nerve surrounded by an infiltration by small round basophilic cells. Hematoxylin–eosin × 48

In patients with atrial arrhythmias, especially atrial fibrillation, the most consistent histological features appear to be: (1) significant alterations of the sinus node; (2) pathological changes in the nervous structures; (3) fibrotic involvement of the atrial wall. Each of these features might, in itself, play a significant role in the genesis of dysrhythmias.

Emphasis on the changes of the sinus node in cases of chronic atrial dysrhythmias has for example already been laid by several investigators[8,9,11,12]. Hudson[9] described the histology in 65 nodes from hearts of patients with cardiac

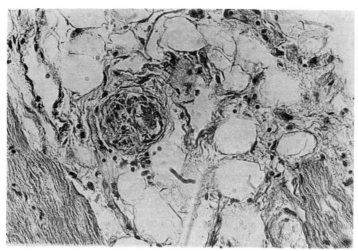

Figure 7.9 This picture shows a diseased ganglion with a definite proliferation of capsular cells (Hematoxylin–eosin × 248)

disease. Extensive damage of the sinus node was found in 15 cases of which 14 had had an atrial arrhythmia, usually atrial fibrillation, during life. Hudson[9] stated that, with rare exceptions, it might be possible, from the appearance of the node, to predict whether an arrhythmia had been present in life or not. This data leads to the hypothesis that a depressed SA node function is a predisposing, if not factor necessary, for the development of sustained atrial fibrillation.

The lesions of the nervous structures are also potentially of cardinal importance, since numerous experimental reports have previously stressed the role of neurogenic influences as contributory factors in the genesis of atrial arrhythmias and fibrillation[13,14].

Finally, the pathological involvement of the atrial wall may also be hypothetized to play a role[15] by giving rise to ectopic pacemakers, or by modifying the electrophysiological properties of the myocardium causing, for example, unequality of refractoriness and conduction in various areas of the atrial chambers. Trautwein and his co-workers[16] studied fragments of diseased human atria obtained at surgery. Their most significant findings was that excitation did not spread radially as they had expected but was confined to limited pathways. Some fibres areas could only be excited by impulses which entered at certain points. The authors assumed that these features were related to partial or complete block, presumably caused by scars and deteriorated tissue. This, indeed, leads to believe that fibrotic lesions embedded in the thin atrial wall can constitute ideal paths for circus movement and re-entrant excitation.

Altogether, the findings in patients with SA disease are not strikingly different from those obtained in the preceding group. The triad made up of nodal destruction, nervous lesions and atrial wall involvement is also encountered in this clinical setting[17-21]. Some particular features however deserve a special comment. First of all, in five of our six patients with SA disease, the nodoatrial muscle junctions were totally replaced by fibrosis. These areas of nodoatrial continuity which represent important structural bridges, have probably not received in the past all the attention they actually deserve. Their partial or total interruption may of course account for the various forms of entrance or exit conduction block to or from the sinus node which are so frequently discovered in SA disease, either during routine electrocardiographic examination, or by programmed atrial stimulation[22]. The same alterations also provide the anatomical substrate for sinus re-entry (echo beats and re-entrant arrhythmias). A second aspect which could be mentioned is that in our small series of patients with SA disease, the lesions of the atrial wall were more often of type III than of type II. This indicates that definite and relatively large anatomical obstacles are present within the auricular myocardium. Whether this may influence the nature of the atrial arrhythmias which develop in this disease and, for example, account for the relatively high incidence of paroxysmal atrial tachycardia[23] still remains to be further investigated.

Putting together these anatomical findings and even without taking into account the pathology of the AV node and infrahisian structures, one can propose a satisfactory correlation between the clinical and anatomical features of SA disease

Table 7.2   Sino-atrial Disease

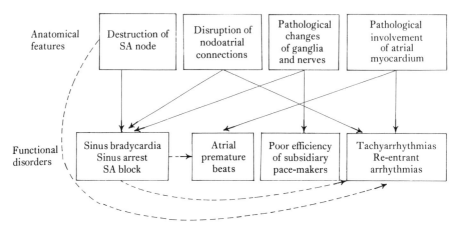

(Table 7.2). However, it is the authors' impression that in this field of cardiology, the anatomical findings considered in isolation will probably always leave some feelings of disappointment. The fact that some patients with normal sinus rhythm exhibit exactly the same alterations as those encountered in the presence of severe dysrhythmias demonstrate that we presently have an idea of the various anatomical conditions which set the stage for the atrial rhythm disturbances but still ignore which precise factor or association of factors can trigger the arrhythmias and permit their persistence.

It is likely that no major contribution will be achieved until completion of studies investigating simultaneously, and site by site, the histological and ultrastructural changes and the electrophysiological properties of specimens of diseased myocardium. In spite of their difficulty, such studies will probably constitute the only possible way to draw satisfactory correlations between the pathological alterations and functional disorders.

References

1. Truex, R. C. (1976). The sinoatrial node and its connections with the atrial tissues. *The Conduction System of the Heart*. H. J. J. Wellens, K. I. Lie and M. J. Janse, (eds.). (Leiden: Stenfert Kroese) p. 209
2. Bachmann, G. (1916). The inter-auricular time interval. *Am. J. Physiol.*, **41**, 309
3. Wenckebach, K. F. (1906). Beitrage zur Kenntnis der Menschlichen Herztätigkeit. *Arch. Anat. Physiol.*, 297
4. Thorel, C. (1909). Vorläufige Mitteilung über eine besondere Muskel-Verbindung zwischen der Cava superior und den Hisschen Bündeln. *Muench. Med. Wochenschr.*, **56**, 2159
5. Bailey, G. W. K., Braniff, B. A., Hancock, E. W. and Cohn, K. E. (1968). Relation of the left atrial pathology to atrial fibrillation in mitral valvular disease. *Ann. Intern. Med.*, **69**, 13
6. Rossi, L. (1969). Pathologic features of cardiac arrhythmias. *Case Editrice Ambrosiana, Milano*
7. Lev, M. (1954). Ageing changes in the human sino-atrial node. *J. Gerontol.*, **9**, 1
8. Sims, B. A. (1972). Pathogenesis of atrial arrhythmias. *Br. Heart J.*, **34**, 336

9. Hudson, R. E. B. (1960). The human pacemaker and its pathology. *Br. Heart J.*, *22*, 153
10. Brooks, Mc, C. and Lu, H. H. (1972). *The sinoatrial pacemaker of the heart.* (Springfield, Ill.: C. C. Thomas Publ.)
11. Doerr, W. (1959). Histopathologie des Reitzbildungs und Reitzeitlungs-systems des Herzens. *Verh. Dtsch. Ges. Inn. Med.*, *65*, 459
12. James, T. N. (1961). Myocardial infarction and atrial arrhythmias. *Circulation*, *24*, 761
13. James, T. N. and Hershey, E. A. (1962). Experimental studies on the pathogenesis of atrial arrhythmias in myocardial infarction. *Am. Heart J.*, *63*, 196
14. Trautwein, W. (1970). Mechanisms of tachyarrhythmias and extrasystoles. Symposium on Cardiac Arrhythmias. E. Sandoe, E. Flensted-Jensen and K. H. Olesen (eds.). *Ab. Astra. Södertalje, Sweden*, p. 53
15. Olesen, K. H., Andersen, M., Flensted-Jensen, E., Fischer-Hansen, J., Steiness, E. and Winkel, P. (1970). Conversion of atrial fibrillation in mitral stenosis. Symposium on Cardiac Arrhythmias, E. Sandoe, E. Flensted-Jensen and K. H. Olesen (eds.). *Ab. Astra, Södertalje, Sweden*, p. 393
16. Trautwein, W., Kassebaum, D. G., Nelson, R. M. and Hecht, H. H. (1962). Electrophysiological study of human heart muscle. *Circ. Res.*, *10*, 306
17. Acar, J., Hammo, J. C. and Diradourian, J. C. (1970). Troubles du rythme et de la conduction et amylose. A propos d'un cas anatomo-clinique. *Ann. Méd. Int.*, *121*, 703
18. Rosen, M. K., Rahimtoola, R. M., Gunnar, R. N. and Lev, M. (1971). Transient and persistent atrial standstill with His bundle lesions. *Circulation*, *44*, 220
19. Kaplan, B. M., Langendorf, R., Lev, M. and Pick, A. (1973). Tachycardia-bradycardia syndrome (so-called 'Sick Sinus Syndrome'). Pathology, mechanisms and treatment. *Am. J. Cardiol.*, *31*, 497
20. Kulbertus, H. E., de Leval-Rutten, F. and Demoulin, J. C. (1973). Sino-atrial disease. A report of 13 cases. *J. Electrocardiol.*, *6*, 303
21. Warembourg, H., Thery, Cl., Lekieffre, J., Delbecque, H. and Gosselin, B. (1974). Blocs sinoauriculaires et blocs auriculo-ventriculaires associés. Etude anatomo-clinique. *Arch. Mal. Coeur, Vaiss.*, *67*, 787
22. Strauss, H. C. and Wallace, A. G. (1970). Direct and indirect techniques in the evaluation of sinus node function. In: *The Conduction System of the Heart*, H. J. J. Wellens, K. I. Lie and M. J. Janse (eds.). (Leiden: Stenfert Kroeoe) p. 227
23. Gurtner, H. P., Lenzinger, H. R. and Dolder, M. (1976). Clinical aspects of the Sick Sinus Syndrome. In: *Cardiac Pacing. Diagnostic and Therapeutic Tools*. B. Lüderitz (ed.). (Berlin, Heidelberg, New York: Springer-Verlag) p. 12

Section III

Re-entrant Arrhythmias Involving the Atrioventricular Junction (With or Without Accessory Pathways)

8
Reciprocating Tachycardia using a Latent Left-sided Accessory Pathway. Diagnostic Approach by Conventional ECG

P. PUECH, R. GROLLEAU and J. CINCA

Service de Cardiologie, Cliniques St Eloi, Montpellier

In recent years, latent pre-excitation, most often left-sided[1-5], has been demonstrated with increasing frequency by means of intracavitary investigations. Careful analysis of conventional electrocardiograms in cases of reciprocating tachycardia incorporating a left-sided bypass, proven by electrophysiologic studies and in a few cases by the successful result of surgery, show that it is sometimes possible to predict the presence of the accessory pathway. The diagnostic criteria are based on the known influence of the sequence of ventricular depolarization upon ventriculo-atrial conduction time[6-9] and on a heretofore undescribed sign based upon the morphology of the retrograde P wave.

The occasional occurrence of a functional bundle branch block during a reciprocating tachycardia may help recognize a latent accessory pathway if the bundle branch block is located on the same side as the bypass. Indeed the cycle length of the circus movement is prolonged in its ventricular part, because of later arrival of the circulating impulse at the ventricular end of the bypass. As a consequence, the cycle length of the reciprocating tachycardia increases. The magnitude of the slowing in tachycardia rate induced by the bundle branch block is related to many factors, including the degree of asynchronism in ventricular activation (incomplete or complete bundle branch block), the site of insertion of the bypass in respect to the ventricular septum and the specific conducting tissue, the transeptal conduction time and the possible existence of multiple accessory pathways. In cases of left-sided Kent bundles, the slowing of the tachycardia by a left bundle branch block is *ca.* 20–60 msec.

Another factor can influence the rate of a reciprocating tachycardia when a functional bundle branch block, ipsilateral to the bypass, develops and, in fact, may reduce or cancel the effect of the bundle branch block: slowing of retrograde conduction (R–P interval) can be compensated by an improvement in antegrade (intranodal) conduction time[10]. If the V–A interval cannot be measured accurately in the surface leads, intracavitary recordings are needed to show that the behaviour of the cycle length depends on the magnitude of the retrograde conduction time and not on A–H or H–V intervals. In contrast to the usual slowing influence of left bundle branch block in cases with left-sided bypass, the inconstancy of the modifications of cycle length in cases of reciprocating tachycardia with right bundle branch block and right-sided pre-excitation has been pointed out[11].

The morphology of the retrograde P wave depends on the topography of the atrial end of the bypass and on the pattern of ventriculo-atrial conduction.

In the course of reciprocating tachycardias using the Kent bundle in antidromic way, the atrial depolarization starts from the area of the bypass input and spreads over the atria without any participation of the nodo-Hisian axis in atrial activation. Thus, the morphology of the retrograde P wave exclusively results from the location of the accessory pathway and may be used as a guide to predict the topography of the Kent bundle. If ectopic ventricular rhythms, either spontaneous or induced by intracavitary stimulation, are considered, the pattern of atrial depolarization is more complex and depends on the respective retrograde refractory periods of the normal and accessory pathways. Thus, the morphology of the retrograde P waves following an ectopic ventricular beat is identical to that of the reciprocating tachycardia in case of exclusive ventriculo-atrial conduction over the accessory pathway; it will be different if ventriculo-atrial conduction occurs over the normal pathway or simultaneously over both pathways, leading to an atrial fusion beat.

A latent left-sided bypass may be suggested to be incorporated in the circuit of a re-entrant tachycardia when retrograde negative P waves are recorded in lead I. This assumption is based on: (1) the correlation between the origin of the atrial activation in the postero-lateral region of the left atrium and the corresponding morphology of the P wave in surface leads; (2) the configuration of the P wave during left atrial stimulation from the great coronary vein and (3) the presence of retrograde negative P waves in lead I in cases of overt left-sided pre-excitation, corresponding to Type A Wolff–Parkinson–White syndrome.

The value of the morphology of the surface P wave, as an index of the area of the primary atrial depolarization has been discussed elsewhere[12–17]. Recently however, the direct study in man of the effect of atrial stimulation by fixed and close epicardial electrodes[18] showed a satisfactory correlation between excitation of the postero-lateral wall of the left atrium, in the vicinity of the inferior pulmonary veins, and P wave negativity in lead I. The mean atrial vector, oriented from the left to the right, has a variable inclination in the frontal plane, ca. $\pm 180°$; it may also be directed downward giving rise to positive P waves in leads II and III. The latter feature relates to the superior location of the most part of the left atrial mass, as compared to the right atrial body.

Left atrial stimulation by an electrode-catheter introduced via the coronary venous system which is close to the posterior margin of the mitral annulus, allows to establish a correlation between the zone of atrial depolarization beginning in the postero-inferior region of the left atrium and the morphology of the resulting P wave[19-21]. The P wave becomes negative in lead I when stimulation is performed in the great coronary vein. The inverted P wave reaches its maximal amplitude when the electrodes are located near the lateral margin of the heart at P–A fluoroscopy. Concomitantly the P wave-negativity in leads II and III, which is deep when stimulation is performed near the coronary sinus ostium, is progressively reduced as the stimulating site is moved toward the lateral wall of the left atrium.

The negativity of the P wave in lead I during reciprocating tachycardia in patients with overt left-sided pre-excitation (Type A Wolff–Parkinson–White syndrome) was obvious in many of our cases, where an accurate analysis of the retrograde P wave was possible, sometimes including amplified recordings of the frontal leads to allow a better recognition of the retrograde atrial activity. In a recent unpublished case (Medvedowsky and Nicolai, personal communication) of a patent postero-lateral left-sided bypass confirmed by epicardial mapping at surgery, clearly negative P waves in lead I appeared during attacks of reciprocating tachycardia.

Another way of demonstrating the retrograde invasion of the Kent bundle in Type A WPW syndrome is to induce progressively earlier ventricular beats until negative retrograde P waves in lead I occur.

During tachycardia, the precise analysis of the morphology of the surface P wave can be difficult, limiting the value of the conventional ECG.

When the negative retrograde P wave is superimposed on the beginning of the T wave, the latter seems inverted. This pseudo-T wave inversion can be recognized by comparing ventricular repolarization from QRS complexes with and without retrograde P wave. Premature atrial beats, given before the arrival of the excitation wave over the accessory pathway, thereby preventing retrograde atrial activation, help to differentiate between an inverted T-wave and the effect of the retrograde P wave on ventricular repolarization.

ILLUSTRATIVE CASES

Case 1. Minor degree of intermittent Wolff–Parkinson–White syndrome. Pre-excitation usually absent (Figure 8.1). Frequent runs of reciprocating tachycardia with always narrow QRS complexes, negative and deep retrograde P waves

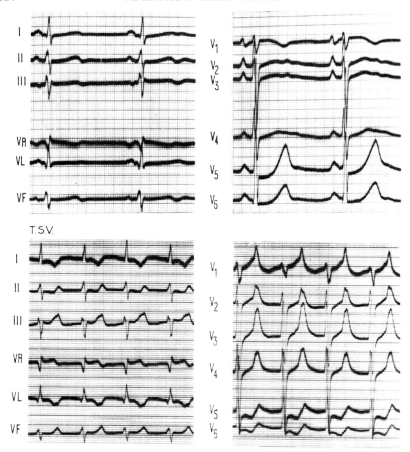

Figure 8.1 (case 1) Upper panel: sinus rhythm showing absence of pre-excitation; left atrial hypertrophy. Lower panel: reciprocating tachycardia (TSV) at a rate of 125/min. Retrograde P wave negative in lead I, VL, V_5 and V_6, positive in leads II and III, dome and dart shaped in V_1

in lead I, mean atrial vector oriented inferiorly and to the right in the frontal plane. In precordial leads, the retrograde P waves are negative in V_5 and V_6 and positive, dome and dart shaped in V_1 (Figure 8.1).

Electrophysiologic investigation demonstrates the presence of an accessory left-sided pathway. Comparative studies of the right and the left atrial stimulation through a patent foramen ovale at increasing pacing rates (Figure 8.2) show that the degree of pre-excitation at a given pacing rate is larger when the left atrium is paced[22,23]. When maximum pre-excitation is reached, Type A WPW syndrome with exclusive R waves in lead V_1 is recorded.

Episodes of reciprocating tachycardia could be elicited and stopped by atrial or ventricular extrastimuli properly timed in the cardiac cycle (Figure 8.3). Atrial mapping during tachycardia, shows the activation of the left atrium to precede that of the low right atrial septum (in the His bundle lead) and of the

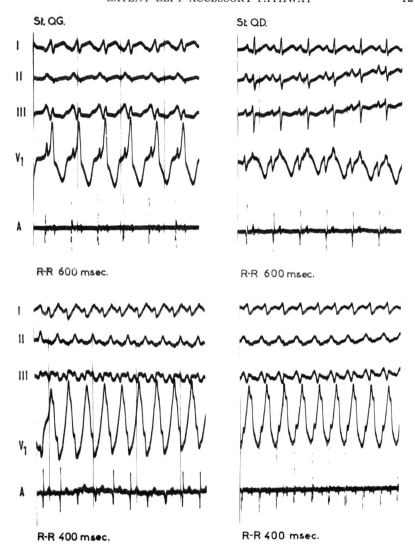

Figure 8.2 (case 1) Stimulation of the left atrium (St. O. G) at a rate of 100/min (left upper panel) produces a higher degree of pre-excitation, as compared to right atrial stimulation (St. OD) (right upper panel) at the same rate. Stimulation of both atria at a rate of 150/min produces maximal pre-excitation with exclusively positive R waves in V_1. The P waves resulting from left atrial stimulation (near the left cardiac border) are negative in lead I, positive in leads II and III, dome and dart shaped in V_1 (left upper panel). (A: intra-atrial recording)

free wall of the right atrium; the latter is activated about 75 msec after the beginning of left atrial depolarization (Figure 8.4). This sequence of atrial excitation is characteristic of a parietal left-sided bypass used in retrograde direction[22]. Ventricular programmed stimulation during the tachycardia allows

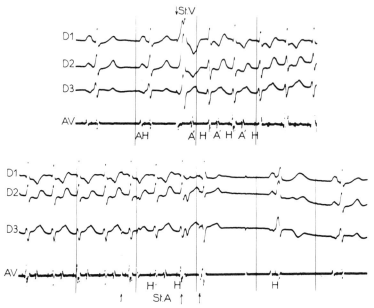

Figure 8.3 (case 1) Upper panel: initiation of reciprocating tachycardia by a single ventricular extrastimulus (St. V.). Lower panel: atrial stimulation stopping the tachycardia. The effective atrial stimulus delivered at the low right atrium gives rise to P waves deeply negative in leads II and III. The last QRS complex of the tachycardia is not followed by a retrograde P wave, making it possible to compare ventricular repolarization with and without superimposed P wave. This shows that the pseudo-negative T wave in lead I is actually due to the inverted retrograde P wave. (AV: His bundle recording)

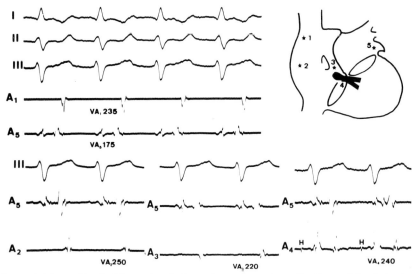

Figure 8.4 (case 1) Atrial mapping during reciprocating tachycardia. Onset of depolarization occurs in the left atrium (position 5), then activation spreads over the atria in the following order: middle part of the interatrial septum (position 3), high right atrium (position 1), low right atrial septum (position 4, corresponding to the His bundle lead) and ending in the free wall of the right atrium (position 2). (A_1 to A_5 all correspond to intra-atrial recordings)

atrial captures at the time when the normal pathway has been depolarized. This represents a further argument in favour of the incorporation of the accessory pathway in the circuit of the reciprocating tachycardia[5,9,10].

Stimulation of the lower part of the right atrium during the tachycardia (Figure 8.3) alters the morphology of the P wave, which becomes deeply negative in leads II and III. The termination of tachycardia after a QRS complex not followed by a retrograde P wave allows the comparison of the ventricular repolarization with and without superimposed retrograde P wave at equivalent cycle lengths, and shows that the pseudo-negative T wave in lead I was actually caused by the retrograde P wave.

Left atrial stimulation, near the projection of the left cardiac border gives rise to P waves, negative in lead I, positive in leads II and III, dome and dart shaped in lead V_1. This morphology is similar to that of the retrograde P waves seen in the course of the reciprocating tachycardia.

Case 2. Repetitive paroxysmal supraventricular tachycardia in a patient who always showed a normal ECG in sinus rhythm (Figure 8.5). During the tachycardia, the P wave is negative in lead I, simulating inversion of the T wave (comparison of the ventricular repolarization in tachycardia and sinus rhythm). The morphology of the retrograde P wave is more difficult to define in the other frontal leads. It seems negative in lead II, less inverted than in lead I and diphasic (−+) in lead III.

Atrial mapping, including coronary sinus and right atrial leads (recordings performed in 1953 by Latour and Puech) shows earlier beginning of left atrial depolarization in respect to the right atrium. The shortest R–P interval (0.10 sec) is recorded in the coronary sinus (Figure 8.6). The presence of a functional

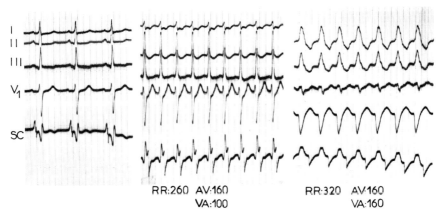

RR:260   AV:160
VA:100

RR:320   AV:160
VA:160

Figure 8.5 (case 2) Simultaneous recordings of surface leads and coronary sinus lead (SC). Left panel: sinus rhythm and absence of pre-excitation. Middle panel: reciprocating tachycardia at a rate of 230/min. Negative retrograde P wave in lead I simulating T wave inversion. Right panel: functional left bundle branch block, slowing the rate of the tachycardia. Lengthening of the cycle (from 260 to 320 msec) is due to prolongation of V–A conduction time (from 100 to 160 msec), the A–V conduction time remaining unchanged (160 msec)

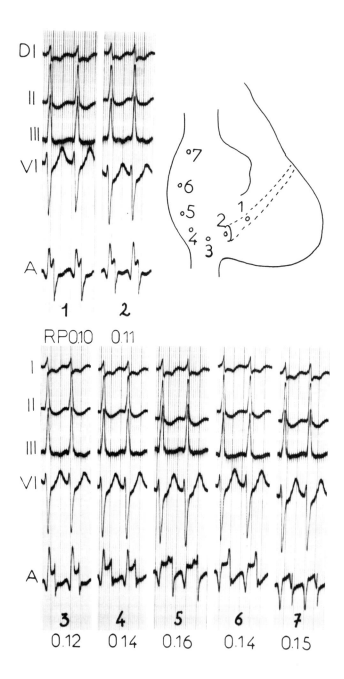

Figure 8.6 (case 2) Atrial mapping during reciprocating tachycardia, showing onset of depolarization in the coronary sinus lead (position 1). Activation of the free wall of the right atrium occurs 60 msec later (position 5)

left bundle branch block, slowing the rate of the tachycardia is, in retrospect, another argument in favour of a latent left-sided accessory pathway (Figure 8.5). When the QRS complexes are narrow, the cycle of the tachycardia is 260 msec and the A–V and V–A conduction times in the coronary sinus lead 160 and 100 msec respectively. When left bundle branch block is present, the cycle length is 320 msec. Lengthening of the R–R interval is caused by prolongation of the V–A conduction time, which increases from 100 to 160 msec, becoming equal to the unchanged A–V interval.

The effect of vagal and pharmacological influences to demonstrate the negative retrograde P wave in lead I and the latent left-sided accessory pathway is worth considering (Figure 8.7). Carotid sinus compression leads to slowing of the rate followed by an alternation in cycle length. The ventricular

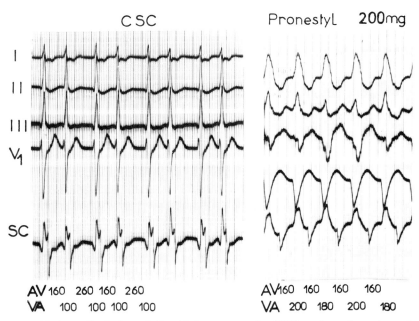

Figure 8.7 (case 2) Left panel. Carotid sinus compression (CSC) produces alternating cycle lengths, due to vagal effect on A–V conduction (A–V intervals of 160 and 260 msec), while retrograde conduction over the concealed Kent bundle is unchanged (100 msec). Right panel. Intravenous injection of 200 mg of procainamide (Pronestyl) during tachycardia with left bundle branch block does not modify A–V conduction (160 msec) but exaggerates the intraventricular conduction disturbance and prolongs the V–A conduction up to 200 msec

repolarization has the same morphology either after the long or the short ventricular cycle, showing that the pseudo-inversion of the T wave (which could be attributed initially to the fast rate of the tachycardia) is really due to the superimposed negative P wave. The vagal effect influences the antegrade conduction (AV node) and results in alternating cycles due to a change in the A–V interval (160 and 260 msec) while retrograde conduction remains unchanged (100 msec). The accessory pathway was insensitive to parasympathetic stimulation. Procainamide had an opposite effect on both pathways. The intravenous injection of 200 mg of Pronestyl, during functional left bundle branch block was followed by a lengthening of the V–A interval (from 160 to 200 msec). On the contrary, antegrade conduction was not influenced by the drug.

Case 3. Recurrent paroxysmal supraventricular tachycardia without overt pre-excitation. During the tachycardia, retrograde P waves are negative in lead I and hardly recognizable in leads II and III. The reciprocating mechanism of the tachycardia is demonstrated by intracardiac stimulation, the tachycardia being elicited and ended by properly timed atrial and ventricular extrastimuli.

Atrial mapping in the course of reciprocating tachycardia favours the hypothesis of a left-sided bypass used for retrograde conduction: atrial depolarization in the coronary sinus lead precedes right atrial activation by an interval of 60 msec; depolarization of the upper and lower parts of the right atrium is nearly simultaneous (Figures 8.8 and 8.9).

Functional bundle branch block recorded at the beginning of most episodes of reciprocating tachycardia provided a further argument for the existence of a latent left-sided accessory pathway (Figure 8.9). The RR intervals are the

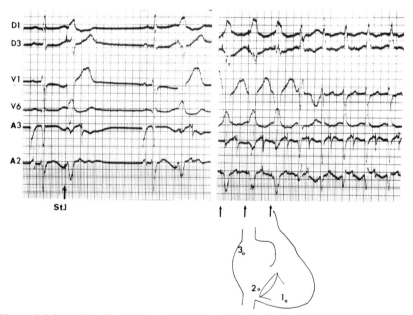

Figure 8.8 (case 3)   Right panel. Right ventricular stimulation (indicated by the arrows) initiates a reciprocating tachycardia with negative retrograde P waves in lead I and nearly simultaneous depolarization of the low (position 2) and high (position 3) right atrium. Left panel. Premature ventricular beats elicited by right ventricular stimulation (position 1) are followed by inverted retrograde P waves in lead I and a right atrial activation pattern identical to that seen during reciprocating tachycardia

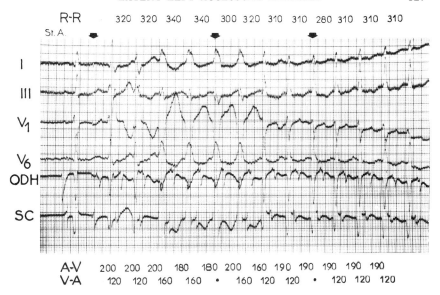

Figure 8.9 (case 3) Initiation of reciprocating tachycardia by programmed atrial stimulation (St. A). The first two QRS complexes of the tachycardia show a functional right bundle branch block and the four subsequent QRS have a pattern of left bundle branch block. During the tachycardia, left atrial depolarization (coronary sinus lead: SC) precedes high right atrial depolarization (ODH) by 60 msec. The V–A conduction time is the same when the QRS complexes are narrow or deformed by the functional right bundle branch block (120 msec) and prolonged when the functional left bundle branch block is present (160 msec). The variations of the RR intervals depend on the slowing effect of the left bundle branch block, on the changes in A–V conduction (between 160 and 200 msec), and on the interference of induced premature atrial beats followed by ventricular captures (atrial extrastimuli indicated by the arrows)

shortest when QRS complexes are narrow (310 msec) and the longest (340 msec) when a functional left bundle branch block is present. Intermediate cycle lengths are observed during functional right bundle branch block (320 msec). However, the value of the retrograde conduction time remains the same (V–A: 120 msec) either if the QRS complexes are narrow or deformed by the functional right bundle branch block. V–A conduction time is longer (160 mec) when left bundle branch block is present.

Ventricular extrastimuli coupled to the sinus rhythm (Figure 8.8) are followed by retrograde P waves, which are negative in lead I. The pattern of right atrial depolarization is the same as during the reciprocating tachycardia, that is, the activation of the top and bottom parts of the right atrium is nearly simultaneous, a finding which differs from that observed during retrograde atrial depolarization from the AV node[24,25].

Ventricular stimulation at increasing rates confirmed the duality of the pathways conducting in retrograde direction. The strip reproduced in Figure 8.10 illustrates the occurrence of two series of retrograde atrial responses

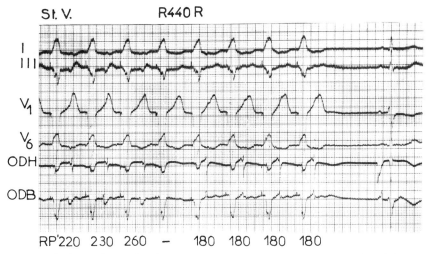

Figure 8.10 (case 3) During right ventricular stimulation (St. V) at a rate of 130/min, two patterns of retrograde conduction are successively observed. (1) First, VA conduction over the normal pathway with (a) a Wenckebach phenomenon; (b) retrograde P waves negative in lead III; (c) depolarization of the low right atrium (ODB) preceding that of the high right atrium (ODH) by 40 msec. (2) Then, V–A conduction over the accessory pathway with (a) shorter and fixed duration of the RP' interval; (b) retrograde P waves negative in lead I; (c) nearly simultaneous depolarization of the low and high right atrium, as in the course of the reciprocating tachycardia

during fixed ventricular stimulation at a rate of 130 beats/min (RR cycle length 440 msec). The first series corresponds to exclusive conduction over the normal pathway: progressive lengthening of the RP interval until a retrograde P wave is dropped (Wenckebach phenomenon in retrograde conduction); negative retrograde P waves in lead III; depolarization of the low right atrium preceding that of the upper right atrium. The second series reflects exclusive conduction over the accessory pathway; shorter and fixed R–P interval (180 msec); negative retrograde P wave in lead I and nearly simultaneous depolarization of the lower and upper parts of the right atrial cavity.

Left atrial premature beats, elicited by stimulation in the great coronary vein, in the vicinity of the left cardiac border (Figure 8.11) give rise to negative P waves in lead I and positive P waves in lead III, confirming the correlation existing between the onset of depolarization in the posterolateral part of the left atrium and the negativity of the P wave in lead I.

CONCLUSIONS

From a practical viewpoint, three conclusions can be drawn:

(1) If Type A Wolff–Parkinson–White syndrome is present during sinus rhythm, retrograde negative P waves in lead I during reciprocating tachycardia

confirm the existence of a parietal left-sided bypass, used in retrograde direction.

(2) Two accessory pathways may exist in patients with overt pre-excitation[2,8,10,26]. An additional bypass may be the explanation for failure of surgery directed to the overt Kent bundle in preventing recurrence of the tachycardia[26]. Thus, if right-sided pre-excitation is present (Type B Wolff–Parkinson–White syndrome) the occurrence of retrograde negative P wave in lead I must suggest a latent left-sided bypass. Denes' case (Reference

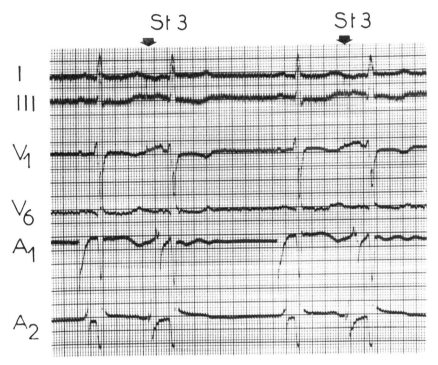

Figure 8.11 (case 3)   Left atrial stimulation elicited by extrastimuli delivered in the great coronary vein (arrows), gives rise to a P wave negative in lead I and positive in lead III. A1: high right atrium. A2: coronary sinus ostium

26, Figure 8.7) is an example of this event, which was confirmed by simultaneous coronary sinus and right atrial recordings.

(3) In the absence of overt pre-excitation, a retrograde negative P wave in lead I, occurring during reciprocating tachycardia, and/or after ventricular stimulation, suggests a parietal left-sided bundle of Kent used in retrograde direction. It must be confirmed by precise electrophysiological studies if surgery is considered for the treatment of recurrent disabling tachycardias.

References

1. Slama, R., Coumel, Ph. and Bouvrain, Y. (1973). Les syndromes de Wolff–Parkinson–White de type A inapparents ou latents en rythme sinusal. *Arch. Mal. Coeur Vaiss.*, **66**, 639

2. Spurrell, R. A. J., Krikler, D. M. and Sowton, E. (1974). Concealed by-pass of the atrioventricular node in patients with paroxysmal supraventricular tachycardias revealed by intracardiac stimulation and verapamil. *Am. J. Cardiol.*, **33**, 590

3. Svenson, R. H., Miller, H. C., Gallagher, J. J. and Wallace, A. G. (1975). Electrophysiological evaluation of the Wolff–Parkinson–White. Problems in assessing antegrade and retrograde conduction over the accessory pathways. *Circulation*, **52**, 552

4. Tonkin, A. M., Gallagher, J. J., Svenson, R. H., Wallace, A. G. and Sealy, W. C. (1975). Antegrade block in accessory pathways with retrograde conduction in reciprocating tachycardia. *Eur. J. Cardiol.*, **3**, 143

5. Wellens, H. J. and Durrer, D. (1975). The role of an accessory atrio-ventricular pathway in reciprocal tachycardia: observations in patients with and without the Wolff–Parkinson–White syndrome. *Circulation*, **52**, 58

6. Coumel, Ph. and Attuel, P. (1974). Reciprocating tachycardia in overt and latent preexcitation. Influence of functional bundle branch block on the rate of the tachycardia. *Eur. J. Cardiol.*, **1**, 423

7. Spurrell, R. A. J., Krikler, D. M. and Sowton, E. (1974). Retrograde invasion of the bundle branches producing aberration of the QRS complex during supraventricular tachycardia studied by programmed electrical stimulation. *Circulation*, **50**, 487

8. Zipes, D. P., De Joseph, R. L. and Rothbaum, D. A. (1974). Unusual properties of accessory pathways. *Circulation*, **49**, 1200

9. Neuss, H., Schlepper, M. and Thormann, J. (1975). Analysis of re-entry mechanisms in three patients with concealed Wolff–Parkinson–White syndrome. *Circulation*, **51**, 75

10. Coumel, Ph. and Attuel, P. (1975). Localization of the circus movement during reciprocating tachycardia in Wolff–Parkinson–White syndrome. In: *His Bundle Electrocardiography and Clinical Electrophysiology*. O. S. Narula (ed.). (Philadelphia: F. A. Davis Company), p. 343

11. Slama, R., Coumel, Ph., Motté, G. and Bouvrain, Y. Tachycardies paroxystiques liées à un syndrome de Wolff–Parkinson–White inapparent. *Nouv. Presse Med.*, **4**, 3169

12. Puech, P. (1956). L'activité électrique auriculaire normale et pathologique. 1. vol. (Paris: Masson)

13. Massumi, R. and Tawakkol, A. A. (1967). Direct study of left atrial P waves. *Am. J. Cardiol.*, **20**, 331

14. Mirowski, M. (1967). Ectopic rhythms originating in the left atrium. *Am. Heart J.*, **74**, 299

15. Harris, B. C., Shaver, J. A., Gray, S., Kroetz, F. W. and Leonard, J. J. (1968). Left atrial rhythm. Experimental production in man. *Circulation*, **37**, 1000

16. Cohen, J. and Scherf, D. (1973). Considerations on impulse formation in the left atrium and its diagnosis by electrocardiogram. *Am. J. Cardiol.*, **31**, 799

17. Waldo, A. L., Vitikainen, K. J., Kaiser, G. A., Malm, J. R. and Hoffman, B. F. (1970). The P wave and PR interval: Effects of the site of origin of atrial depolarization. *Circulation*, **42**, 653

18. MacLean, W. A. H., Karp, R. B., Kouchoukos, N. D., James, Th. N. and Waldo, A. L. (1975). P waves during ectopic atrial rhythms in man. A study utilizing atrial pacing with fixed electrodes. *Circulation*, **52**, 426

19. Lancaster, J. F., Leonard, J. J., Leon, D. F., Kroetz, F. W. and Shaver, J. A. (1965). Experimental production of coronary sinus rhythm in man. *Am. Heart J.*, **70**, 89

20. Lau, S. H., Cohen, S. I., Stein, E., Haft, J. I., Rosen, K. M. and Damato, A. N. (1970). P waves and P loops in coronary sinus and left atrial rhythms. *Am. Heart J.*, **79**, 201

21. Puech, P. (1974). The P wave: correlation of surface and intra-atrial electrograms. In: *Complex Electrocardiography*, vol. 2, Ch. Fisch (ed.). Cardiovascular clinics, vol. 6, (Philadelphia: F. A. Davis Company), p. 43

22. Gallagher, J. J., Gilbert, M., Svenson, R. H., Sealy, W. C., Kasell, J. and Wallace, A. G. (1975). Wolff–Parkinson–White syndrome. The problem, evaluation and surgical correction. *Circulation,* **51,** 767

23. Touboul, P., Clément, C., Porte, J., Chulliat, J. C., Bons, J. P. and Dalahaye, J. P. (1973). Etude comparée des effets de la stimulation auriculaire gauche et droite dans le syndrome de Wolff–Parkinson–White. *Arch. Mal. Coeur Vaiss.,* **66,** 1027

24. Agha, A. S., Befeler, B., Castellanos, A. M., Sung, R. J., Castillo, A., Myerburg, R. J. and Castellanos, A. (1976). Bipolar catheter electrograms for study of retrograde activation pattern in patients without pre-excitation syndrome. *Br. Heart J.,* **38,** 641

25. Amat-y-Leon, F., Dhingra, R. C., Wu, D., Denes, P., Wyndham, C. and Rosen, K. M. (1976). Catheter mapping of retrograde atrial activation. Observations during ventricular pacing and AV nodal re-entrant paroxysmal tachycardia. *Br. Heart J.,* **38,** 355

26. Denes, P., Amat-y-Leon, F., Wyndham, Ch., Wu, D., Levistsky, S., Rosen, K. M. (1976). Electrophysiologic demonstration of bilateral anomalous pathways in a patient with Wolff–Parkinson–White syndrome (Type B pre-excitation). *Am. J. Cardiol.,* **37,** 93

9

Unusual Re-entrant Tachycardias Associated with Accessory Pathways

P. TOUBOUL, A. GRESSARD, R. M. VEXLER,
and M. T. CHATELAIN

Laboratory of Clinical Electrophysiology,
Hôpital Cardiovasculaire et Pneumologique, Lyon

The understanding of arrhythmias associated with accessory pathways syndromes has made important progress owing to the development of electrophysiologic techniques in man. Use of the extrastimulus method has stressed the importance of re-entry mechanisms in the genesis of the tachyarrhythmias. The ability to initiate and terminate a tachycardia by electrically induced premature atrial and ventricular stimuli is accepted as proof that a circus movement of excitation is occurring within the atrioventricular (AV) junction[1-3]. Given the presence of accessory tracts bypassing some or all of the normal AV conduction system, ventricular pre-excitation syndromes offer an anatomical basis for re-entry.

Several different types of bypasses have been elucidated[4]:

(1) Atrio–His bundle connections (James fibres), thought to be the basis for the short P–R interval syndrome, which is rarely associated with episodes of reciprocal tachycardia[5].

(2) Paraspecific fibres described by Mahaim as originating from the AV node, the His bundle or the bundle branches, and inserting into the ventricular myocardium. It has recently been suggested that these fibres may play a role in the genesis of circus movement[6].

(3) Direct connections between atria and ventricles (Kent bundle). Such bypass tracts are noted in the most common form of pre-excitation, the Wolff–Parkinson–White (WPW) syndrome.

The existence of large dimension re-entry circuits (macro-re-entry) was first established in the WPW syndrome[7-9]. According to classical concepts, the impulse travels from atria to ventricles via the normal pathway only and subsequently returns to its point of origin via the accessory fibres. Thus, the QRS complexes do not exhibit evidence of pre-excitation. These junctional tachycardias are much more frequent than other types of tachyarrhythmias.

From our own series other varieties of reciprocating rhythm associated with the WPW syndrome will be examined. In addition, we will provide data favouring a circus movement between Mahaim fibres and the His bundle as a possible mechanism for reciprocating tachycardia.

UNUSUAL RECIPROCATING RHYTHMS DURING THE WPW SYNDROME

The data herein presented are taken from a series of 49 cases of WPW investigated by means of electrophysiologic techniques. In more than 80% of the cases (29/35), the usual type of reciprocal rhythm existed with antegrade conduction via normal A–V pathways and retrograde conduction by way of a Kent bundle. Exceptions to this rule occurred: (1) by an inversion of the circus movement (antidromic reciprocating rhythm) or (2) because fast pathways were implied in antegrade and retrograde conduction.

Inverted or antidromic reciprocating tachycardia (two cases)

In this mode of conduction, the impulse reaches the ventricles by the accessory pathway and returns to the atria via the His bundle and AV node. The rarity of such inverted reciprocal rhythms is supported by the following observations:

(1) In order to initiate an antidromic circus movement, a premature atrial depolarization must be blocked in the normal A–V pathway and conducted exclusively by accessory fibres. Such a sequence of events implies that the effective refractory period of the Kent bundle is shorter than that of the normal A–V conduction system. But in 4/5 of our cases, the opposite was seen. It follows, therefore, that the difference in refractory periods of the two pathways does not usually lend itself to creation of inverted reciprocating rhythms. Even in the favourable situation, the refractory state induced in the AV node by concealed conduction of the premature beat offers an obstacle to re-entry. One can imagine that the appearance of echo beats is favoured by high-level blockade of the initiating impulse in the atrionodal zone.

(2) The initiation of tachycardia by ventricular extrastimuli (one case) suggests several analogous points. Since it is blocked in the Kent pathway, the premature depolarization is conducted exclusively to the atria by the normal AV system. It can then return to the ventricles via the accessory fibres. The retrograde refractory period of the Kent bundle must exceed that of the normal pathways, which was the case in less than 1/3 of our patients; in the others, the

retrograde effective refractory period of the specialized AV tissue was the longest.

Inverted reciprocating tachycardias exhibit wide QRS complexes with an exaggeration of the WPW phenomenon. There is a 1:1 ventriculo-atrial (VA) response in which septal activity (as recorded by the His bundle catheter) precedes the electrogram recorded in the high right atrium[10]. The R–P' retrograde interval is longer than the P'–R. A His potential can occasionally be seen: in Figure 9.1, it is visible towards the end of the ventricular electrogram. Episodes of tachycardia are generally of short duration, lasting several seconds.

The diagnosis of antidromic reciprocal rhythm leaves room for discussion. One must first exclude low atrial tachycardia with pre-excitation QRS com-

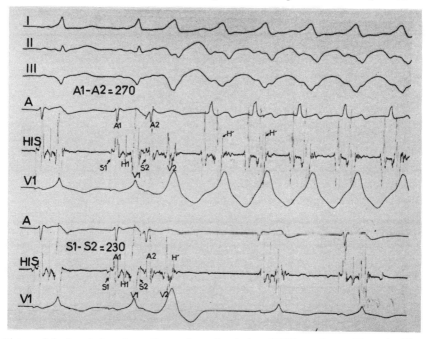

Figure 9.1 Inverted reciprocating tachycardia during WPW syndrome Type A. The extrastimulus method is used at a basic cycle length of 600 msec. A premature atrial response A_2, induced at a coupling interval of 270 msec, is followed by a WPW beat with increased pre-excitation pattern. Then a tachycardia is initiated, exhibiting antegrade conduction through the accessory pathway (upper panel). A 1:1 inverted atrial activity accompanies each QRS complex: the R–P' interval is longer than P'–R. A His bundle activity (H') is apparent at the end of the ventricular electrogram. A circus movement involving the Kent bundle for A–V transmission and the AV node. His pathway for retrograde conduction is likely to occur. However AV nodal reciprocating tachycardia or atrial tachycardia cannot be excluded (for further details see text). A shorter coupling intervals (lower panel), no tachycardia appears. The His potential accompanying the ventricular premature beat is to be related to concealed retrograde invasion of the common bundle by the re-entrant impulse. A: right atrial electrogram. His: His bundle lead. S: stimulus artefact. A and V: respectively atrial and ventricular activity recorded in the His bundle lead. Basic and premature responses are labelled 1 and 2. The values are in milliseconds

plexes. The initiation by a premature ventricular beat favours the concept of AV junctional re-entry. On the other hand, the differentiation is less certain when the tachycardia follows an atrial premature beat. A strong argument in favour of reversed circuits is the ability to interrupt episodes of tachycardia by induced ventricular depolarizations. Such a response is even more convincing when these premature beats are not conducted to the atria. Finally, reciprocating activity within the AV node still remains an alternative possibility. Figure 9.2 shows in a diagrammatic way a similar situation. The impulse leaving the AV nodal re-entry circuit reaches the atria and enters the Kent pathway. The same impulse is permanently blocked in the normal AV pathways which are kept refractory by concealed retrograde conduction of the anomalous excitation. However, it must be admitted that this latter concept does not provide the simplest explanation for the observed phenomena.

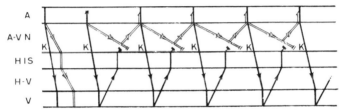

Figure 9.2 Diagrammatic representation of a reciprocating AV nodal tachycardia associated with anomalous AV conduction. The circus movement involves the AV node. The excitation emerging from the circuit reaches the atrial end of the accessory pathway and is transmitted to the ventricles. On the other hand, propagation through the normal pathway is permanently blocked as a consequence of repetitive concealed retrograde conduction of the ventricular excitation. A: atrium; A–V N: atrioventricular node; V: ventricle; K: Kent bundle

Circus movement with bidirectional abnormal conduction

Accelerated atrio–His bundle conduction and re-entry via Kent bundle (three cases)

The association of WPW with an atrio–AV nodal or atrio–Hisian bypass is suggested by the following characteristics[11]: (1) The pre-excitation pattern is of minor degree or completely absent in sinus rhythm; (2) The A–H interval is relatively short (average 60 msec) and increases little during rapid pacing (Figure 9.3). It may abruptly lengthen at a critical rate suggesting the sudden exclusion of a fast pathway; (3) Premature atrial stimulation gives similar results. Reduction of the coupling interval produces little change in the A–H or the delta wave. Occasionally, an increase in the pre-excitation pattern develops in spite of the absence of significant A–H delay (atypical concertina phenomenon). This can be explained by slowing of conduction in the His–Purkinje tissue (Figure 9.4).

The involvement of partial bypass tracts in orthodromic reciprocating rhythms results in the absence of significant A–H interval prolongation and fits

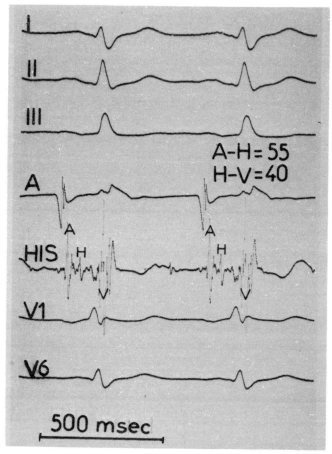

Figure 9.3   WPW type A with possible co-existence of James fibres. Note the short A–H interval (55 msec) in sinus rhythm

well with the very rapid rates of these tachyarrhythmias (generally >200/min). In the case illustrated by Figure 9.5, it is apparent that the A–H interval remains remarkably short during the tachycardia, at 60 msec. Two patients exhibited during tachycardia an alternation of long and short cycles with concomitant variations in A–H intervals as if the fast pathway was blocked during every other beat. The reciprocating tachycardia could also manifest two different rates in the same patient. Such a sequence is shown in Figure 9.6. The cycle length during the tachycardia abruptly shortens from 320 to 260 msec while A–H is reduced from 130 to 70 msec. This change might follow a brief burst of rapid ventricular stimulation, suggesting that, initially, block in the fast pathway was linked to concealed retrograde conduction. By inducing a premature depolarization of this pathway, ventricular extrastimuli were able to shift its recovery, thus allowing the antegrade impulse to conduct. The rapid

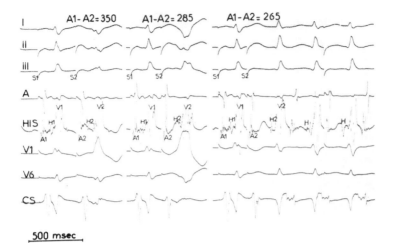

Figure 9.4 Same patient as in Figure 9.3. During the extrastimulus method, the pre-excitation aspect is exaggerated despite the absence of A–H prolongation (left) or minimal increase (middle panel). One must assume that the concertina effect is mainly due to conduction delay within the His–Purkinje system. Premature stimulation at 265 msec (right panel) is accompanied by a sudden lengthening of A–H (from 105 to 195 msec). The WPW pattern is suppressed and a reciprocating tachycardia is initiated. The cycle length is 330 msec. As shown in the coronary sinus lead (CS), the retrograde atrial depolarization begins in the left atrium

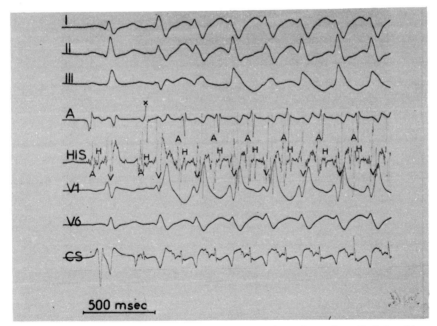

Figure 9.5 Same patient as in Figures 9.3 and 9.4. Reciprocating tachycardia induced by a spontaneous premature beat (X) originating in the left atrium. Retrograde conduction clearly involves a left lateral Kent bundle. The left atrial electrogram precedes the septal and right atrial activity by 40 and 80 msec, respectively. The high rate (240/min) is associated with a functional right bundle branch block. The A–H interval remains remarkably short (65 msec) suggesting that antegrade conduction is occurring through a bypass of the AV node

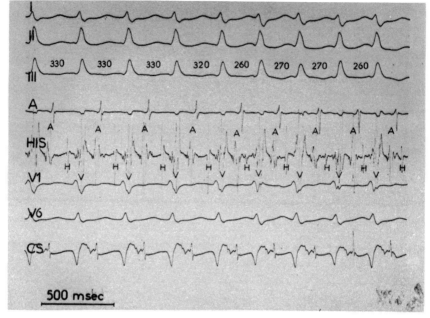

Figure 9.6   Same patient as in Figures 9.3, 9.4 and 9.5. Attack of reciprocating tachycardia showing two different rates. One can see that the tachycardia cycle abruptly shortens by 60 msec with relevant diminution of the A–H interval. Simultaneously a slight change in the QRS morphology is noticed. The sudden increase in rate might be related to the intervention of a fast pathway in antegrade conduction

rate then persisted which eliminates a transitory sympathetic effect on A–V nodal conduction. As for V–A conduction, it was occurring through a left-sided Kent bundle.

Re-entry circuit composed of two Kent bundles (one case)
One patient in this series, referred to our department following an episode of tachycardia, showed during sinus rhythm, a WPW Type B pattern. Several days later, an electrocardiogram revealed WPW Type A associated with a coronary sinus rhythm (Figure 9.7). During the electrophysiological studies, both patterns could be produced successively by stimulation of the right atrium and coronary sinus. Paired stimulation of the right atrium failed to elicit increasing ventricular pre-excitation as the coupling interval was reduced. Then, abruptly, at a coupling interval of 280 msec, a WPW Type A appeared accompanied by a lengthening of the S–delta interval from 60 to 75 msec (Figure 9.8). The effective refractory period of a right-sided accessory pathway was reached while the anomalous conduction persisted only by way of a left-sided Kent pathway. This latter tract was itself refractory at a coupling interval of 270 msec; thereupon normal A–V conduction ensued with an H potential preceding the

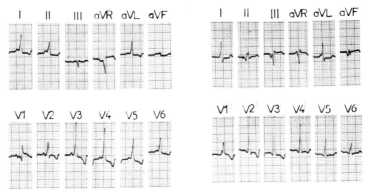

Figure 9.7 WPW syndrome. In sinus rhythm (left panel), the QRS complexes exhibit a Type B pattern. The morphology is changed in Type A when the pacemaker is shifted to the coronary sinus area (right panel)

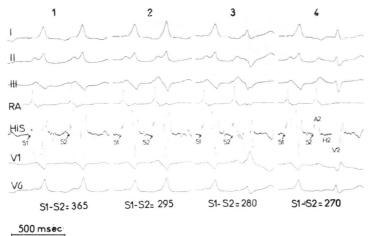

Figure 9.8 Same patient as in Figure 9.7. Extrastimulus method in the right atrium. The electrical impulses are delivered to the septum. The Type B WPW pattern is exaggerated. Reducing the coupling interval to 295 msec does not change the pre-excitation aspect. Such a response supports the view that the QRS complex is entirely dependent on the anomalous conduction (panels 1 and 2). At 280 msec (panel 3), a Type A WPW beat becomes manifest and the S2–R interval is slightly prolonged. The effective refractory period of the right-sided accessory pathway is reached. Now the anomalous conduction only occurs through a left-sided Kent bundle. At 270 msec pre-excitation disappears; the His bundle electrogram precedes QRS by 40 msec. The ventricular response exhibits an incomplete right bundle branch block pattern (panel 4). RA: right atrial electrogram

QRS by 40 msec. Rapid ventricular pacing produced retrograde conduction to the atria. The V–A interval remained fixed up to the highest pacing rate used, 240/min (Figure 9.9). Thus, retrograde conduction via an accessory pathway must be assumed[12,13]. Likewise, there was no increase in V–A time with the induction of increasingly premature ventricular extrastimuli. However, at short

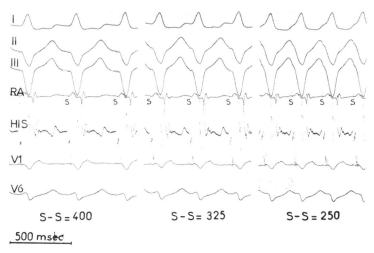

Figure 9.9   Same patient as in Figure 9.7 and 9.8. Incremental right ventricular pacing. The V–A conduction time remains fixed up to the highest pacing rate (240/min). Transmission of the retrograde impulse by way of a bypass tract (Kent bundle?) is likely

coupling intervals (250 msec), a sudden lengthening of V–A time was noted. Figure 9.10 shows that this sequence initiated a reciprocating tachycardia with antegrade conduction via the left-sided accessory pathway, as proved by the WPW Type A complexes. Meanwhile, the retrograde atrial sequence changed clearly after the third beat and at the same time, the right atrial electrogram exhibited the same morphology as that seen during ventricular pacing. Therefore, at this point, the retrograde impulse appeared to be taking an accessory pathway, in all likelihood, the right-sided Kent bundle. Concurrently, the cycle length of the tachycardia lengthened slightly. One could also explain these phenomena using a circuit composed of a left-sided A–V accessory pathway and, for retrograde transmission, an atrio-Hisian bypass. However, this hypothesis appears to be further from the observed facts.

RE-ENTRANT TACHYCARDIA VIA MAHAIM FIBRES

Such a mechanism was invoked in a 21-year-old patient who presented with episodes of paroxysmal tachycardia with wide QRS complexes. No evidence of pre-excitation was noted during sinus rhythm. However, His bundle electrography revealed an abnormally short H–V interval of 30 msec. Using the extrastimulus technique in the right atrium, as illustrated in Figure 9.11, we noticed that increasing stimulus prematurity produced concomitant lengthening of the S–R and S–H intervals. Subsequently, while S–R continued to prolong, the H spike became incorporated in the QRS. The latter manifested a left bundle branch block pattern identical to that seen during tachycardia.

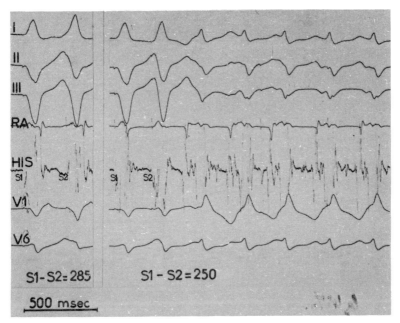

Figure 9.10.   Same patient as in Figure 9.7, 9.8 and 9.9. Premature stimulation of the right ventricle. At a coupling interval of 285 msec, the ventricular premature beat does not exhibit any prolongation of the V–A time (left panel). The right panel shows the sequence of events at a shorter coupling interval (250 msec). The atrial activity accompanying the basic ventricular beat (S_1) is of sinus origin. The premature beat S_2 is followed by a long V–A conduction interval. Then a tachycardia ensues with Type A WPW beats. After the third beat, the retrograde atrial sequence clearly changes and the morphology of the right atrial electrogram is again similar to that seen during ventricular pacing. One can assume that we are dealing with a circus movement involving the left-sided Kent bundle for antegrade conduction. As for retrograde conduction, it occurs at first through the normal pathways (first two beats) and then by the use of the right-sided Kent bundle

These phenomena suggested the existence of Mahaim fibres connecting the AV node and right ventricular myocardium. Initially, the premature impulse slowed in an AV nodal area above the emergence of the anomalous tract. Then, a supplemental zone of block appeared below, delaying progressively the arrival of the excitation at the His bundle. The anomalous QRS complex was due to the increasingly important role played in ventricular activation by the Mahaim fibres.

Bursts of tachycardia identical to the spontaneous arrhythmia were produced by premature ventricular stimulation. In Figure 9.12, it can be seen that the beat initiating a tachycardia is followed by prolongation of the V–A time. A His potential appears separated from the end of the QRS complex, the V–H interval accounting for retrograde delay. During tachycardia H becomes incorporated in the QRS complex which itself manifests major pre-excitation. A 1:1 inverted atrial activity is present. Suppression of these episodes by atrial or

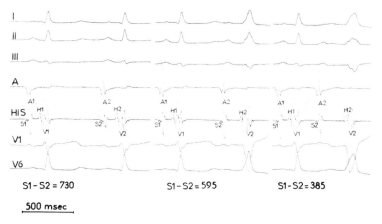

S1-S2 = 730   S1-S2 = 595   S1-S2 = 385

500 msec

Figure 9.11 Pre-excitation of the Mahaim type. Extrastimulus method. The right atrium is paced at a rate of 66/min. Note the absence of pre-excitation pattern in the basic beats: nevertheless the H–V interval is short (30 msec). An atrial premature depolarization elicited at a coupling interval of 730 msec is followed by a slight prolongation of the SR and SH intervals, without change in HV (left panel). At 595 msec, the A–V conduction time continues to lengthen. Now HV is shorter (20 msec) and the QRS complex is altered (middle panel). At shorter coupling intervals (285 msec), the His bundle electrogram is recorded 10 msec after the onset of QRS. Concurrently the ventricular complex develops a left bundle branch block pattern (for explanation see text)

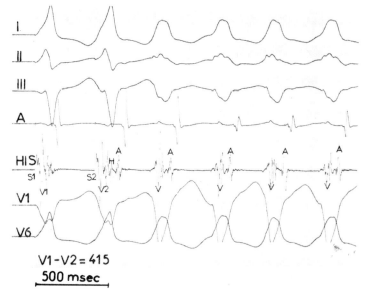

V1–V2 = 415
500 msec

Figure 9.12 Same patient as in Figure 9.11. Tachycardia induced by ventricular premature stimulation. Increase in V–A conduction seen on the initiating premature beat is based upon a V–H delay. The tachycardia exhibits wide QRS complexes identical to those recorded during atrial pacing (see Figure 9.10). The His activity then becomes incorporated into the ventricular electrogram. A circus movement involving Mahaim fibres (antegrade conduction) and the His bundle (retrograde conduction) is likely.

ventricular stimuli provided further evidence for a reciprocal mechanism. The most plausible explanation for these phenomena is that of a circus movement involving Mahaim fibres in an antegrade direction and the His bundle retrogradely. A reversed circuit could explain reciprocating tachycardias with normal QRS complexes. Proof that such a mechanism may exist remains to be shown.

References

1. Bigger, J. T., Jr. and Goldreyer, B. N. (1970). The mechanism of paroxysmal supraventricular tachycardia. *Circulation*, **42**, 673
2. Coumel, P., Motté, G., Gourgon, R., Fabiato, A., Slama, R. and Bouvrain, Y. (1970). Les tachycardies supraventriculaires par rythme réciproque en dehors du syndrome de Wolff–Parkinson–White. *Arch. Mal. Coeur Vaiss.*, **63**, 35
3. Wellens, H. J. (1971). *Electrical Stimulation of the Heart in the Study and Treatment of Tachycardias.* (Baltimore: University Park Press)
4. Lev, M. (1966). Anatomic consideration of anomalous AV pathways. In: *Mechanisms and Therapy of Cardiac Arrhythmias.* L. S. Dreifus and W. Likoff (eds.). (New York: Grune and Stratton) p. 665
5. Coumel, P., Waynberger, M., Slama, R. and Bouvrain, Y. (1972). Le syndrome du PR court avec complexe QRS normal: particularités électrocardiographiques. *Arch. Mal. Coeur Vaiss.*, **65**, 161
6. Tonkin, A. M., Dugan, A. P., Svenson, R. H., Sealy, W. C., Wallace, A. G. and Gallagher, J. J. (1975). Coexistence of functional Kent and Mahaim-type tracts in the pre-excitation syndrome: Demonstration by catheter technique and epicardial mapping. *Circulation*, **52**, 193
7. Durrer, D., Schoo, L., Schuilenburg, R. M. and Wellens, H. J. (1967). The role of premature beats in the initiation and the termination of supraventricular tachycardia in the Wolff–Parkinson–White syndrome. *Circulation*, **36**, 644
8. Durrer, D., Schuilenburg, R. M. and Wellens, H. J. (1970). Pre-excitation revisited. *Am. J. Cardiol.*, **25**, 690
9. Grolleau, R., Dufoix, R., Puech, P. and Latour, H. (1970). Les tachycardies par rythme réciproque dans le syndrome de Wolff–Parkinson–White. *Arch. Mal. Coeur Vaiss.*, **63**, 74
10. Wellens, H. J., Schuilenburg, R. M. and Durrer, D. (1971). Electrical stimulation of the heart in patient with Wolff–Parkinson–White syndrome, Type A. *Circulation*, **43**, 99
11. Coumel, P., Waynberger, M., Fabiato, A., Slama, R., Aigueperse, J. and Bouvrain, Y. (1977). Wolff–Parkinson–White syndrome: Problems in evaluation of multiple accessory pathways and surgical therapy. *Circulation*, **45**, 1216
12. Narula, O. S. (1974). Retrograde pre-excitation: comparison of antegrade and retrograde conduction intervals in man. *Circulation*, **50**, 1129
13. Wellens, H. J. and Durrer, D. (1974). Patterns of ventriculo-atrial conduction in the Wolff–Parkinson–White syndrome. *Circulation*, **49**, 22

10
Atypical Initiation of Reciprocating Tachycardia in the Wolff–Parkinson– White Syndrome

D. KRIKLER and P. CURRY

Cardiovascular Division, Royal Postgraduate Medical School, Hammersmith Hospital, London

Reciprocating atrioventricular (AV) tachycardias, whether involving the AV node alone or in association with an extranodal bypass, depend on the existence of two separate functional (or anatomic) pathways that can constitute a circuit that permits reciprocation – the persistent transmission of an impulse anterogradely in the one direction and retrogradely in the other[1,2]. Classically such tachycardias are initiated by extrasystoles that induce an anterograde block in one pathway, with P–R prolongation[3], and occur in the form of intermittent episodes of varying duration, usually infrequently, but sometimes sufficiently often to be labelled repetitive[4]. It is only recently that a specific 'incessant' form of reciprocating AV nodal tachycardia has been recognized and its features clarified[5,6]. This arrhythmia tends to affect children rather than adults, classically shows inverted P' waves in leads II, III and aVF (with R–P' longer than P'–R) and is initiated *not* by P–R prolongation but by a critical shortening of the P–P interval in sinus rhythm. We have now recognized that this last mechanism, namely, critical shortening of the P–P interval, can induce reciprocating tachycardia in the Wolff–Parkinson–White (WPW) syndrome, especially though not invariably in response to the administration of various antiarrhythmic agents and reported six cases that illustrate its features[7]. In another eight patients initiation of the tachycardia depended neither on the occurrence of premature beats nor on antecedent cycle-length shortening; seven of these cases have already been reported[8]. In six (five already reported) occurrence of escape beats in the bundle of His (five times in the presence of sinoatrial disease, and twice after ajmaline) activated the tachycardia circuit, but in the other two there were unusual mechanisms related to bradycardia-dependent block in the anomalous pathway, and delayed response to anterograde conduction delay, respectively. Careful assessment of such mechanisms is essential for the correct choice of antiarrhythmic prophylactic therapy.

Electrophysiological studies were carried out by recognized techniques of intracardiac recording and programmed stimulation[9], the patients or their guardians having given consent after proper explanation; sedation was not used and all medications were discontinued for at least 72 hours before investigation. The main features of the 14 cases are indicated in Table 10.1.

Table 10.1

Case	Age (years)	Sex	Mechanism of initiation	Factors	Bypass location
1	2	Male	cycle shortening	isoprenaline	right
2	18	Male	cycle shortening	spontaneous; ajma-line	left
3	42	Male	cycle shortening	ajmaline	right
4	31	Male	cycle shortening	ajmaline	right
5	5	Male	cycle shortening	spontaneous; ajma-line	right
6	58	Female	cycle shortening	lignocaine + practolol + digoxin	left (retrograde only)
7	35	Female	cycle lengthening	ajmaline	left
8	45	Male	anterograde block	slow atrial pacing	right
9	43	Male	His bundle escape	sinoatrial disease	left
10	75	Female	His bundle escape	sinoatrial disease	uncertain, usually latent
11	60	Female	His bundle escape	sinoatrial disease	left (concealed)
12	68	Female	His bundle escape	sinoatrial disease	left
13	67	Male	His bundle escape	ajmaline	left, usually latent
14	18	Female	His bundle escape	ajmaline	right

A typical example of incessant tachycardia complicating the Wolff–Parkinson–White syndrome is shown in Figure 10.1 (case 4). The pre-excitation pattern is suppressed in panels A and B due to the influence of ajmaline, but can be seen in alternate cycles during sinus rhythm in panel C, once the effect of the drug had decreased. In the upper two panels, reciprocating tachycardia is stopped by single ventricular stimuli; in all three panels, resumption of tachycardia is not dependent on extrasystoles or P–R lengthening, but rather on changes in the response to sinus beats. This can be seen in panels A and C as re-initiation of tachycardia following gradual, indeed sometimes barely perceptible, shortening of the sinus cycle length. In case 3 (Figure 10.2), following termination of the tachycardia, the cycle length was sufficiently short following the second sinus beat for tachycardia to restart.

Analysing conventional electrocardiograms, Katz and Pick[10] and Kistin[11] at-

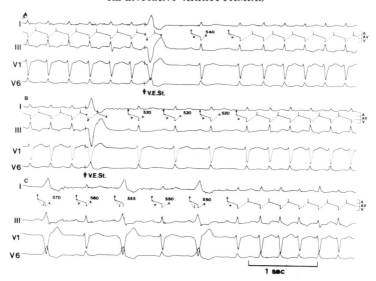

Figure 10.1 (Case 4). ECGs (leads I, III, V_1 and V_6); A and B are within 10 min and C, 15 min, after ajmaline (0.75 mg/kg body weight i.v.). *(a)* Reciprocating tachycardia stopped by a ventricular extrastimulus; tachycardia re-initiated by the second of the subsequent sinus beats, neither of which showed pre-excitation; *(b)* as in A but tachycardia re-initiated by fourth sinus beat; *(c)* in sinus rhythm there is alternating nodal/bypass conduction, with re-initiation of tachycardia by a sinus beat with A–V nodal conduction. Note that the first R–R interval during tachycardia is longer than those in subsequent beats.

tributed repetitive paroxysmal tachycardia to a re-entry mechanism. Focal left atrial tachycardia is sometimes suggested by the relative closeness of the first P′ wave to the first QRS of tachycardia and the inverted P′ waves in leads II, III and aVF[11-13] or, in these chronic intranodal tachycardias[5] there may be confusion with the usual mechanism for the initiation of reciprocating junctional tachycardia[14,15]. Using progressively accelerated atrial pacing, it is possible to show that a critical P–P interval can be reached in order to initiate the tachycardia[6]. Castellanos and Myerburg[16] may well be hinting at this mechanism when they indicate that marked sinus arrhythmia may act like extrasystoles in inducing reciprocating AV tachycardia.

Our cases with pre-excitation differ in several important ways from these chronic intranodal tachycardias. Most important, the P′–R interval was always longer than R–P′, instead of the converse, and R–P′ was constant and uninfluenced by vagal or drug effects. The relatively short and constant R–P′ in our present cases conforms with the use of a bypass tract retrogradely during tachycardia. Also, the first cycle length (R–R) of tachycardia in cases 1, 2 and 4 was longer than the cycle lengths in successive beats (Figure 10.1), by which time anterograde intranodal conduction had speeded in proportion to the heart rate; the first cycle length in the intranodal form is often shorter, in keeping with the presence of an initial common pathway. Classically, of course, the intranodal tachycardias

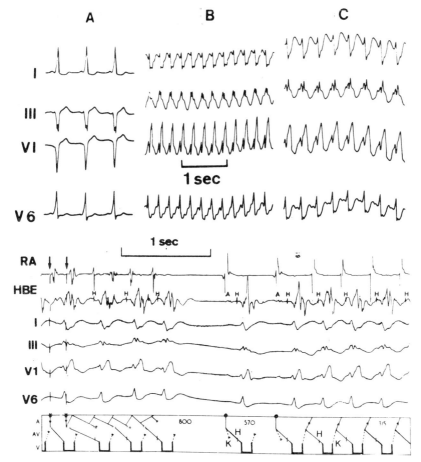

Figure 10.2   (Case 3). Panels A, B and C: ECG (leds I, III, V_1 and V_6). H = bundle of His; K = bundle of Kent. *(a)* WPW syndrome type B; *(b)* Reciprocating tachycardia (240/min), with RBBB; *(c)* Same as in B, but after ajmaline (0.75 mg/kg body weight i.v.), showing slower rate (180/min) with additional QRS widening; *(d)* Intracardiac and surface electrocardiograms, after ajmaline: following two atrial premature beats (arrows) introduced during the tachycardia, a localized irregular atrial tachycardia developed as the reciprocating tachycardia terminated; the two subsequent beats are sinus in origin, showing no evidence of anterograde bypass conduction, but are conducted with RBBB. Tachycardia starts after the second sinus beat at a critical and reproducible P–P interval of 570 msec but without previous lengthening of the anterograde conduction time (AH = 120 msec)

originate in infancy and persist for long periods, even decades; we now, however, describe briefer, perhaps ephemeral, phenomena which are usually drug induced.

In assessing mechanisms of the initiation of incessant tachycardia in the WPW syndrome, the same basic prerequisite obtains as with reciprocating tachycardias of the more usual variety affecting the AV junction or complicating the WPW syndrome: unidirectional block must exist in one pathway.

If the refractory period of the accessory pathway is long in the anterograde direction, all that may be required for the sinus impulse to encounter this situation may be a minor increase in the heart rate (shortening of sinus cycle length) so that it is conducted to the ventricles slowly via the AV node. Alternatively, anterograde unidirectional block in the accessory pathway may already exist, the pre-excitation being latent or concealed in the anterograde direction[17]. The second prerequisite follows from this: the time for conduction of the sinus beat through the AV node, when there is unidirectional block in the anomalous pathway, must be sufficiently long to permit the atrium to recover from activation by the preceding sinus beat; a possible corollary may be the need for the accessory pathway to recover from concealed anterograde conduction from the preceding sinus beat, if this had occurred.

Should these conditions be met, an atrial echo may occur when the sinus rate speeds up sufficiently for the refractory period of the anomalous pathway to be reached in the anterograde direction, this pathway now being conductive retrogradely; this may allow a burst of tachycardia to occur whenever the sinus cycle length is sufficiently short. On the other hand, when there is established unidirectional block in the anterograde pathway, speeding of the sinus rate may shorten the atrial and anomalous pathway refractory periods sufficiently to permit retrograde conduction up the anomalous pathway to the atrium, with an echo beat and tachycardia. The reciprocating AV tachycardia (whether intranodal or complicating pre-excitation) induced by exercise, in which sinus tachycardia is converted to paroxysmal tachycardia when a critical rate is reached, clearly has a similar mechanism; continuous monitoring may reveal this mechanism and exclude exercise-induced extrasystoles as the initiating factors[18].

In the three individuals aged 18 years or under, exactly similar incessant attacks of tachycardia have occurred spontaneously, or during febrile illnesses or exertion (cases 1, 2 and 5), in all three being more obvious after drugs (Table 10.1). Cases 3 and 4 only showed the situation under the influence of ajmaline, and in case 6 it had occurred when she received several drugs in rapid succession and was not reproduced during the study. In case 3, incremental atrial pacing failed to initiate tachycardia until ajmaline was given, when it became incessant during the effect of the drug. Case 4 presented similar features in that, under the influence of ajmaline, which abolished anterograde bypass conduction, tachycardia was incessant; after its effect had worn off, premature stimuli were needed in order to initiate tachycardia. The classical features of incessant tachycardia were seen in case 6 when she received vigorous antiarrhythmic therapy; the situation was not duplicated with ajmaline and verapamil during electrophysiological study.

For the electrocardiographic diagnosis of the WPW syndrome to be made in sinus rhythm, it is necessary for both the normal and anomalous pathways to function anterogradely, thus producing the characteristic fusion beat of the WPW syndrome. It is now becoming more and more obvious that in many cases there is intermittent or even permanent anterograde block in the anomalous pathway, causing the syndrome to be intermittent or indeed latent or concealed[19-21]. Unless this is appreciated, it is possible for cases of incessant junctional tachycardia to be considered to be AV nodal in origin: only cases 3 and 4 consistently showed evidence of the WPW syndrome during sinus rhythm, it being intermittent in cases 1, 2 and 5 (only appearing at the age of 4 years in the latter even though tachycardia was present from early infancy). Case 6 never showed evidence of anterograde bypass conduction on surface ECGs, electrophysiological investigation being necessary. As is the case in incessant AV nodal reciprocating tachycardias, cycle-length dependent reciprocation in the WPW syndrome mainly affects younger individuals, the situation only having occurred in case 6 on a single occasion when she received a variety of medications in rapid succession. There may however, as in case 5, be spontaneous improvement in the clinical condition and the frequency and severity of the arrhythmias may wane with increasing age.

Although the mechanism may be easy to detect when it is specifically sought, the cycle length shortening may be very subtle, and perhaps impossible to affirm on conventional ECGs, but be demonstrated by appropriate electrophysiological studies. When there is no cycle length shortening one can only speculate that unknown factors curtail the atrial refractory period, thus permitting concealed retrograde conduction into the bypass to become manifest and establish a reciprocating circuit. This is perhaps analogous to the finding that atropine permitted re-entry to become established at an A–H interval that had not provoked tachycardia before it had been given[21]; we feel that two of these cases may have concealed pre-excitation.

In some cases of reciprocating tachycardia complicating the WPW syndrome, apparent failure to respond to therapy may reflect the fact that the agents enhance the discrepancy between the respective refractory periods of the AV node and bypass and thus enhance the opportunity for tachycardia to occur. This should be borne in mind and the patient assessed by thorough electrophysiological study before it is concluded that antiarrhythmic drug therapy has failed.

In eight cases other mechanisms produced atypical initiation. *Block in the accessory pathway,* however produced, led to tachycardia in all our cases; this had been produced pharmacologically (cases 13 and 14); by phase 4 block due to an increase in the rate of the stimulation (case 12); or by phase 3 block undoubtedly due to a fatigue phenomenon, the rate of stimulation not having been increased (cases 8 and 9). The situation in case 7 was highly unusual, in that the block was paradoxical, due to prolongation of the atrial cycle length, in association with concealed as opposed to overt anterograde conduction in the accessory pathway.

Even if P–R prolongation was present, as in cases 8, 9 and 12, tachycardia started without additional prolongation, the accessory pathway being blocked in case 8; the onset was seen in cases 9 and 12 when atrial stimulation was interrupted. In addition, these latter two cases, as well as case 14, show that P–R lengthening is by no means essential, since the tachycardia could be initiated by His bundle escape beats, without prolongation of the conduction time.

Escape beats within the re-entry circuit constitute an important mechanism for the initiation of attacks (cases 9, 11, 13 and 14) (Figure 10.3) but this still conforms with the requirements for re-entry. Thus, in case 8 the escape beats failed to provoke tachycardia in the presence of concealed retrograde conduction into the normal pathways; similarly, as in cases 10 and 12, concealed anterograde conduction of the P waves also prevented the onset of tachycardia. On the other hand, lack of atrial activation, as indicated by the absence of a P wave, could enable an incessant tachycardia to start (cases 13 and 14). We have

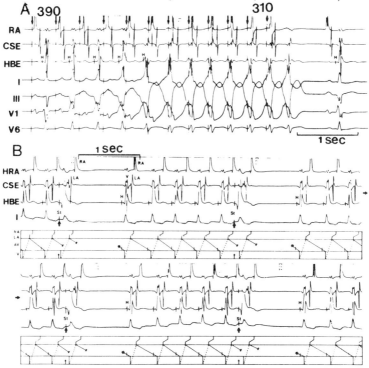

Figure 10.3 (case 13). *(a)* RA, coronary sinus electrogram (CSE), HBE and leads I, III, V$_1$ and V$_6$ bringing out the pre-excitation as the pacing rate was progressively increased (intervals between stimuli decreased from 390 to 330 msec); *(b)* Continuous tracings (HRA, CSE, HBE and lead I), showing termination of tachycardia by ventricular stimuli (St) and immediate re-initiation by His bundle escape beats.

been able to demonstrate the presence of the WPW syndrome in these cases, but this does not mean that this phenomenon cannot occur in nodal re-entry; it does however appear to us much less likely because under those circumstances the escape occurs *outside* the circuit.

That nodal–His bundle escape beats, originating as they do within the substrate for the circuit, are able to induce tachycardias with ease is evident in six of our patients, often in the context of sinoatrial disease, itself an important mechanism for the occurrence of paroxysmal tachycardia. Sinoatrial disease was present or considered highly likely in three of our patients (cases 9, 11 and 12), but His bundle escape beats also occurred when it was not possible to affirm its presence (cases 10, 13 and 14). It is self-evident that for tachycardia to occur His bundle escape beats must be conducted anterogradely better than retrogradely, thus leaving the AV node ready for the circus wave once it has reached the atrium via the bypass.

These phenomena are of interest in that they may explain the occurrence of tachycardias complicating pre-excitation in the absence of premature beats, and without immediately antecedent conduction delay in the blocked pathway. Nodal–His escape beats are potentially of great importance but other mechanisms are more complex and each atypical case needs the most careful scrutiny in order to define possible causes for tachycardia. That this is of therapeutic as well as academic significance is shown by case 12, in whom drug therapy proved unhelpful by producing further depression of the SA node, leading to syncope, as well as a consequent increased tendency to tachycardia induced by the junctional escape beats[23]. That more than one mechanism may apply in a patient is well shown by the same case, who had tachycardia initiated both by progressive atrial pacing and by the junctional escape beats.

While these atypical types of tachycardia are unusual, they are by no means rare, and may apply particularly to older subjects in whom the junctional escape beats, perhaps originating in the bundle of His, occur more frequently as a consequence of disease affecting proximal physiological pacemaking cells, e.g. sinoatrial disease. It is important to remember that depressant antiarrhythmic drugs may paradoxically induce incessant tachycardias in this way; elucidation of apparent paradoxical responses of this sort may be of practical importance as well as indicating the reason for the apparent failure of treatment. Finally, it is in cases like this that long-term pacing may be particularly helpful in the prevention of attacks[24].

Acknowledgements

This presentation is derived from two articles[7,8] and we are grateful to our co-authors and the editor and publisher of the *British Heart Journal* for permission to quote from the text and to reproduce illustrations. That part of this work carried out in London received generous support from the British Heart Foundation.

References

1. Mendez, C. and Moe, G. K. (1966). Demonstration of a dual A–V nodal conduction system in the isolated rabbit heart. *Circ. Res.*, **19**, 378
2. Janse, M. J., Van Capelle, F. J. L., Freud, G. E. and Durrer, D. (1971). Circus movement within the AV node as a basis for supraventricular tachycardia as shown by multiple microelectrode recording in the isolated rabbit heart. *Circ. Res.*, **28**, 403
3. Goldreyer, B. N. and Damato, A. N. (1971). The essential role of atrioventricular conduction

delay in the initiation of paroxysmal supraventricular tachycardia. *Circulation*, **13,** 679

4. Parkinson, J. and Papp, C. (1947). Repetitive paroxysmal tachycardia. *Br. Heart J.*, **9,** 241

5. Coumel, Ph., Cabrol, C., Fabiato, A., Gourgon, R. and Slama, R. (1967). Tachycardie permanente par rythme réciproque. I. Preuves du diagnostic par stimulation auriculaire et ventriculaire. II. Traitement par l'implantation intracorporelle d'un stimulateur cardiaque avec entraînement simultané de l'oreillette et du ventricule. *Arch. Mal. Coeur Vaiss.*, **60,** 1830, 1850

6. Coumel, Ph. (1975). Junctional reciprocating tachycardias. The permanent and paroxysmal forms of A–V nodal reciprocating tachycardias. *J. Electrocardiol.*, **8,** 79

7. Krikler, D., Curry, P., Attuel, P. and Coumel, Ph. (1976). Incessant tachycardias in Wolff–Parkinson–White syndrome. I. Initiation without antecedent extrasystoles or PR lengthening with reference to reciprocation after shortening of cycle length. *Br. Heart J.*, **38,** 885

8. Coumel, Ph., Attuel, P., Slama, R., Curry, P. and Krikler, D. (1976). Incessant tachycardias in Wolff–Parkinson–White syndrome. II. Role of atypical cycle length dependency and nodal–His escape beats in initiating reciprocating tachycardias. *Br. Heart J.*, **38,** 897

9. Curry, P. V. L. (1975). Fundamentals of arrhythmias: modern methods of investigation. In: *Cardiac Arrhythmias: The Modern Electrophysiological Approach*, Krikler and Goodwin (eds.). (London: W. B. Saunders Co.) p. 39

10. Katz, L. N. and Pick, A. (1956). *Clinical Electrocardiography. I: The Arrhythmias.* (Philadelphia: Lea and Febiger)

11. Kistin, A. D. (1965). Atrial reciprocal rhythm. *Circulation*, **32,** 687

12. Keane, J. E., Plauth, W. H. and Nadas, A. S. (1972). Chronic ectopic tachycardia of infancy and childhood. *Am. Heart J.*, **84,** 748

13. Von Bernuth, G., Belz, G. G. and Schairer, K. (1973). Repetitive paroxysmal tachycardia originating in the left atrium. *Br. Heart J.*, **35,** 729

14. Gettes, L. S. and Yoshonis, K. F. (1970). Rapidly recurring supraventricular tachycardia: a manifestation of reciprocating tachycardia and an indication for propranolol therapy. *Circulation*, **41,** 689

15. Rosen, K. M. (1973). Junctional tachycardia: mechanisms, diagnosis, differential diagnosis, and management. *Circulation*, **47,** 654

16. Castellanos, A., Jr. and Myerburg, R. J. (1975). Repetitive supraventricular tachycardias in context. *Am. Heart J.*, **90,** 131

17. Krikler, D. M. (1975). The Wolff–Parkinson–White and related syndromes. I. Presentations and implications. In: *Cardiac Arrhythmias. The Modern Electrophysiological Approach.* Krikler and Goodwin, (eds.). (London: W. B. Saunders Co.) p. 144

18. Krikler, D. M. and Curry, P. V. L. (1976). The paroxysmal supraventricular tachyarrhythmias. In: *Progress in Cardiology, V.* Goodwin and Yu (eds.). (Philadelphia: Lea and Febiger)

19. Wilson, F. N. (1915). A case in which the vagus influenced the form of the ventricular complex of the electrocardiogram. *Arch. Intern. Med.*, **16,** 1008

20. Slama, R., Coumel, Ph. and Bouvrain, Y. (1973). Les syndromes de Wolff–Parkinson–White de type A inapparents ou latents en rythme sinusal. *Arch. Mal. Coeur Vaiss.*, **66,** 639

21. Spurrell, R. A. J., Krikler, D. M. and Sowton, E. (1974). Retrograde invasion of the bundle branches producing aberration of the QRS complexes during supraventricular tachycardia studied by programmed electrical stimulation. *Circulation*, **50,** 487

22. Akhtar, M., Damato, A. N., Batsford, W. P., Caracta, A. R., Ruskin, J. N., Weisfogel, G. M. and Lau, S. H. (1975). Induction of atrioventricular nodal re-entrant tachycardia after atropine. Report of five cases. *Am. J. Cardiol.*, **36,** 286

23. Krikler, D., Curry, P., Coumel, Ph. and Oakley, C. (1977). Wolff–Parkinson–White syndrome type A obscured by left bundle branch block. *Eur. J. Cardiol.*, **5,** 49

24. Krikler, D., Curry, P. and Buffet, J. (1976). Dual-demand pacing for reciprocating atrioventricular tachycardias. *Br. Med. J.*, **1,** 1114

11
Modes of Initiation of Circus Movement Tachycardia in 139 Patients with the Wolff–Parkinson–White Syndrome Studied by Programmed Electrical Stimulation

H. J. J. WELLENS

University Department of Cardiology, Wilhelmina Gasthuis, Amsterdam

The introduction of programmed electrical stimulation of the heart into clinical cardiology opened the way to study mechanisms of tachycardia directly in the human heart[1]. The first group of patients investigated by this technique suffered from the Wolff–Parkinson–White syndrome. It was shown that in these patients with two connections between atrium and ventricle tachycardias could be initiated and terminated by critically timed premature stimuli.

It was postulated that a critically timed atrial or ventricular premature beat created block in one of the two atrioventricular connections enabling the impulse to traverse a circuit consisting of atrium – first AV connection–ventricle–second AV connection–atrium, etc.[1].

The validity of this theory could be confirmed by epicardial activation studies and results of surgery. While the basic concept of circus movement (CM) tachycardia is a simple one, the electrophysiological properties of the different constituents of the tachycardia circuit may lead to several different modes of initiation of CM tachycardia.

This article will attempt to review the different mechanisms by which CM tachycardias can be initiated in patients with the Wolff–Parkinson–White syndrome. It is based upon observations from stimulation studies, in 139 patients. In all patients both single test stimulation and regular pacing at increasing rates was done from the atrium and ventricle. The location of the intracavitary catheters has been given elsewhere[2]. Based upon the criteria given in Table 11.1, 87 of these patients used their accessory pathway during CM tachycardia (Table 11.2). Fifteen different mechanisms of initiation of CM tachycardia could be identified.

Table 11.1   Criteria suggestive for Incorporation of an Accessory Atrioventricular Pathway in the Circuit of a CM Tachycardia

(1) Activation of low left atrium (in case of a left-sided accessory pathway) or activation of low-right atrium (if a lateral right-sided accessory pathway is present) prior to atrial activation in the His bundle recording.

(2) Slowing in rate of tachycardia following bundle branch block to ventricle in which accessory pathway inserts.

(3) V–A conduction time of induced ventricular beat during tachycardia equal to or less than V–A conduction time following QRS complex of tachycardia ($A-A_e$ interval less than or equal to $V-V_e$ interval).

(4) An $A-A_e$ interval longer than $V-V_e$ interval, but less than A–A interval following an induced ventricular beat during tachycardia, with no effect of the induced ventricular beat on the antegrade His bundle electrogram.

(5) Equality in V–A conduction time of tachycardia initiating ventricular premature beat and V–A conduction time during basic paced ventricular rhythm.

(6) Termination of tachycardia following block in or distal to the bundle of His.

(7) Inability to initiate tachycardia or slowing of conduction in the tachycardia circuit outside the AV node, following the administration of drugs affecting the accessory pathway

(1) Initiation of CM tachycardia by an atrial premature beat on reaching the effective refractory period of the accessory pathway in A–V direction

In these patients QRS during tachycardia is narrow or shows a typical bundle branch block configuration. An example is given in Figure 11.1. Characteristically the tachycardia zone (the zone of premature beat intervals initiating tachycardia) extends from the effective refractory period of the accessory pathway in A–V direction to the effective refractory period of the AV node in A–V direction. This pattern was found in 32 patients.

(2) Initiation of CM tachycardia by an atrial premature beat on reaching the effective refractory period of the AV node in A–V direction

QRS during tachycardia is wide because ventricular activation occurs exclusively over the accessory pathway[2]. The width of the tachycardia zone corresponds to the difference between the effective refractory period of the AV node in A–V direction and the effective refractory period of the accessory pathway in AV direction. This type of tachycardia which was present in four of our patients has to be differentiated from a tachycardia originating in the atrium with A–V conduction exclusively or predominately over the accessory pathway. Puech and Latour[3] pointed to the value of drugs blocking conduction

Table 11.2 Type of Tachycardia initiated during Programmed electrical Stimulation in 139 patients with the WPW Syndrome

CM tachycardia incorporating AP	87
Atrial tachycardia	3
AV nodal tachycardia	8
Ventricular tachycardia	1
Undetermined	15

AP = Accessory Pathway
CM = Circus Movement

over the accessory pathway in the distinction between these two types of tachycardia. A tachycardia originating in the atrium will persist with disappearance of A–V conduction over the accessory pathway while the other type of tachycardia will be terminated.

(3) *Initiation of CM tachycardia by an atrial premature beat given after an interval much shorter than the length of effective refractory period of the accessory pathway*

An example is given in Figure 11.2. A variant is shown in Figure 11.3. Essential for initiation of CM tachycardia by an atrial premature beat in these patients is delay in AV nodal transmission sufficiently long to enable the impulse to be conducted over the accessory pathway in V–A direction. In patients with a relatively long effective refractory period of their accessory pathway it is important to differentiate CM tachycardia with V–A conduction over the accessory pathway from AV nodal re-entrant tachycardia[4]. Criteria for differentiation between these two types of tachycardia have been given elsewhere[5]. These

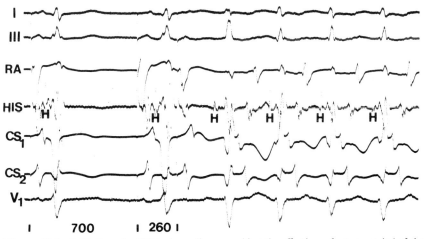

Figure 11.1 Initiation of a CM tachycardia on reaching the effective refractory period of the accessory pathway by an atrial premature beat given after 260 msec in a patient with left-sided WPW. Note that during tachycardia atrial activation starts close to a lead in the distal coronary sinus (CS_1), followed by activation of the lead proximal in the coronary sinus (CS_2) low right atrium (His) and high right atrium (RA).

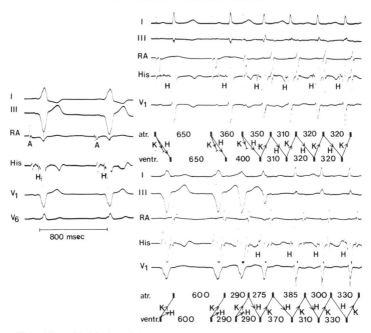

Figure 11.2 Type 3 initiation of CM tachycardia. As shown on the left during sinus rhythm right-sided WPW syndrome is present. Pacing the atrium at rates above 90/min results in complete block in the accessory pathway in AV direction. During pacing of the atrium with a basic cycle length of 650 msec an atrial premature beat given after 360 msec initiates tachycardia. As shown in the right lower panel mode of initiation of tachycardia by a ventricular premature beat during ventricular pacing (absence of increase in V–A conduction time following the premature beat) reveals that during tachycardia V–A conduction occurs over an accessory A–V pathway.

patients with a long effective refractory period of their accessory pathway in A–V direction and CM tachycardia form an intermediate group between patients of Type 1 and patients with complete block in their accessory pathway in AV direction who because of their ability to conduct over the accessory pathway in V–A direction suffer from CM tachycardia (so-called 'concealed' WPW syndrome[5-8]). Nine of our patients showed Type 3 tachycardia.

(4) *Initiation of CM tachycardia by an atrial premature beat following slow conduction in the A–V conduction system distal to the A–V node*

As shown in Figure 11.4 (which was recorded from a patient during treatment with amiodarone) on shortening the atrial premature beat interval gradual prolongation of the H–V interval occurred. At a critical H–V interval the impulse following activation of the ventricle, was retrogradely conducted to the atrium over the accessory pathway followed by tachycardia[9]. Shortening of the premature beat interval resulted in further lengthening of the HV interval, leading to prolongation of the refractory period of the conduction system distal to the bundle of His and block of the re-entrant impulse in this area (Figure

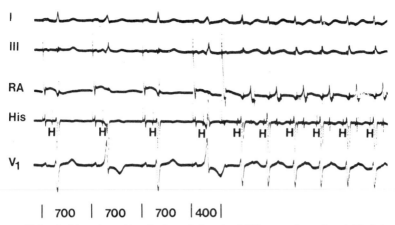

Figure 11.3 Atrial pacing with a basic cycle length of 700 msec shows 2 to 1 block in the accessory pathway in a patient with a left-sided WPW syndrome. A tachycardia is initiated by an atrial premature beat given after 400 msec. Slowing in heart rate during tachycardia following the development of left bundle branch block (not shown) supported incorporation of a left-sided accessory pathway in the tachycardia circuit.

11.4). One patient showed (only after administration of amiodarone) this type of initiation of CM tachycardia.

(5) *Initiation of CM tachycardia by an atrial echo beat following a critically timed atrial premature beat*

Figure 11.5 shows that an atrial premature beat given after 260 msec is followed by an atrial complex with a high–low sequence of atrial activation (possibly re-entry in the sinus node area). This atrial echo is conducted towards the ventricle over the AV node (QRS showing right bundle branch block). Following ventricular activation the impulse (as shown in the coronary sinus lead) returns to the atrium over the accessory pathway. This sequence of activation is thereafter repeated twice. This pattern was seen in only one patient.

(6) *Initiation of CM tachycardia during sinus rhythm without a triggering mechanism of an atrial or ventricular premature beat*

Figure 11.6 demonstrates the initiation of CM tachycardia after six sinus beats of which two are conducted over both the AV node and a left-sided accessory pathway, while the remaining four sinus beats are conducted over the AV node only. As shown, prior to initiation of tachycardia, there is no acceleration of sinus nodal discharge rate. Initiation of reciprocal tachycardia during sinus rhythm without a precipitating extrasystole has been described by Coumel et al.[10] in the so-called 'permanent' or 'incessant' form of AV junctional tachycardia and by Sung et al.[11] in a patient with a concealed WPW syndrome. In the patients described[10,11] acceleration of the sinus rate usually preceded initiation of tachycardia. This was not the case in the patient shown in Figure 11.6. However changes must have occurred in the electrophysiological properties of the tachycardia circuit resulting in a critical arrival time of the impulse

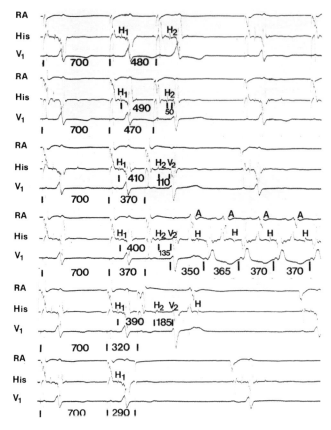

Figure 11.4 Initiation of tachycardia by an atrial premature beat during atrial pacing on reaching a critical delay in the AV nodal–His pathway distal to the AV node. See the text

at the ventricular end of the accessory pathway to be conducted through this structure to the atrium to initiate tachycardia. Two of our patients showed initiation of CM tachycardia during sinus rhythm without an atrial or ventricular premature beat as triggering mechanism.

(7) *Initiation of CM tachycardia on reaching a critical heart rate during regular pacing of the atrium*

This mode of initiation of CM tachycardia can be considered a variant of Type 1. It is based upon block in the accessory pathway at a critical atrial pacing rate. Ventricular activation by way of exclusive A–V conduction over the AV node–His pathway is followed by V–A conduction over the accessory pathway and CM tachycardia. Nine patients showed this pattern of initiation of CM tachycardia. Theoretically, because of lengthening of the effective refractory period of the AV node and shortening of the effective refractory period of the accessory pathway, on increasing atrial pacing rate[12], it should be possible also, depending upon the electrophysiological properties of the two A–V con-

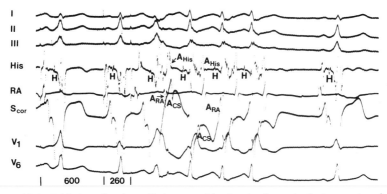

Figure 11.5   Initiation of tachycardia by an atrial echo. As shown in the intracavitary leads (His bundle recording) (His), high right atrial (RA) and coronary sinus lead (Scor) an atrial premature beat given after 260 msec is followed by an atrial complex with a high–low sequence of atrial activation. This atrial complex is conducted over the AV node–His pathway only, initiating a short burst of tachycardia. Note that during tachycardia atrial activation in the coronary sinus lead precedes atrial activation in His bundle and right atrial lead indicating V–A conduction during tachycardia over a left-sided accessory pathway

nections in the individual patient to initiate CM tachycardia with A–V conduction over the accessory pathway by atrial pacing at increasing rates.

(8) *Initiation of CM tachycardia by a ventricular premature beat on reaching the effective refractory period of the His–AV node pathway in V–A direction*

Figure 11.7 gives an example of this type of initiation of tachycardia. Note that in this patient *(a)* the V–A conduction time of the premature beat is identical to the V–A conduction time during basic ventricular pacing and *(b)* tachycardia is initiated up to the refractory period of the accessory pathway.

Lengthening of V–A conduction time on increasing the prematurity of the test pulse during ventricular pacing does not exclude V–A conduction over the accessory pathway[5]. It is essential however to record as closely as possible to the accessory pathway to be accurately informed about V–A conduction time over this structure[13]. 29 patients showed Type 8 initiation of CM tachycardia.

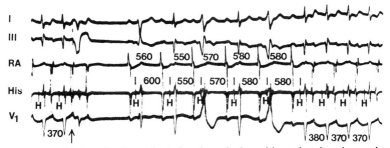

Figure 11.6   Initiation of tachycardia during sinus rhythm without the triggering mechanism of a premature beat. In this patient following termination of tachycardia by an induced ventricular beat (arrow) tachycardia always recurred after a few sinus beats. See the text

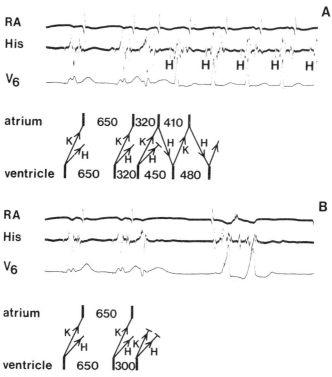

Figure 11.7 Initiation of tachycardia by a ventricular premature beat during ventricular pacing. Note (1) no difference in V–A time following the tachycardia initiating premature beat and following QRS complexes during basic rhythm (upper panel) (2) initiation of tachycardia until the effective refractory period of the accessory pathway in V–A direction is reached (lower panel)

(9) *Initiation of CM tachycardia by a ventricular premature beat on reaching the effective refractory period of the accessory pathway in V–A direction*

During tachycardia QRS shows exclusive ventricular activation by way of the accessory pathway. This mechanism was observed in one patient and has been published previously[14].

(10) *Initiation of CM tachycardia by a ventricular echo beat following a critically timed ventricular premature beat*

Figure 11.8 shows block in V–A conduction over the accessory pathway on reaching a premature beat interval of 380 msec. As demonstrated in Figure 11.9 further shortening of the premature beat interval results in the occurrence of a ventricular echo beat on reaching a premature beat interval of 310 msec. V–A conduction over the accessory pathway is followed by tachycardia. The site of the ventricular re-entrant beat may be close to the site of stimulation, in the bundle branch system, the bundle of His or in the AV node[2]. The ventricular

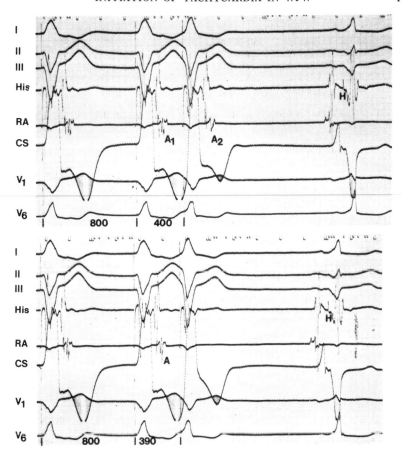

Figure 11.8 On pacing the ventricle with a basic cycle length of 800 msec the effective refractory period of the accessory pathway in VA direction is found to measure 400 msec

re-entrant beat therefore may or may not be preceded by activation of the bundle of His (see also Figure 11.11). Nine patients showed type 10 initiation of tachycardia.

(11) *Initiation of CM tachycardia by a ventricular premature beat on reaching the effective refractory period of the AV node in spite of retrograde penetration into the subnodal conduction system*

An example is given in Figures 11.10 and 11.11. On shortening the premature beat interval a tachycardia is initiated by a ventricular premature beat given after an interval of 440 msec. Further shortening of the premature beat interval reveals that the impulse is not only retrogradely conducted towards the atrium over the accessory pathway but also retrogradely activates the bundle of His. The finding that following the premature beat given after 320 msec the AH interval preceding the first QRS complex of the tachycardia is

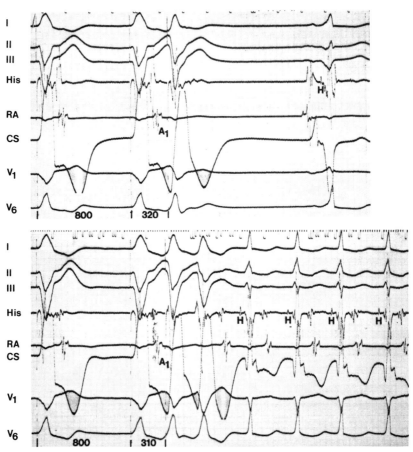

Figure 11.9 Same patient as Figure 11.8. On further shortening of the ventricular premature beat interval to 310 msec a ventricular echo beat occurs. This is followed by V–A conduction over the accessory pathway and initiation of tachycardia

longer than the AH interval following the premature beat given after 440 msec (Figure 11.10) even suggests concealed retrograde penetration into a part of the AV node.

At a premature beat interval of 310 msec (Figure 11.11) the timing of retrograde activation of the bundle of His and possibly concealed retrograde penetration into the distal AV node created refractoriness for the impulse re-entering from the atrium thereby preventing initiation of tachycardia.

Characteristically these patients on shortening the premature beat interval, in contrast to patients with Type 8, show inability to initiate tachycardia on reaching a critical premature beat interval. This mechanism of initiation of CM tachycardia was observed in eight patients. Six of these patients showed a second tachycardia zone when further shortening of the premature beat interval

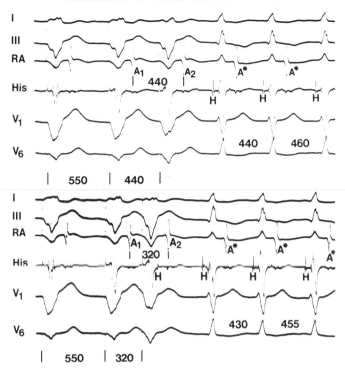

Figure 11.10 Initiation of tachycardia by a ventricular premature beat in spite of retrograde penetration into the subnodal conduction system. As shown in the upper part of the figure the latest premature beat able to initiate tachycardia could be given after an interval of 440 msec. On increasing the prematurity of the test pulse activation of the bundle of His is seen without increase in V–A conduction time, indicating V–A conduction over the accessory pathway but also retrograde activation of the bundle of His

resulted in the genesis of a ventricular re-entrant beat initiating tachycardia (lower part of Figure 11.11).

(12) *Initiation of CM tachycardia by a ventricular premature beat because of a 'gap' in V–A conduction over the His–AV node pathway*

One patient showed initiation of CM tachycardia by a ventricular premature beat in a premature beat interval range from 370 to 340 msec (Figures 11.12 and 11.13). The intracavitary recordings demonstrated during this interval range exclusive V–A conduction over the accessory pathway (Figure 11.13 and 11.14) suggesting that only during a 'gap' in V–A conduction over the accessory pathway a CM tachycardia could be initiated.

(13) *Initiation of CM tachycardia by a ventricular beat because of exclusive VA conduction over the accessory pathway*

Two patients showed initiation of CM tachycardia as soon as ventricular pacing was started, the most likely explanation being V–A conduction during ventricular pacing over the accessory pathway only, enabling the impulse after

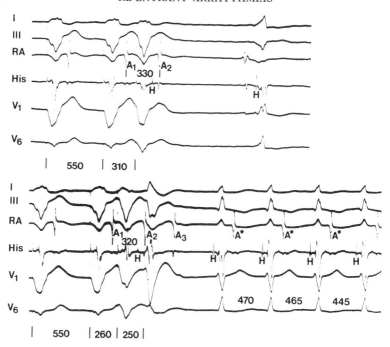

Figure 11.11   Same patient as Figure 11.10. At a premature beat interval of 310 msec the atrial activation wave resulting from V–A conduction over the accessory pathway on coming down through the AV node encounters refractory tissue in the lower AV node or bundle of His and tachycardia is not longer initiated (upper panel). Further shortening of the premature beat interval results in a ventricular echo which is exclusively conducted towards the atrium over the accessory pathway thereby again initiating tachycardia (lower panel)

activating the atrium to return to the ventricle over the AV node–His pathway. As soon as the atrial activation wave following V–A conduction of the ventricular beat is able to pass the AV node in A–V direction, CM tachycardia ensues.

   (14) *Initiation of a CM tachycardia by an atrial echo beat elicited by a ventricular premature beat which is conducted to the atrium*

As shown in Figure 11.15 on increasing the prematurity of the ventricular premature beat during ventricular pacing V–A conduction over the accessory pathway evokes an atrial complex. The configuration of this atrial complex suggests the possibility of a sinus node re-entrant beat. This atrial complex is conducted to the ventricle exclusively over the AV node–His pathway thereby initiating tachycardia. This mode of initiation was seen in one patient.

   (15) *Initiation of CM tachycardia by regular ventricular pacing on reaching a critical pacing rate*

An example is given in Figure 11.16. This mechanism may be based upon *(a)* reaching the refractory period of the AV node in V–A direction at a critical

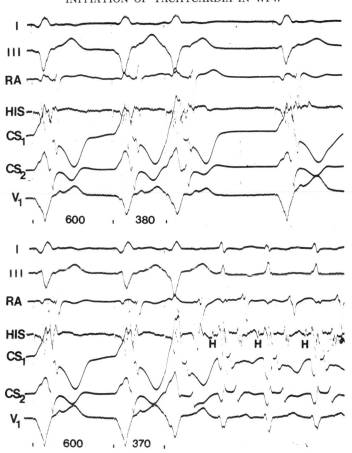

Figure 11.12 Initiation of tachycardia by a ventricular premature beat because of a 'gap' in V–A conduction over the His–AV node pathway. As shown in the lower part of this figure on reaching a premature beat interval of 370 msec exclusive V–A conduction over a left-sided accessory pathway is followed by tachycardia. CS$_1$ = distal recording from the coronary sinus. CS$_2$ — proximal recording from the coronary sinus

pacing rate or *(b)* concealed retrograde penetration of the impulse into the AV node at decreasing depths of penetration. Both mechanisms will eventually result in exclusive V–A conduction over the accessory pathway followed by tachycardia. This pattern of initiation was seen in six patients.

The mechanism of initiation of CM tachycardia by an AV nodal escape beat followed by V–A conduction over the accessory pathway, reported by Harper *et al.*[15], was not seen in our patients. We also did not observe a possible mechanism suggested by Neuss *et al.*[16]. They described a double ventricular response to an atrial extra stimulus. The second ventricular response, which is the result of exclusive activation over the AV node–His pathway, may when retrogradely conducted over the accessory pathway initiate a CM tachycardia.

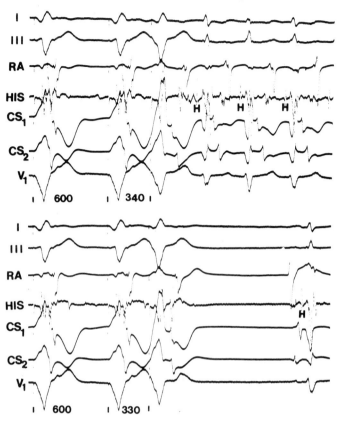

Figure 11.13   Same patient as Figure 11.12. Over a premature beat interval range of 30 msec (from 370 to 340 msec) the same pattern of initiation is seen as shown in the lower part of Figure 11.12. A premature beat given after 330 msec however shows in the intracavitary recordings a pattern of V–A conduction indicating fusion between activation over the accessory pathway and the His-AV node pathway. Obviously at this time no tachycardia can be initiated

Therefore at least 17 different mechanisms of initiation of CM tachycardia are possible in patients suffering from the WPW syndrome.

Role of basic pacing rate and drugs on modes of initiation of CM tachycardia

The electrophysiological properties of the different components of the tachycardia circuit will be influenced by basic heart rate and will also be affected by the administration of drugs

While the effective refractory period of the AV node lengthens on increasing heart rate, the effective refractory periods of the other components of the tachycardia circuit tend to shorten. This may lead to widening of the tachycar-

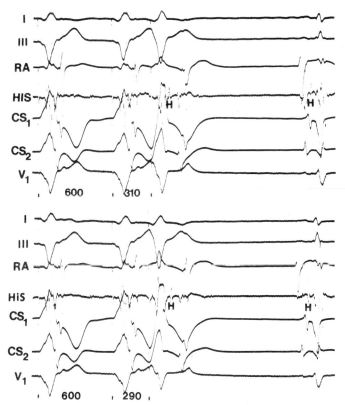

Figure 11.14 Same patient as Figures 11.12 and 11.13. Further shortening of the premature beat interval reveals VA conduction over the His–AV node pathway only. A 'gap' in V–A conduction over the His–AV node pathway could explain the sequence seen in Figures 11.12, 11.13 and 11.14

dia zone of patients with Type 8 initiation of CM tachycardia. It was also observed that in eight of our patients different types of initiation of CM tachycardia occurred depending upon basic pacing rate.

Drug administration may also result in changes in mechanism of initiation of CM tachycardia[9,17]. This phenomenon can be the reason for an increased incidence of arrhythmias during drug treatment. Our observations demonstrate that interplay of sometimes complex electrophysiological mechanisms underlies initiation of CM tachycardia in the WPW syndrome. They support the use of stimulation studies before and after drug administration to come to a correct choice of antiarrhythmic agent.

References

1. Durrer, D., Schoo, L., Schuilenburg, R. M. and Wellens, H. J. J. (1967). The role of premature beats in the initiation and termination of supraventricular tachycardia in the Wolff–Parkinson–White syndrome. *Circulation*, **36,** 644

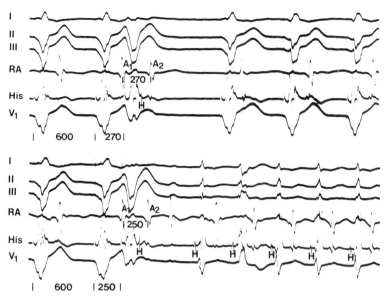

Figure 11.15   Initiation of tachycardia by a ventricular premature beat evoking an atrial re-entrant beat. On pacing the ventricle with a basic cycle length of 600 msec ventricular premature beats are conducted to the atrium over the accessory pathway but also retrogradely activate the bundle of His (upper panel). A premature beat given after 250 msec is retrogradely conducted to the atrium over the accessory pathway and followed by an atrial complex showing an intermediate axis in the frontal plane. This atrial complex is conducted exclusively over the AV node His pathway to the ventricle and initiates a tachycardia.

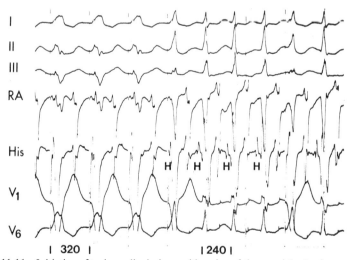

Figure 11.16   Initiation of tachycardia during rapid pacing of the ventricle. As shown on terminating ventricular pacing with a basic cycle length of 320 msec tachycardia supervenes. Block in the His–AV node pathway, at a critical pacing rate, with exclusive V–A conduction over the accessory pathway is the mechanism of initiation of tachycardia

2. Wellens, H. J. J. (1975). Contribution of cardiac pacing to our understanding of the Wolff–Parkinson–White syndrome. *Br. Heart J.*, **37**, 231

3. Puech, P. and Grolleau, R. (1972). L'activité du faisceau de His normale et pathologique. (Paris: Ed. Sandoz)

4. Rosen, K. M. (1973). A–V nodal re-entrance: an unexpected mechanism of paroxysmal tachycardia in patients with pre-excitation. *Circulation*, **47**, 1267

5. Wellens, H. J. J. and Durrer, D. (1975). The role of an accessory atrio-ventricular pathway in reciprocal tachycardia. *Circulation*, **52**, 58

6. Coumel, Ph. and Attuel, P. (1974). Reciprocating tachycardia in overt and latent pre-excitation. *Eur. J. Cardiol.*, **1**, 423

7. Zipes, D. P., De Joseph, R. L. and Rothbaum, D. A. (1974). Unusual properties of accessory pathways. *Circulation*, **49**, 1200

8. Neuss, H., Schlepper, M. and Thormann, J. (1975). Analysis of re-entry mechanisms in three patients with concealed Wolff–Parkinson–White syndrome. *Circulation*, **51**, 75

9. Wellens, H. J. J., Lie, K. I., Bär, F., Wesdorp, J., Dohmen, H. J. M. and Düren, D. (1976). Effect of amiodarone in the Wolff–Parkinson–White syndrome. *Am. J. Cardiol.*, **38**, 189

10. Coumel, Ph. (1975). Junctional reciprocating tachycardias. The permanent and paroxysmal forms of AV-nodal reciprocating tachycardia. *J. Electrocardiol.*, **8**, 79

11. Sung, R. J., Castellanos, A., Gelband, H. and Myerburg, R. J. (1976). Mechanism of reciprocating tachycardia initiated during sinus rhythm in concealed Wolff–Parkinson–White syndrome. Report of a case. *Circulation*, **54**, 338

12. Wellens, H. J. J. and Durrer, D. (1974). Relation between refractory period of the accessory pathway and ventricular frequency during atrial fibrillation in patients with the Wolff–Parkinson–White syndrome. *Am. J. Cardiol.*, **33**, 178

13. Svenson, R. H., Miller, J. C., Gallagher, J. J. and Wallace, A. G. (1975). Electrophysiological evaluation of the Wolff–Parkinson–White syndrome. Problems in assessing antegrade and retrograde conduction over the accessory pathway. *Circulation*, **52**, 552

14. Wellens, H. J. J. and Durrer, D. (1974). Patterns of ventriculo-atrial conduction in the Wolff–Parkinson–White syndrome. *Circulation*, **49**, 22

15. Harper, R., Peter, T., Vohra, J., Hunt, D. and Sloman, G. (1974). Sinus node dysfunction and carotid sinus syncope associated with a Wolff–Parkinson–White syndrome. *Eur. J. Cardiol.*, **2**, 207

16. Neuss, H., Schlepper, M. and Spies, H. F. (1974). Double ventricular response to an atrial extrasystole in a patient with WPW syndrome Type B. A possible mechanism triggering tachycardia. *Eur. J. Cardiol.*, **2**, 175

17. Wellens, H. J. J. and Durrer, D. (1974). Effect of procaine amide, quinidine and ajmaline on the Wolff–Parkinson–White syndrome. *Circulation*, **50**, 114

12

Junctional Reciprocating Tachycardia. The Permanent Form

P. COUMEL, P. ATTUEL and J. MUGICA

Hôpital Lariboisière, 2 Rue Ambroise-Paré, Paris

While an important literature has been devoted for about ten years to the paroxysmal forms of junctional reciprocating tachycardias (JRT), it is rather surprising that little attention has been paid to the particularities of the permanent, or the incessant, the repetitive or rapidly recurring form of these tachycardias. Still, the clinical pattern of this tachycardia was described, and its reciprocating mechanism was suspected 50 years ago by Gallavardin[1,2] Again, Parkinson and Papp in 1947[3] clearly defined its clinical pattern, and several authors[4-7] have proved its mechanism by analysis of the ordinary electrocardiograms. In 1967, we confirmed this mechanism[8] by adopting stimulation techniques similar to those used by Moe *et al.*[9] in animal experiments.

The relative rarity of the permanent form as compared to the high incidence of the paroxysmal form (either intra-nodal or WPW) is probably one of the reasons why it has been neglected. Another reason is certainly that its main electrophysiological characteristic (a normal P–R interval at the onset of the tachycardia) tends at first glance to rule out the reciprocating mechanism and to label this tachycardia atrial rather than AV junctional. Indeed, we are inclined since Moe's studies[9] to believe that the creation of a circus movement requires three conditions: (1) a circuit of conduction; (2) a unidirectional block in this circuit, and (3) a slowed conduction. This third condition, in case of paroxysmal JRT is not only the most apparent, but also the triggering mechanism of the tachycardia: an atrial premature beat responsible for the prolongation of P–R (and eventually the disappearance of the WPW pattern if present) usually precedes the onset of the tachycardia. But the *absence* of this prolonged P–R in *some* cases of paroxysmal JRT[10,11] and in *all* cases of the permanent form may be explained easily on the basis of a conduction speed in the circuit *already slow enough* to allow re-entry, provided unidirectional block occurs. In other words, in this form, condition (2) becomes the triggering mechanism of the tachycardia, instead of condition (3).

CLINICAL PATTERN AND SURFACE ECG

We have studied 20 cases of the permanent form of JRT, which is relatively more frequent in children[12,13] than in adults (beginning of course during childhood in the latter). By comparison, during the same period of time, i.e. about ten years, we have observed *ca.* 250 cases of the paroxysmal form. The electrocardiographic pattern is always the same (Figure 12.1): an almost permanent supraventricular tachycardia, ending from time to time, particularly at rest, and starting again after the interposition of a few sinus beats. A rather characteristic feature is the abortive onset of tachycardia by an isolated atrial echo beat. The analysis of both pattern and timing of the P-waves is very

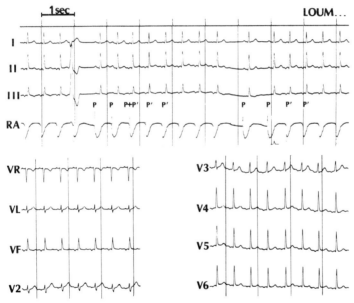

Figure 12.1 Typical permanent reciprocating tachycardia. In the upper trace (standard leads and right atrial bipolar electrogram) a ventricular premature beat interrupts the tachycardia which recurs after two beats. The run of tachycardia stops spontaneously after a few beats, and starts again, justifying the term of incessant rather than permanent tachycardia in this patient. The retrograde pattern of the P' waves is clearly visible in standard and unipolar leads. The intra-atrial lead confirms the inverted polarity of sinus P waves with respect to P' waves, and the possibility of fusion beats at the beginning of this rather slow tachycardia. Abbreviations: RA = right atrial bipolar electrogram. P = sinus P waves. P' = retrograde P waves. P + P' = atrial fusion beats

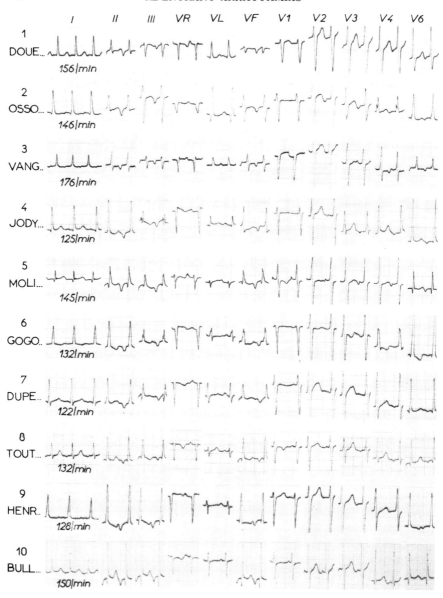

Figure 12.2 Typical feature of the surface ECG in permanent reciprocating tachycardia. The surface tracings of ten patients have been gathered to show the uniformity of the ECGs, making them easily recognizable. P' waves are clearly of retrograde origin, negative in leads II, III and VF. To be noted that they are also positive in VI, negative in left precordial leads, with a transitional zone in V_2. In spite of the variable rate, the P'–R interval is always shorter than R–P', or at best equal (third patient Vang . . .)

valuable in the diagnosis because of their constant characteristics. This is shown in Figure 12.2 in which tracings from ten patients are gathered: P waves display the 'classical' pattern of retrograde activation of the atria, with negativity in leads II, III and aVF. In addition, P waves are also negative in precordial leads from V_2 to V_6, making the tachycardia sometimes wrongly qualified as originating in the left atrium[14]. P waves occur closer to the succeeding QRS than to the preceding one, but the apparent P–R interval is not necessarily short as its absolute value depends on the cardiac rate. The cardiac frequency is never less than 120/min and can be as high as 250/min. In the same patient it can vary by 20–30 beats/min, depending on the activity. In short, the mean ratio of the R–P' interval to the cycle length R–R is 2/3 (with P'–R/R–R = 1/3), the extremes being 3/4 for R–P'/R–R, and 1/2.

In this presentation, we have chosen to study the different electrophysiological phenomena of the tachycardia (mode of onset and termination, localization of the circuit, treatment by stimulation) in two demonstrative patients. With a few small variations, the same phenomena may be demonstrated in all patients, some of them having been already published elsewhere[13,15–17].

THE MODE OF INITIATION OF THE TACHYCARDIA

Figure 12.3 verifies, as we have stated above, that the onset of the tachycardia does not require any prolongation of either P–R or A–H. In this patient the cardiac rate is relatively slow (because of depressive drug treatment), and after four beats the tachycardia is interrupted by a spontaneous atrial premature beat. Then the sinus rhythm is resumed, with an A–H interval of 80 msec not only for the first, but also for the second beat after which the tachycardia recurs. In some cases, where only two sinus beats are visible between the episodes of tachycardia, it may happen that a relative prolongation of P–R (or

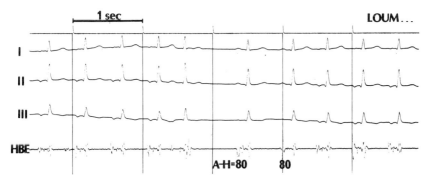

Figure 12.3 Constancy of the A–H interval at the beginning of the tachycardia. The tachycardia stops after four beats thanks to a spontaneous atrial premature beat. It starts again after the second sinus beat, the A–H interval of which is 80 msec, as for the first sinus beat (see the text for explanation). Abbreviations: (same as in Figure 12.1) HBE = His bundle electrogram

A–H) is present in the second beat as compared to the first one, although the absolute value of the A–V conduction remains within the normal limits. In those cases, it is usually not difficult to prove that in fact the A–H interval of the first beat is only apparent, artificially more or less shortened by a His bundle escape beat occurring relatively earlier than the sinus P wave after the pause.

We have already discussed the explanation for the normal P–R interval at the beginning of the tachycardia, i.e. the existence of an already slow enough conduction speed in the retrograde pathway of the circuit, a condition particularly obvious in the patient of Figure 12.3. The problem remains to determine the reason why the tachycardia recurs after a few beats or even a single one (cf. Figure 12.5), or on the contrary may keep quiescent during some minutes or even hours, particularly at rest.

In all patients, the tachycardia starts every time the sinus frequency reaches a definite value, rarely less than 60/min and more than 100/min. The 'critical' value of the P–P cycle length triggering the tachycardia is relatively constant in a given patient, provided the circumstances are unchanged. But the activity (exercise or rest), the drug received, and even the ratio between the cycle immediately triggering the tachycardia and the preceding one, all these conditions may slightly modify this critical value of P–P. In other words this value is related to the rate, in the same way as the prematurity of the atrial stimulation necessary for starting a paroxysmal form of JRT is itself rate related.

Figure 12.4A shows the spontaneous initiation of the tachycardia, due to the progressive acceleration of the sinus frequency (P–R interval remaining constant at 160 msec: the P–P interval decreases progressively from 960 to 930 msec (beats 4 to 5)). Beat 6 is the first of the tachycardia and *not* a spontaneous atrial extrasystole supposedly triggering a paroxysmal form of JRT. In this case, 930 msec is the time interval during which an unidirectional anterograde block is present in the retrograde (beta) pathway of the circuit after the preceding P wave. This block makes it possible for the atrial impulse P_5 to traverse the anterograde pathway (alpha) and to re-enter the alternate one retrogradely. The reason why P_1 to P_4 do not trigger the tachycardia is obviously that atrial impulses are allowed to penetrate anterogradely both pathways (concealed anterograde conduction in the β-path).

Figure 12.4B does confirm the reciprocating mechanism of the tachycardia and shows the principle of its prevention by an artificial ventricular 'pre'-stimulation. Atrial cycles 1–2 to 4–5 are equal, so that P waves labelled 2–4 should trigger the tachycardia. The reason why it is only started by P_5 is that the coupling interval between the onset of the sinus P and the electrically-induced activation of the ventricle is progressively delayed from P_1 (60 msec) to P_3 (110 msec). During the first four beats, the artificial ventricular impulse reaches the circuit early enough: (1) to collide in the α-pathway with the anterograde atrial impulse and (2) to penetrate the β-pathway during its refractory period so that it is not conducted up to the upper junction of the cir-

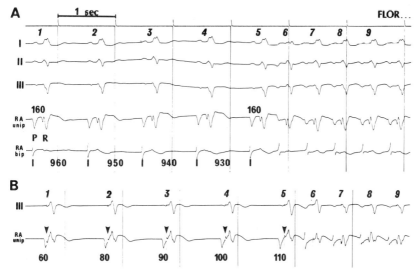

Figure 12.4 Mode of initiation of the tachycardia. (A) The tachycardia starts (without prolongation of PR) after beat 5, and results from the progressive shortening of the P–P interval to 930 msec. To be noted in this patient a constant left bundle branch block is present. (B) Limitations of the prevention of tachycardia by an artificial right ventricular pre-excitation. The ventricular stimulation (arrows) triggered by sinus P waves is progressively delayed from 60 to 100 msec. When the coupling interval reaches 110 msec (beat 5) the ventricular impulse is conducted retrogradely and initiates again the tachycardia (see the text for explanation). Abbreviations: (same as in the preceding figures) RA unip – right atrial unipolar electrocardiogram. RA bip – right atrial bipolar electrogram

cuit. The ventricular stimulation given 110 msec after P_5 is conducted retrogradely: the retrograde P_6 appears more premature than P_6 was in Figure 12.4A, and re-enters the α-pathway, starting the reciprocating tachycardia.

We have stated above that P'_6 was not a coincidental spontaneous atrial premature beat, but the first retrograde P' of the tachycardia. One can verify that the morphology of both spontaneous P'_6 in Figure 12.4A and retrogradely induced P'_6 in Figure 12.4B are quite identical.

LOCALIZATION OF THE CIRCUIT

Determining whether the circus movement is either intra-nodal or related to the presence of an accessory pathway is always a difficult problem in the paroxysmal forms of JRT. Several articles have shown recently[18-20] that the absence of a WPW pattern during sinus rhythm is not a reliable argument to eliminate the possibility of an extra-nodal accessory pathway. As stimulation methods become more and more sophisticated, more and more so-called intra-nodal reciprocating tachycardias are found to be related to either Kent bundles, or Mahaim fibres, or atrio–His bypasses[21]. Thus the fact that we have never seen any WPW pattern in our patients with a permanent JRT does not prove that an accessory pathway is not in use. Nor does it prove that the circuit is strictly intra-nodal.

However, the possibility of a bundle of Kent responsible for the retrograde conduction (β-pathway) can be ruled out with accuracy in our patients: (1) we have seen that the R–P' is always longer than P'–R, and such a pattern would be highly surprising (though not quite impossible) in case of direct V–A accessory pathway; (2) the retrograde conduction time is always rate-dependent in those patients, suggesting that a decremental (AV nodal) conduction is present in at least a portion of the retrograde pathway. Figure 12.5 shows that the spontaneous termination of the episodes is related to the

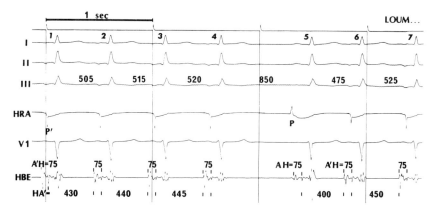

Figure 12.5   Spontaneous termination and recurrence of the tachycardia. The cycle length increases progressively from 505 520 msec between beats 1 and 4. The increment is not related to the anterograde conduction time A'H constant at 75 msec, but to the retrograde one H–A' which increases from 430 to 445 msec. The end of the tachycardia results from the block of the retrograde impulse. The first cycle of the tachycardia (beats 5 to 6) shorter than the others, and the constancy of the A'H interval with respect to A–H, support the hypothesis of an initial common pathway between the atrium and the circuit (see the text for explanation). Abbreviations: (same as in the preceding figures) HRA = High right atrial bipolar electrogram

progressive increase of the H–A' interval up to the blockage of the retrograde impulse. On the other hand, though less frequently, we have seen examples of spontaneous termination of the tachycardia preceded by a slight increase of the A'–H interval, suggesting that the AV node was involved, at least in part, by the anterograde impulse. In short, it appears that manifestations of decremental conduction are present in both anterograde and retrograde pathways: to state things more precisely, they are generally more marked for the retrograde than for the anterograde conduction.

The possibility of an atrio–Hisian accessory pathway (so-called James fibres) may be excluded by using about the same arguments. Indeed, either P–R or A–H intervals are never short in our patients during sinus rhythm, and the duration of the R–P' interval during the tachycardia excludes the presence of an atrio–Hisian accessory pathway used retrogradely. An additional observation is made in some patients, and confirms the probability of an upper junction of the circuit situated below the atrial level: the first cycle of the tachycardia is usually *shorter* than the following ones. An example of this phenomenon is shown in Figure 12.5. In this tracing, the tachycardia ends spontaneously after beat 4. It starts again after a single sinus beat No. 5. The shortness of the first atrial cycle A_5–A'_6 is obviously explained by a retrograde conduction speed H_5–A'_6 (400 msec) faster during the first cycle than during the following ones (450 msec) according to the rate. But such an explanation cannot be applied to the ventricular cycle R_5–R_6 (475 msec) as the conduction velocity in the anterograde pathway (P'_6–R_6 or A'_6–H_6) has been necessarily slowed accordingly to the prematurity of the first re-entrant impulse. Therefore, the first ventricular interval of the tachycardia should be longer than the first atrial one. In other words, the first A'–H interval (75 msec in beat 6) is surprisingly not longer than the A–H interval of the sinus beat 5. The paradoxically short duration of the first atrial cycle (or the absence of prolongation of A'–H) cannot be explained other than by the existence of an upper junction of the circuit situated *below* the atrium: thus the first ventricular cycle is shortened with respect to the following ones by the conduction time within the initial common pathway[22].

The fact that no delta wave is ever visible in our patients, and that both Kent bundle or James fibres blocked anterogradely are certainly eliminated does not allow us to conclude with accuracy that the circus movement is confined to the node. Conceivably it might well be constituted in its upper part by the AV node, with an upper junction situated below the atrium, but the lower junction of the circuit has to be localized precisely. Using the methods previously described[18], we have been able in most of our patients to prove that the level of the lower junction was certainly *extranodal:* probably intra-Hisian and, in at least two cases, intraventricular. One of these cases is presented in Figures 12.6 and 12.7.

The demonstration is based upon the careful study of atrial captures during the tachycardia by stimulating precise areas of the right ventricle. In Figure 12.6, the proximal pair of contacts (1 cm apart) of a quadripolar electrode records the bipolar electrogram of the right ventricular septum (labelled RV sept) while the two distal contacts are situated at the apex: a signal in the lowest lead (labelled Stim. apex) indicates either that the demand system of the stimulator has been triggered by the local depolarization of the apex, or that a stimulus has been delivered in that area. During the tachycardia, the cycle length is perfectly constant at 505 msec and the successive depolarizations of the low right atrium (A'), the high right atrium (P'), the His bundle, the right ventricular septum and the apex are recorded. Just before the occurrence of R_4, a stimulation is delivered at the apex with a coupling interval of 415 msec with respect to the preceding signal recorded at that site. If we consider what happens at the right ventricular septum, the fourth depolarization is premature

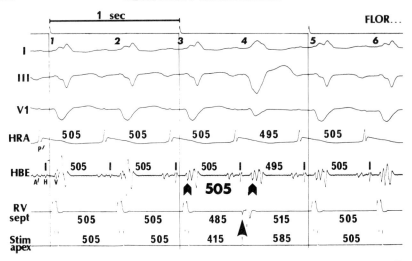

Figure 12.6 Atrial capture by right ventricular apex stimulation. During the tachycardia a right ventricular apex stimulation (4th beat) makes premature the depolarization of the septum, but *not* the occurrence of the 'V' wave in the His bundle electrogram. However, the P' wave is captured (P'₅) proving that the lower junction of the circuit is distal to the His bundle (see the text for discussion). Abbreviations: (the same as in the preceding Figures) RV sept: bipolar electrogram from the right ventricular septum recorded by the proximal pair of contacts of a quadripolar electrode-catheter located at the right ventricular apex. Stim apex = the distal pair of contacts of the same quadripolar electrode either senses the local depolarization at the apex (great deflections) or stimulates it (small deflection with an arrow)

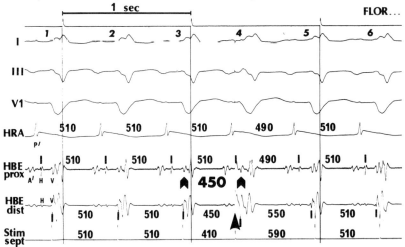

Figure 12.7 Atrial capture by septal stimulation (compare to Figure 12.6.) The quadripolar electrode has been slightly withdrawn from the apex, so that the proximal pair of electrodes records a distal His bundle electrogram (HBE dist), and that the distal pair either senses or stimulates the septum (Stim sept), in the same way as in Figure 12.6. This time, the V₄ wave in the 'proximal' His bundle electrogram (HBE prox) is premature by 60 msec while P'₅ is premature by only 20 msec (see the text for discussion)

by 20 msec (505 − 485 = 20 msec); the inverted R wave in this lead confirms that the spread of activation has been modified. In fact, the important phenomenon is that in the HBE lead the morphology of beat 4 remained absolutely unchanged: this is not surprising for both A'_4 and H_4 which *precede* the rather late stimulation, but it is also true for V_4, the timing (505 msec) and the pattern of which are quite similar to V_3. This fact clearly indicates that the depolarization of the uppermost part of the septum has not been influenced by the apex stimulation occurring too late in the cycle. However, the next P′ (P'_5) as well as A′ are premature by 10 msec (505 − 495 = 10 msec). That fact proves that the stimulated impulse has captured the atrium *without* involving either the upper part of the septum or the His bundle. Thus, the lower junction of the circuit is necessarily situated within the ventricle, a fact which cannot be explained other than by the presence of a bypass taking off somewhere in the ventricle to reach the AV node (a Kent bundle having been previously excluded). In other words, Mahaim fibres are certainly present in this case, and they are conductive only retrogradely as the H–R interval is normal during sinus rhythm.

Figure 12.7 confirms the preceding fact. It shows that a ventricular stimulation given higher in the septum (i.e. in principle nearer to the circuit if it had been intranodal or intra-Hisian) more hardly captures the atrium. The quadripolar electrode has been slightly withdrawn, so that its proximal pair of electrodes records a distal HBE while the distal one stimulates the septum. This time the cardiac cycle is 510 msec, and the stimulation is given slightly earlier than in Figure 12.6: the coupling interval is such that the stimulation coincides exactly with H, and that V_4 occurs 450 msec after V_3, i.e. with a prematurity of 60 msec, (510 − 450 = 60 msec). The prematurity of the next P′ is only 20 msec ($P'_4 − P'_3 = 490$ instead of 510 msec). Thus it is clear that the atrial capture is much easier to provoke by stimulating the ventricular apex (Figure 12.6) than the ventricular septum: consequently, the latter is electrophysiologically 'farther' from the circuit than the former.

To summarize, the electrophysiological findings in our cases of permanent JRT are remarkably uniform:

(1) normality of the P–R interval at the onset of the tachycardia, due to the unidirectional block in one pathway: a concealed, unapparent triggering mechanism, with a critical value of the cardiac rate for its occurrence.

(2) A closed circuit of conduction involving both antero- and retrogradely the AV node at least in part, but not entirely confined to it: the lower junction may be situated either within the His bundle in some cases (longitudinal dissociation of the His bundle?) or within the ventricle itself (Mahaim fibres).

(3) The intra-nodal level of the upper junction explains the constant 'retrograde' pattern of P′ waves and their time-relationship with R waves: these two characteristics are quite different from those observed in the paroxysmal forms of JRT in which direct atrio–His or A–V connective accessory pathways are frequently present.

TREATMENT

The evolution, and the drug responsiveness of these tachycardias are also very particular. While it is quite easy to stop the tachycardia by any depressive drug, the problem is in fact to prevent it. One can conceive why this is difficult because the problem is to depress one of the pathways sufficiently to make it unresponsive. While such an effect can easily be induced by any drug given intravenously, in practice it is impossible to get the same effect orally. Another way to prevent the tachycardia is to slow the sinus rate, so that the 'critical', i.e. the triggering value of the cardiac rate cannot be reached. This is hardly possible by depressive drugs, particularly β-blocking agents given alone or associated with digitalis. Usually the effect is transient, only obtained at rest. In our experience, the only effective drug is amiodarone, associated or not with digitalis. In truth, it is more effective in children than in adults, but it should be stressed that the former tolerate less well the long-term tachycardia than the latter, and more frequently develop congestive heart failure. It is very interesting to discuss the mechanism of action of amiodarone. Amiodarone prevents the tachycardia not by slowing the cardiac frequency under the critical rate, but by *shortening* the critical value of the P–P interval. In other words, amiodarone apparently shortens the duration of the unidirectional block after each P wave, an effect quite paradoxical for a drug known as particularly depressive. An electrophysiological explanation for such a paradoxical phenomenon ought to be paradoxical itself. This fact is probably the consequence of the 'disinhibition' phenomenon recently described by Cranefield[23]. It supposes that the β-pathway, in its upper (AV nodal) part, is constituted in fact by two depressed branches that we may label 'a' and 'b', joining to form the beta pathway itself in its lower part (Figure 12.8). Then conceivably anterograde block of the β-pathway, in the non-treated patient, results from an inhibition phenomenon: the impulse propagating within the branch 'b' may be blocked distal to the junction with the branch 'a', that is within the β 'common' pathway.

Thus this block prevents the impulse involving branch 'a' from being conducted downward if it reaches the junction *after* the impulse 'b'. But, this inhibition can be prevented ('disinhibition') by further depressing branch 'b' so that the impulse 'a' can reach the junction and the β-pathway *before* the 'blocking' impulse 'b'.

When the tachycardia is poorly tolerated and not responsive to treatment, the prevention of the tachycardia by means of long-term stimulation should be considered. We have described above (Figure 12.4B) the principle of this treatment: by creating artificial pre-excitation of the ventricle after every P wave, the retrograde ventricular impulse permanently penetrates and blocks the pathway. The effectiveness of this type of stimulation is verified in Figure 12.9. In A, the first four beats are artificially pre-excited: the stimulus is triggered by the spontaneous P wave with a minimal delay of 10–15 msec (Figure 12.4C).

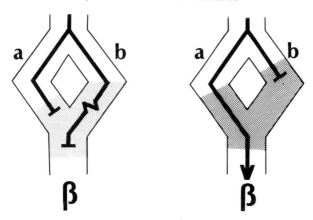

Figure 12.8 The phenomenon of 'disinhibition' (from reference 23). The β-pathway is supposed to divide and reunite. In the left diagram, (basic conditions) the impulse travelling along the depressed branch 'b' reaches the point of convergence *before* the impulse travelling in branch 'a'. It dies out leaving refractoriness behind it so that the impulse involving the branch 'a' is blocked: none of the two impulses 'a' and 'b' has been conducted, and the β-pathway is blocked anterogradely, setting the stage for re-entry. In the right diagram, a depressive treatment is supposed to prevent the phenomenon of inhibition, and to re-establish paradoxically the anterograde conduction in the β-pathway. If the impulse 'b' is further depressed by the drug it will not reach the junction of the two branches, leaving the branch 'a' open to the anterograde impulse

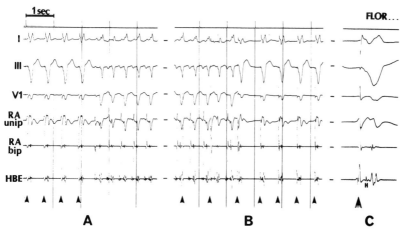

Figure 12.9 Prevention of the tachycardia by artificial 'pre-excitation'. Pre-operative study. *(a)* four ventricular stimuli are triggered by spontaneous P waves. The tachycardia recurs as soon as the stimulation is stopped; *(b)* the third random ventricular stimulation stops the tachycardia, and the artificial pre-excitation is resumed; *(c)* at faster paper speed (100 mm/sec) the very beginning of sinus P waves is visible in RA unip and HBE (see the text for discussion)

After the fourth beat the stimulation is switched off, and the next sinus beat is followed by the onset of the tachycardia. In B the ventricular stimulation is applied randomly; the third stimulus falls early in the diastole and stops the tachycardia. Then the artificial 'pre'-stimulation is resumed, preventing again recurrence of the tachycardia. On the basis of these results, an implantable pacemaker has been specially designed for this patient.

Two pick-up electrodes have been implanted surgically in the right atrium; the stimulating circuit is triggered by the P waves, thus permitting a physiologically varying cardiac rate, and activates the right anterior ventricular wall with a minimal delay. Figure 12.10 is a post-operative tracing; after the first three beats, a magnet is applied on the implanted pacemaker and inhibits the triggered stimulation. The escape rate of the pacemaker (60/min) then appears during the time the magnet is maintained. Relief of the magnet shows how the tachycardia is automatically stopped; the retrograde P' following beat 14 triggers the pacemaker which delivers the stimulation early enough to be effective. Again the escape rate of the pacemaker appears in beats 16 and 17 because of a sinus pause. We have now three patients treated this way, with a satisfactory long-term result after respectively 9 years, 3 years and 6 months.

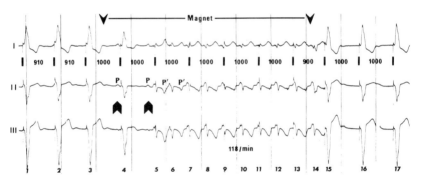

Figure 12.10 Effect of the magnet on the implanted pacemaker. Applying the magnet on the implanted pacemaker allows us to verify the effectiveness of the method: the escape rhythm of 60/min no longer prevents the tachycardia which is automatically interrupted by releasing the magnet

References

1. Gallavardin, L. and Gravier, L. (1921). Bradycardie nodale permanente. Etude du rythme atrioventriculaire. *Arch. Mal. Coeur Vaiss*, **14**, 71
2. Gallavardin, L. and Veil, P. (1927). Deux cas de tachycardie en salve chez de jeunes sujets. *Arch. Mal. Coeur Vaiss*, **20**, 1
3. Parkinson, J. and Papp, C. (1947). Repetitive paroxysmal tachycardia. *Br. Heart J.*, **9**, 241
4. Naim, M. (1945). Paroxysmal auricular tachycardia due to reciprocal rhythm. *Am. Heart J.*, **29**, 398
5. Bix, H. H. (1951). Various mechanisms in reciprocal rhythm. *Am. Heart J.*, **41**, 448
6. Katz, L. N. and Pick, A. (1956). *Clinical Electrocardiography. The Arrhythmias.* (Philadelphia: Lea and Febiger)

7. Kistin, A. D. (1959). Mechanisms determining reciprocal rhythm initiated by ventricular premature systoles. Multiple pathways of conduction. *Am. J. Cardiol.*, **3**, 365

8. Coumel, Ph., Cabrol, C., Fabiato, A., Gourgon, R. and Slama, R. Tachycardie permanente par rythme réciproque. *Arch. Mal. Coeur Vaiss*, **60**, 1830

9. Moe, G. K. and Mendez, C. (1945). Physiological basis of reciprocal rhythm. *Am. Heart J.*, **29**, 398

10. Coumel, Ph., Attuel, P., Slama, R., Curry, P. and Krikler, D. (1976). 'Incessant' tachycardias in Wolff–Parkinson–White syndrome. II. Role of atypical cycle length dependency and nodal His escape beats in initiating reciprocating tachycardias. *Br. Heart J.*, **38**, 897

11. Krikler, D. M., Curry, P. V. L., Attuel, P. and Coumel, Ph. 'Incessant' tachycardias in Wolff–Parkinson–White syndrome. I. Initiation without antecedent extrasystoles or PR lengthening with reference to reciprocation after shortening of cycle length. *Br. Heart J.*, **38**, 885

12. Keane, J. F., Plauth, W. H. and Nadas, A. S. (1972). Chronic ectopic tachycardias in infancy and childhood. *Am. Heart J.*, **84**, 748

13. Coumel, Ph., Fidelle, J., Cloup, M., Toumieux, M. C. and Attuel, P. (1974). Les tachycardies réciproques à évolution prolongée chez l'enfant. *Arch. Mal. Coeur Vaiss.*, **67**, 23

14. Mirowski, M. (1966). Left atrial rhythm. Diagnostic criteria and differentiation from nodal arrhythmias. *Am. J. Cardiol.*, **17**, 203

15. Coumel, Ph., Motté, G., Gourgon, R., Fabiato, A., Slama, R. and Bouvrain, Y. (1970). Les tachycardies supraventriculaires par rythme réciproque en dehors du syndrome de Wolff–Parkinson–White. *Arch. Mal. Coeur Vaiss.*, **63**, 35

16. Coumel, Ph. and Barold, S. (1975). Mechanisms of supraventricular tachycardias. In *His Bundle Electrocardiography and Clinical Electrophysiology*, O. S. Narula, (ed.). (Philadelphia: F. A. Davis Comp. Publ.), p. 203

17. Coumel, Ph. (1975). Junctional reciprocating tachycardias. The permanent and paroxysmal forms of A–V nodal reciprocating tachycardias. *J. Electrocardiol.*, **8**, 79

18. Coumel, Ph., Attuel, P., Motté, G., Slama, R. and Bouvrain, Y. (1975). Les tachycardies jonctionnelles paroxystiques. Evaluation du point de jonction inférieur du circuit de réentrée. Démembrement des 'rythmes réciproques intra-nodaux'. *Arch. Mal. Coeur Vaiss.*, **68**, 1255

19. Wellens, H. J. J. and Durrer, D. (1975). The role of an accessory atrioventricular pathway in reciprocal tachycardia. Observations in patients with and without the Wolff–Parkinson–White syndrome. *Circulation*, **52**, 58

20. Curry, P. V. L. and Krikler, D. M. (1976). Cycle length alternation during drug treatment in supraventricular tachycardias. *Br. Heart J.*, **38**, 882

21. Durrer, D., Schuilenburg, R. M. and Wellens, H. J. J. (1970). Pre-excitation revisited. *Am. J. Cardiol.*, **25**, 690

22. Coumel, Ph. (1975). Supraventricular tachycardias. In *Cardiac Arrhythmias*, D. M. Krikler and J. F. Goodwin, (eds.). (London: W. B. Saunders), p. 116

23. Cranefield, P. F. (1975). *The Conduction of the Cardiac Impulse.* (Mount Kisco, NY.: Futura Publishing Comp.), p. 71

13
Mechanisms underlying Sudden Changes in Heart Rate during Paroxysmal Supraventricular Tachycardia

M. SCHLEPPER

Kerckhoff—Klinik of the Max Planck Society, Bad Nauheim, West Germany

In supraventricular paroxysmal tachycardias insignificant changes in heart rate are often observed, when a tracing is carefully evaluated. The heart rate may change with respiration and immediately following initiation of the tachycardia there may be a 'warming up' period. The latter phenomenon was thought to be a characteristic of supraventricular tachycardias of focal origin[1]. However, in patients with tachycardias initiated and terminated by properly timed atrial and/or ventricular premature depolarizations – and hence more likely to be of re-entrant nature – these phenomena can also be observed. During paroxysmal supraventricular tachycardias we found a 'warming up' period in *ca.* 21% of the patients with and without electrocardiographic signs of pre-excitation[2]. All these alterations in heart rate occur gradually, and therefore are not the subject of this presentation.

Sudden changes in heart rate may occur, when, under the bombardment of rapid excitations of the atria, atrial fibrillation develops causing tachy-arrhythmias, which in the presence of an anomalous pathway may lead to a life threatening situation. However, suddenly noticeable changes in heart rate during SVPT, in which a regular rate is maintained are indeed rare events and have been reported only in a few cases[3].

In a re-entrant tachycardia the resulting excitation interval and hence the heart rate equals the sum of conduction velocity values in each of the structures forming the re-entry circuit. This interval has to be longer than the refractoriness in the different structures of the re-entry circuit, so that the excitation wave always finds excitable tissue. Considering this basic concept certain predictions can be made regarding sudden changes in heart rate during re-entrant tachycardia. The excitation interval will lengthen, when a conduction delay occurs in a part of the re-entry circuit.

If the re-entry circuit includes part of the ventricular myocardium as in the presence of accessory A–V connections the myocardium at the ventricular insertion of the accessory pathway may be reached anterogradely via a bundle branch. When bundle branch block occurs during a tachycardia the excitation reaches the insertion in a roundabout way traversing the free ventricular myocardium. Even if conduction velocity does not change, the circuit will lengthen and the excitation interval increases. It is well established that in patients with Type A and Type B WPW syndrome the development of LBBB or RBBB respectively results in an increase of cycle length during the tachycardia[4].

Furthermore, the occurrence or disappearance of intraventricular conduction disturbances associated with sudden changes in the RR-interval may give first diagnostic clues for the presence of concealed WPW syndromes in an otherwise normal electrocardiogram[5-7].

In a 16-year-old boy without evidence of pre-excitation in the ECG (Figure 13.1) an atrial extra stimulus with a coupling interval of 250 msec initiated a supraventricular tachycardia with an unusual HQ-prolongation from 55 to 140 msec. The first five QRS complexes show RBBB and retrograde conduction time, as measured by the QA' interval is 200 msec, the R–R distance 340 msec. When intraventricular conduction normalizes, there is a sudden decrease in retrograde conduction time to 130 msec and cycle length is reduced to 300

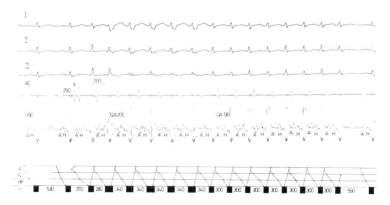

Figure 13.1 Original recording from a 16-year-old boy. Top to bottom: ECG I–III, Atrial EG (AE), His bundle EG (HBE). After the initiation of the tachycardia by a PAD with a coupling interval of 250 msec RBBB is present. During block the Q–A' interval is 200 msec and decreases to 130 msec when intraventricular conduction becomes normal. Ladder diagram illustrates the sequences of activation. All numbers in msec (see the text)

msec. During RBBB therefore the ventricular insertion of the right-sided accessory pathway – responsible for retrograde conduction – is reached with delay.

If a re-entry circuit is confined to proximal structures of the specific conduction system appearance and disappearance of block distal to the site of re-entry alters the ventricular rate.

In a 15-year-old boy with WPW syndrome Type A tachycardias with different heart rates were observed. Such a tachycardia was initiated by a single premature atrial depolarization with a coupling interval of 270 msec at a basic driven heart rate of 120/min (Figure 13.2A). The atrial extra stimulus was exclusively conducted via the accessory pathway and the resulting QRS complex showed complete pre-excitation, followed by an atrial echo with retrograde atrial conduction time of 35 msec. The next QRS was of normal configuration, but the sequence of retrograde atrial excitation remained identical. The next two QRS complexes showed LBBB configuration and following these a 2:1 block below the bundle of His occurred with the ventricular rate dropping from 200/min to 100/min, while the frequency of atrial depolarization remained at 200/min. In the course of the tachycardia (Figure 13.2B) 1:1 A–V conduction was restored and again block occurred for one excitation sequence following the QRS with left bundle branch block configuration (Figure 13.2). Then 1:1 A–V-conduction was maintained with a ventricular rate of 200/min. The occurrence of a block below the bundle of His proves that the re-entry circuit was confined to nodal structures and that the anomalous pathway did not participate in the re-entry circuit, neither for anterograde nor for retrograde conduction.

This was further proved by electrophysiological data. At certain coupling intervals normal conduction failed and ventricular activation was completely over the anomalous pathway. This critical coupling interval increased with augmentation of heart rate (340 msec in sinus rhythm, 370 msec at a driven basic rate of 120/min and 410 msec at a heart rate of 135/min). At these frequency ranges a further shortening of the coupling interval of *ca.* 20–40 msec elicited an atrial echo and a re-entry tachycardia. With further shortening of the coupling interval down to 240 msec there was an abrupt normalization of the QRS complex at all heart rates and the normalization was accompanied by a sudden increase of the A–H interval to 300 msec, which further lengthened, when the coupling interval was decreased. A–V conduction was limited by refractoriness of the atria. When refractoriness of V–A conduction was proved by premature depolarizations applied to the apex of the right ventricle anomalous conduction, as measured by the stimulus–A' interval remained at 145 msec down to a coupling interval of 350 msec. Then a gradual increase in retrograde conduction velocity occurred with shortening of the coupling interval, indicating nodal conduction.

From these data it can be assumed that three pathways were used for anterograde conduction, one nodal pathway with a long refractoriness and a fast conduction velocity. When this pathway became refractory, the bypass

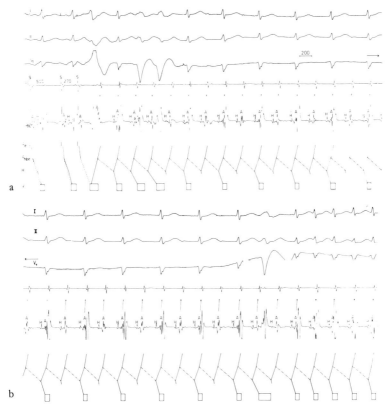

Figure 13.2 (a) Original recording: ECG, cranial atrial EG (AE), His bundle EG (HBE) and ladder diagram to illustrate the mode of excitation. Tachycardia is initiated by a PAD coupled to the foregoing atrial depolarization with 270 msec. The first QRS complex is of WPW morphology. Following the second QRS with LBBB configuration block below the bundle of His occurs. (b) 1:1 A–V conduction is restored and again block occurs for one excitation after the occurrence of LBBB (numbers in msec; see the text)

tract was traversed and after its refractoriness was reached, conduction took place over a nodal pathway with short refractoriness and slow conduction velocity. While in the first tachycardia with an R–R interval between 330 and 300 msec the re-entry circuit seemed to be confined to nodal structures without participation of the accessory pathway the boy exhibited a second type of tachycardia (Figure 13.3). In this second type of SVTP with an R–R interval of about 240 msec the QRS complexes were bizarre, showing complete pre-excitation with no foregoing H potentials before ventricular activation. However, the sequence of retrograde atrial activation remained equal and the interval between the nodal and the cranial atrial depolarization was still 35 msec. This type of tachycardia was elicited at sinus rhythm by PADs with a coupling interval between 270 and 235 msec.

The boy, however, alternated between the two types of tachycardia. While

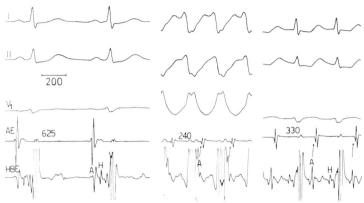

Figure 13.3   Original recording from the same patient as in Figure 13.2. During sinus rhythm only a small degree of pre-excitation is present, the H-spike appears well before the Δ-wave (left panel). In the middle panel a tachycardia with QRS complexes of WPW morphology without foregoing H-potentials is illustrated, cycle length 240 msec. The right panel demonstrates the other type of tachycardia with H potentials before the ventricular depolarizations and an R–R interval of 330 msec. In both types of tachycardia the sequence of retrograde atrial excitation was identical

the tachycardia with normal QRS complexes was well tolerated, the tachycardia with anterograde conduction over the accessory pathway had dangerous hemodynamic effects. In Figure 13.4 such a sudden change is shown. At a basic driven heart rate of 120/min a PAD with a coupling interval of 220 msec led to an A–H prolongation of 300 msec and immediately after A–H prolongation an atrial echo occurred starting the tachycardia. The fifth QRS in that trace was of left bundle branch configuration. Probably because of a rate dependent increase in refractoriness caused by that conduction delay the next excitation was blocked below the bundle of His and from now on anterograde conduction occurred over the accessory pathway with an R–R interval of 260 msec soon 'warming up' to 240 msec.

The sudden shift from one type of tachycardia to the other was associated with a conduction block below the bundle of His, and it can only be assumed that during the tachycardia with normalized QRS complexes there was concealed penetration into the ventricular outlet as well as into the atrial insertion of the accessory pathway, leading to physiological interference of the two excitation waves. When block of the bundle of His occurred excitation failed to reach the ventricular insertion, so that anterograde conduction over the accessory pathway now became possible. The new re-entry circuit with different conduction properties was responsible for the second type of tachycardia, showing QRS complexes with complete pre-excitation.

However, why this happened in one instance and that shift did not occur in the other traces with block below the bundle of His remains unclear.

Unusual re-entry mechanisms in the presence of WPW-syndromes have been described by us and others[8–11], and at least in the case reported by Spurrell *et*

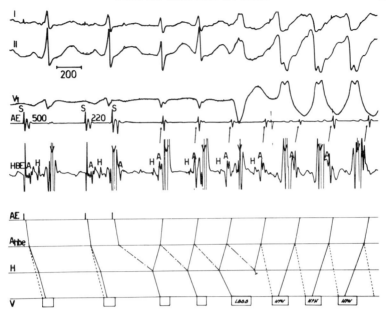

Figure 13.4   Trace from the same patient as in Figures 13.2 and 13.3 demonstrating a sudden shift from one type of tachycardia to the other. Following a QRS with LBBB-configuration anterograde conduction is blocked below the bundle of His and then is via the accessory pathway (see the text, numbers in msec)

al.[10] physiological interference in the accessory path was assumed, thus resembling the findings in this boy. If more than one anterograde pathway is present they may be used alternately thus leading to a sequence of shorter and longer R–R intervals[10,11], but this does not lead to a sudden change in the rate of tachycardia.

In this context it is, however, noteworthy that more than one anomalous pathway may be present in WPW and related syndromes[12,13].

As in this example different re-entry circuits may then exist at the same level of the conduction system especially at the AV junction. In the presence of multiple pathways in one junction the re-entry circuit may differ in length and/or conduction properties. The various circuits, however, are always composed of parts of the structures forming other circuits as well.

However, independent re-entry circuits may exist at different levels of the conduction pathways and one may trigger the other. A 49 year-old female patient had a history of paroxysmal tachycardias mostly with a heart rate of *ca.* 120/min, but sometimes with a heart rate of *ca.* 180/min. The two types occurred independently of each other, but sometimes the tachycardia with the low heart rate abruptly changed to that tachycardia with a higher frequency. Electrophysiological studies revealed a rate dependent 'break phenomenon' at the nodal level. A PAD (Figure 13.5) with a coupling interval of 290 msec led to

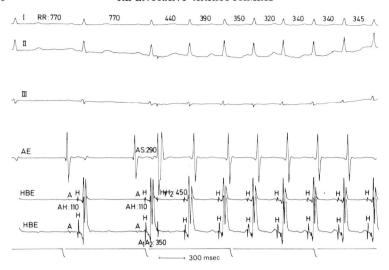

Figure 13.5   Recording from a 49-year-old female patient. ECG, cranial atrial EG and two bundle of His EGs (HBE) are shown (top to bottom). A PAD with a coupling interval of 290 msec is propagated with an A–H interval of 260 msec. A nodal type of supraventricular tachycardia is initiated (see the text; numbers in msec)

an A–H prolongation from 110 to 260 msec starting a supraventricular tachycardia with retrograde atrial activation. The nodal atrial depolarizations were invisible in the V-potentials. When at the same sinus rate the coupling interval of the PAD was 320 msec, there was only an increase in the A–H interval to 190 msec (Figure 13.6). Again a tachycardia was started, but this time anterograde conduction was normal. The cranial atrial depolarizations appeared with the same interval of 25 msec before the nodal atrial depolarizations. In the further course of the tachycardia the A–H interval decreased from 190 to 140 and finally to 120 msec. Both types of tachycardias could be stopped with appropriately placed premature atrial depolarizations, thus fulfilling important requirements for the diagnosis of re-entrant tachycardia. According to the diagnostic criteria as outlined by Narula[14] the tachycardia with undisturbed anterograde atrionodal conduction may be considered due to a sinoatrial re-entry. In the course of such a sinoatrial re-entry tachycardia (Figure 13.7) a sudden prolongation of the A–H interval became apparent and at a certain A–H interval atrial echoes appeared initiating a self-sustaining nodal re-entrant tachycardia.

For the shift from one re-entry circuit to the other changes in the tone of the autonomous nervous system may be responsible but this is rather speculative.

The cases presented here exemplify various electrophysiological mechanisms underlying sudden changes of heart rate in supraventricular paroxysmal tachycardias.

(1) Conduction delay or block in one of the structures forming the re-entry

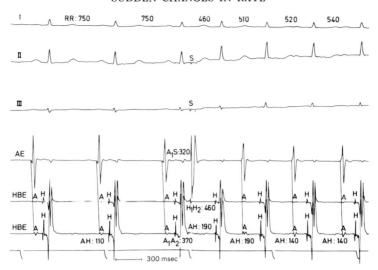

Figure 13.6 Traces from the same patient as in Figure 13.5. A PAD with a coupling interval of 320 msec initiates a tachycardia, during which the normal anterograde atrionodal conduction is maintained. The extrastimulus is propagated with an A–H interval of 190 msec (see the text; numbers in msec)

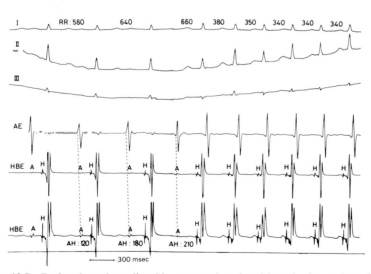

Figure 13.7 During the tachycardia with anterograde atrionodal conduction prolongation of the A–H interval occurs, and at an interval of 210 msec an atrial echo appears starting a tachycardia of nodal type (see the text; tracing from the same patient as in Figure 13.5 and 13.6, numbers in msec)

circuit may be responsible for changes in cycle length. This applies also to ventricular re-entrant tachycardias, in which different bundle branches can be blocked or used for impulse transmission[15].

(2) In re-entrant tachycardias with a circuit confined to a proximal level, block below the common final pathway may alter ventricular rate. When block occurs below or in the bundle of His, this is strong evidence that the re-entry circuit is confined to the AV-node.

(3) Different pathways for anterograde and retrograde conduction may exist at one junction in the conduction system (preferably in the AV junction) and the pathways can be used alternately thus forming re-entry circuits of different length and with different conduction properties.

(4) Re-entry circuits may exist at different levels and one may trigger the other, so that a re-entrant tachycardia is shifted from one circuit to another.

References

1. Goldreger, B. N., Gallagher, J. J. and Damato, A. N. (1973). The electrophysiological demonstration of atrial ectopic tachycardia in man. *Am. Heart J.*, **85**, 205
2. Schlepper, M. Unpublished observation
3. Zipes, D. P., De Joseph, R. L. and Rothbaum, D. A. (1974). Unusual properties of accessory pathways. *Circulation*, **49**, 1200
4. Durrer, D. and Wellens, H. J. (1974). The Wolff–Parkinson–White syndrome anno 1973. *Eur. J. Cardiol.*, **1**, 347
5. Slama, R., Coumel, P. and Bouvrain, Y. (1973). Les syndromes des Wolff–Parkinson–White de type A inapparents ou latents en rythme sinusal. *Arch. Mal. Coeur Vaiss.*, **66**, 639
6. Coumel, P. and Attuel, P. (1974). Reciprocating tachycardia in overt and latent pre-excitation. *Eur. J. Cardiol.*, **1**, 423
7. Neuss, H., Schlepper, M. and Thormann, J. (1975). Analysis of re-entry mechanisms in three patients with concealed Wolff–Parkinson–White syndrome. *Circulation*, **51**, 75
8. Neuss, H. and Schlepper, M. (1974). Unusual re-entry mechanisms in patients with the Wolff–Parkinson–White syndrome. *Br. Heart J.*, **38**, 880
9. Rosen, K. M. (1973). AV–nodal re-entrance. An unexpected mechanism of paroxysmal tachycardia in a patient with pre-excitation. *Circulation*, **47**, 1267
10. Spurrell, R. A. J., Krikler, D. and Sowton, E. (1973). Two or more intra AV-nodal pathways in association with either a James or Kent extra-nodal bypass in three patients with paroxysmal supraventricular tachycardia. *Br. Heart J.*, **35**, 113
11. Friedberg, H. D. and Schamroth, L. (1973). Three atrioventricular pathways. Reciprocating tachycardia with alternation of conduction time. *J. Electrocardiol.*, **6**, 159
12. Coumel, P., Waynberger, M., Slama, R. and Bouvrain, Y. (1972). Intérêt de l'enregistrement des potentiels hisiens au cours du syndrome de Wolff–Parkinson–White. A propos de six observations. *Acta Cardiol.*, **26**, 188
13. Ramachandran, S. (1972). Wolff–Parkinson–White Syndrome: Conversion of type A to type B electrocardiographic changes. *Circulation*, **45**, 529
14. Narula, O. S. (1974). Sinus node re-entry. A mechanism for supraventricular tachycardia. *Circulation*, **50**, 1114
15. Wellens, H. J., Schuilenburg, R. M. and Durrer, D. (1972). Electrical stimulation of the heart in patients with ventricular tachycardia. *Circulation*, **46**, 216

Section IV

Ventricular Arrhythmias (With Special Reference to Rhythm Disorders Related to Ischaemic Heart Disease)

14

The Effect of Acute Ischaemia on Transmembrane Potentials in the Intact Heart. The Relation to Re-entrant Mechanisms

M. J. JANSE and E. DOWNAR

Department of Cardiology and Clinical Physiology,
The Inter-University Institute of Cardiology, Amsterdam

Knowledge of the nature and time course of changes in cardiac transmembrane potential following coronary artery occlusion would be helpful in understanding the mechanisms underlying the arrhythmias occurring during myocardial ischaemia. Previous workers[1-3] have recorded with microelectrodes from intact hearts following coronary artery occlusion. Only relatively minor changes were reported, such as a slight shortening in action potential duration and loss of resting membrane potential, and it would be difficult to explain the arrhythmias associated with the initial stages of myocardial ischaemia on the basis of these slight changes. *In vitro* studies, in which injured parts of the heart were resected some time after coronary artery occlusion (varying from 30 min to several days), and maintained by superfusion in a tissue bath revealed more striking changes in cardiac action potentials[4-6]. In these studies, the earliest intracellular recordings could be made some 15 min after resection. Thus, information about the behaviour of the cardiac transmembrane potential in the very early stages of myocardial ischaemia is lacking. By combining techniques previously described[1,7], we have followed the changes in transmembrane potential from the subepicardium of both *in situ* and isolated perfused pigs' hearts immediately after coronary occlusion for a period of 30–60 min. The purpose of this paper is firstly to describe the effects of ischaemia on action potential configuration and excitability; secondly to show that ischaemic myocardium releases substances which are able to produce the same electrophysiological effects in normal myocardium; and finally to try to relate the ischaemic changes in transmembrane potential to re-entrant mechanisms.

METHODS

A detailed description of the methods can be found elsewhere[8,9], and only the most relevant points will be mentioned here. Experiments were performed on both *in situ* pig hearts and isolated hearts perfused according to Langendorf. The perfusion fluid consisted of the pig's own blood, mixed with an equal amount of a modified Tyrode solution to which glucose, insulin, dextran and heparin was added. The left anterior descending artery was dissected free so that it could be occluded by a broad clamp, release of which would instantly result in reperfusion. The epicardium was removed from the anterior aspect of the left ventricle to facilitate microelectrode impalement. Conventional microelectrodes with a very short shaft were mounted on chlorided silver wire spirals in order to be able to follow the movements of the heart[7]. In the *in situ* experiments, where contractions were usually more vigorous than in the perfused hearts, a device by Czarnecka *et al.*[1] was used. It involved a perspex ring sutured onto the heart and held rigidly. The ring was filled with agar to further dampen the movements of the heart and to prevent breaking of microelectrode tips. In order to minimize interference from the extrinsic electrocardiogram a differential method of recording was used in which the local extracellular electrogram was subtracted from the intracellular signal. The extracellular signal was obtained from an extracellular microelectrode positioned as closely as possible to the intracellular microelectrode. In the illustrations only the differentially recorded signals are shown. Often, because of the contraction of the heart, impalements were less than ideal causing action potential amplitude to be subnormal. Also movement artefacts sometimes distorted the potentials. In some illustrations therefore, voltage calibrations are absent, and potentials with distorted baselines are shown.

RESULTS

Ischaemic changes '*in situ*'

Figure 14.1 shows recordings of subepicardial ventricular transmembrane potentials from an *in situ* pig heart before and after occlusion of the left anterior descending coronary artery. The heart was paced from a remote ventricular site at a basic length of 390 msec. Following coronary artery occlusion, the action potential shortens, and its amplitude and upstroke velocity diminish. There is delay of activation and loss of resting membrane potential. After 9 min

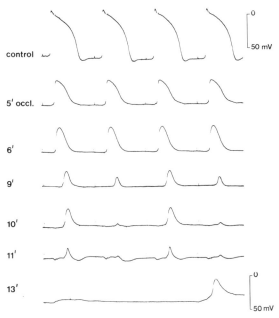

Figure 14.1 Action potentials from a subepicardial ventricular cell in an *in situ* pig heart by means of a floating microelectrode before and after occlusion of the left anterior descending artery. The ventricle was paced at a cycle length of 390 msec. In lowest panel pacing was stopped to introduce a long diastolic pause. Note progressive shortening in action potential duration, and alternation leading to 2:1 responses, until after 11 min of coronary artery occlusion the fibre is virtually irresponsive (reproduced from reference 9 by permission of the authors and the publishers)

of ischaemia, alternation occurs, which evolves into 2:1 responses. The moment of activation is delayed by some 100 msec, and the duration of the response is in the order of 100 msec. After 12 min of ischaemia, irresponsiveness occurs. Initially, as shown in the lowest panel, a sufficiently long pause is able to restore a fairly large response from a previously irresponsive cell, but later the cell is totally irresponsive regardless of pauses. Reperfusion could rapidly restore electrical activity in fibres that had become irresponsive, provided the occlusion had not lasted longer than 30–40 min. Within a few beats after release of coronary artery occlusion, action potentials of near normal configuration could be restored. Very often, ventricular fibrillation occurred shortly after the beginning of reperfusion (Figure 14.2). If the occlusion had lasted longer than an hour, cells in the centre of the ischaemic zone could not be revived by reperfusion. Return of electrical activity in irresponsive fibres could also be accomplished by flushing 20 ml of saline bubbled with nitrogen into the coronary artery distal to the occlusion, as shown in Figure 14.3. The fact that the mere injection of saline could, temporarily, restore near normal action potentials, suggests that at least in some cells the ischaemic changes in

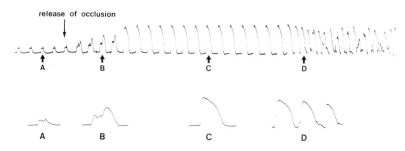

Figure 14.2   Rapid re-establishment of near normal action potential in ischaemic cell following reperfusion. In the lower panel the time base is expanded. Note ventricular fibrillation following release of occlusion

transmembrane potential are due to accumulation of substances in the extracellular space of the ischaemic compartment. Such substances may diffuse out into the region where there is still some blood flow, and may affect the electrical behaviour of cells which in principle are still viable.

'In vitro' effects of ischaemic blood

To test whether ischaemic tissue releases substances capable of influencing the electrophysiology of normal cells, coronary venous blood was collected from a local vein draining an ischaemic region, and its effects upon action potentials recorded from an isolated strip of normal ventricular myocardium was studied[8].

A few ml of so-called 'ischaemic' blood was collected on release of a coronary

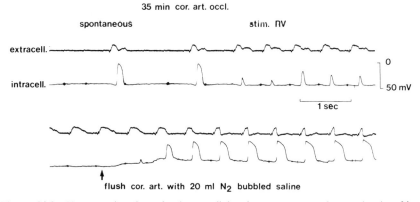

Figure 14.3   Upper tracing shows local extracellular electrogram, very close to the site of intracellular recordings of lower trace. In upper panel there is AV block after 35 min of coronary artery occlusion and fairly large action potentials are recorded with a slow upstroke and no overshoot. Pacing of the right ventricle results in small action potentials, which disappear altogether a few seconds later (lower panel). During total irresponsiveness, the extracellular electrogram is a mono-phasic potential. Flushing the occluded coronary artery with nitrogenated saline results in rapid re-establishment of near normal action potentials. Note deflections in extracellular electrogram coinciding with intracellular potentials

artery occlusion, the duration of which varied between 5 and 20 min. The isolated preparation was taken either from the moderator band, or from the right ventricular outflow tract. It was placed in a tissue bath, superfused with Tyrode solution and electrically stimulated. When the preparation was immersed in a few ml of 'ischaemic' blood, the action potentials shortened and the amplitude and upstroke velocity decreased, until within 12 min of incubation, the preparation became totally irresponsive at resting membrane potential levels of about -50 mV (see Figure 14.4).

These changes were reversible when the ischaemic blood was washed out, and superfusion with Tyrode solution resumed. During incubation of the preparation in stagnant non-ischaemic blood for a similar time period, action potentials remained stable.

Thus, the same changes in transmembrane potential that were observed in the ischaemic area of a heart *in situ* could be reproduced *in vitro* by 'ischaemic' blood. Thus far, attempts to identify the substances present in 'ischaemic' blood responsible for the effects have failed. However, it could be demonstrated that several likely candidates, such as elevated potassium concentration, low pH, low glucose level, and low pO_2, could not account completely for the observed effects[8]. Addition of excess glucose to ischaemic blood did not prevent its effects. The average K^+ concentration in ischaemic blood was 7 mM, but could be as low as 5 mM. Such K^+ concentrations are not high enough to produce irresponsiveness. The combined effects of elevated K, low pH and low pO_2 were studied by abnormalizing samples of non-ischaemic coronary venous blood in such a way as to achieve values for K, pH and pO_2 similar to those of ischaemic blood. These abnormalized samples did not produce irresponsiveness, as did ischaemic blood, but only resulted in some shortening of the action potential duration and the development of some degree of post-repolarization refractoriness. Only when K concentrations in abnormalized blood samples were raised to levels around 15 mM, irresponsiveness occurred in the same way as during incubation in ischaemic blood with K concentration of 6–7 mM. Thus, it would seem that additional substances, as yet unknown, are released by ischaemic myocardium which have potent effects on the electrical activity of normal myocardium, ranging in scope from action potential shortening to complete inexcitability.

Changes in excitability

In order to correlate changes in action potential configuration with changes in excitability we estimated local refractory periods in perfused hearts, using a floating stimulating electrode. This consisted of a thin double spiral wire insulated except at the tips with an interelectrode distance of 0.5 mm. It could be positioned very close to the recording microelectrode, usually within 1 mm. The heart was paced via this electrode and test stimuli of four times diastolic threshold strength were given after every seventh basic stimulus to determine

EFFECTS OF "ISCHEMIC BLOOD"
(13 min occlusion)

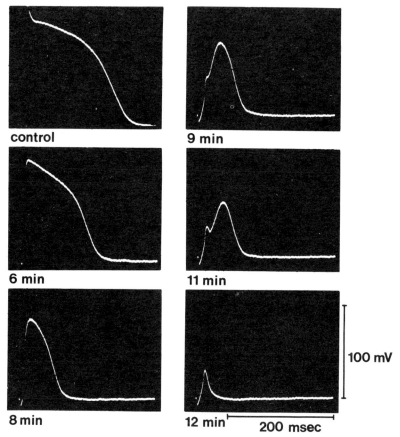

Figure 14.4 Action potentials recorded in tissue bath from an isolated strip of normal myocardium. In control situation, the preparation had been incubated in stagnant normal coronary venous blood for 12 min. So-called 'ischaemic blood' was collected from a local coronary vein on release of a coronary artery occlusion of 13 min duration. The preparation was immersed in 2 ml of 'ischaemic blood', and within minutes action potentials shortened, and became smaller, until after 12 min of incubation the preparation became totally irresponsive, at a resting membrane potential of *ca.* −50 mV (zero potential level is not indicated)

local refractory periods. In order to minimize stimulus artefacts in the microelectrode recordings we usually stimulated bipolarly. However, to exclude the possibility that some effects were due to anodal stimulation, we also used unipolar cathodal stimuli, using as an anode a large clip attached to the aortic root. Both modes of stimulation gave identical results.

In Figure 14.5 two simultaneously recorded action potentials are shown recorded with two pairs of microelectrodes. Stimuli were applied close to the

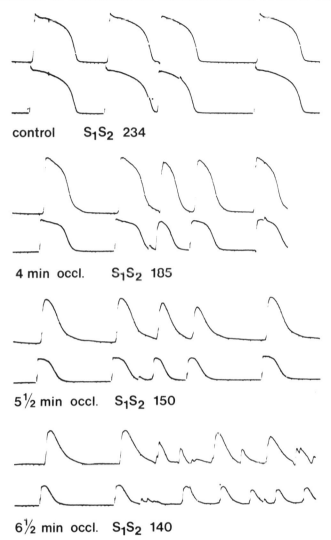

Figure 14.5 Two simultaneously recorded action potentials from cells 1 cm apart. Stimuli were applied close to lower cell. Note shortening in refractory periods following coronary artery occlusion. Note difference in latency of test stimuli delivered 185 and 150 msec after basic stimulus (2nd and 3rd panel). In lowest panel the test pulse does not result in a regenerative response in lower cell but must have excited a more remote cell from which activity proceeded towards upper cell. The inhomogeneity in activation may have been responsible for the ensuing ventricular activation

cell of the lower trace in each panel. In the control situation, local refractory period was 234 msec. Within 1 min of coronary artery occlusion, the refractory period lengthened by 20 msec (not shown) and subsequently shortened, as did action potential duration to a value of 185 msec after 4 min of ischaemia. After

5.5 min the refractory period had further shortened to 150 msec. However, the latency between premature stimulus and response had increased considerably to *ca*. 75 msec suggesting that the stimulating current first had excited a more remote fibre having a shorter refractory period. The premature action potential of the cell in the lower trace would then be a propagated response, originating in the more remote fibre. The suggestion that in the small area surrounding the stimulating electrode fibres exist with different refractory periods is borne out by the lowest panel, in which a test pulse given after 140 msec did not excite the lower cell but must have excited a more distal element from which activity proceeded towards the upper cell.

The lower cell was excited after a very long interval and the ensuing ventricular fibrillation may have been due to the inhomogeneity in refractory periods in closely adjacent areas and the resulting inhomogeneity in spread of activation following the premature stimulus.

Another example of inhomogeneity in refractory periods is given in Figure 14.6. In nearly every experiment we have seen alternation in action potential

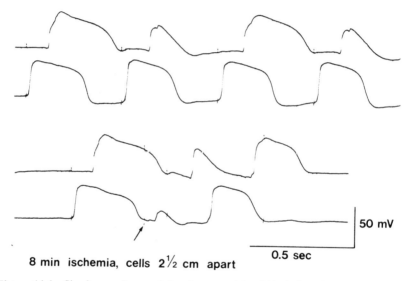

8 min ischemia, cells 2½ cm apart

50 mV

0.5 sec

Figure 14.6 Simultaneously recorded action potentials within ischaemic zone. Upper panel: alternation in upper cell. Lower panel: premature stimulus delivered close to lower cell (arrow). Note increased delay in activation of upper cell and occurrence of non-stimulated, possibly re-entrant beats. See text

duration, occurring between 5 and 10 min of ischaemia. In some fibres this alternation occurs earlier than in others (Figure 14.6, upper panel). Refractory periods alternate also, the difference between alternate beats being of the order of 60 msec, whereas refractory periods of non-alternating cells are stable. During this phase of alternation, runs of ventricular tachycardia and ventricular

fibrillation are very easily elicited by premature stimuli, and also frequently occur spontaneously. In the lower panel of Figure 14.6, a premature stimulus
delivered close to the lower cell (arrow) elicits a very small and short response,
while the upper cell is activated after an enormous delay of 240 msec (activation delay of the basic stimulus was 110 msec), well after recovery of excitability of the lower cell. It is tempting to suggest that the following non-stimulated
responses are re-entrant in nature.

The alternation between long and short action potentials, and larger and
smaller responses, suggests that in this stage refractory periods begin to lag
behind full repolarization. Figure 14.7 gives an example of this so-called post-
repolarization refractoriness, which can be best demonstrated when the
phase of alternation is over. In the control situation, recovery of excitability

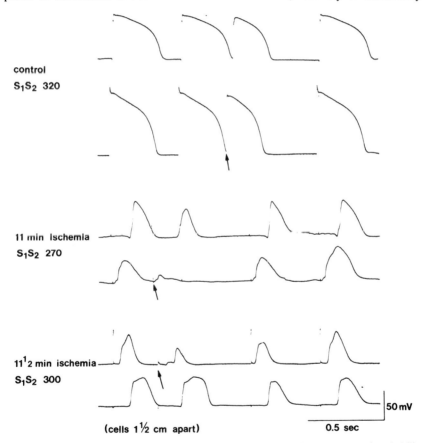

Figure 14.7 Post-repolarization refractoriness. In control situation, recovery of excitability
follows time course of repolarization. After 11 minutes of ischaemia earliest successful test pulse
(arrow) occurs well after repolarization is complete. When stimuli are given close to upper cell
(lowest panel, arrow) the post-repolarization refractoriness is even more pronounced, and the
long latency suggests that a more remote fibre with shorter refractory period was excited first

closely followed the time course of repolarization, and the refractory period was 320 msec. After 11 min of ischaemia, the action potentials of both cells had shortened from *ca.* 330 to *ca.* 200 msec. The refractory period of the lower cell was 270 msec, of the upper cell 300 msec. The salient feature of this figure is that the earliest premature response occurs long after repolarization is complete. In the lowest panel, there is a long latency between stimulus and response, indicating that close to the site of stimulation other fibres with shorter refractory periods were excited earlier.

In summary, the changes in excitability that occur during acute ischaemia are as follows: in the first two minutes of ischaemia there is a slight increase in refractory period duration synchronous to lengthening of the action potential, presumably due to cooling of the subepicardium as a consequence of reduced blood flow[10]. After 2 min, action potentials and refractory period begin to shorten. In the most severely affected areas alternation in action potential duration and refractory period occurs, at *ca.* 5–10 min of ischaemia. With the development of post-repolarization refractoriness, refractory periods begin to lengthen, and 2:1 responses begin to occur at *ca.* 10 min of ischaemia, leading eventually to total irresponsiveness at 12–15 min in the centre of the ischaemic zone. At that time, refractory periods of less injured cells are more stable; cells close to the irresponsive zone have short action potentials, low resting membrane potentials and have post-repolarization refractoriness. Cells closer to the border with normal myocardium have normal action potentials with durations shorter than those of normal myocardium, and the refractory period of these cells follows the time course of repolarization. An example of such a border cell is shown in Figure 14.8A.

Changes following reperfusion

As already shown in Figures 14.2 and 14.3, reperfusion, or even the mere flushing with nitrogenated saline, can rapidly restore electrical activity in previously irresponsive cells. Changes in excitability occur too rapidly to be determined by premature stimulation, but occur probably concomitantly with changes in action potential duration. Reperfusion has different effects on cells in the border zone. In Figure 14.8B, two action potentials of cells in the border zone are shown. After 39 min of ischaemia, a test pulse given after 205 msec was without effect. Two seconds later, the coronary artery occlusion was released and 10 sec later a test pulse given after 202 msec did elicit a response. After 2.5 min of reperfusion, the action potential of the upper cell had shortened considerably, as did the refractory period which now was 152 msec, whereas the action potential duration of the other cell had remained constant. The ventricular fibrillation that followed the test stimulus may have been the result of the rapid changes in refractory period in both the border zone and the more central ischaemic area. It seems evident that the restoration of electrical activity in previously irresponsive fibres must be due partly to the availability

cells in border of infarct

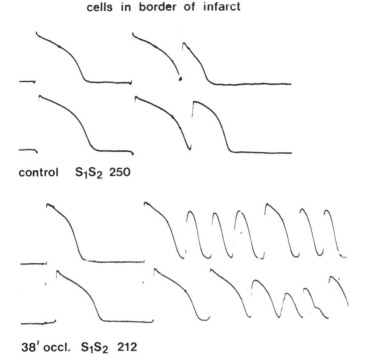

control   S₁S₂ 250

38′ occl. S₁S₂ 212

Figure 14.8A   Action potentials from cells in border of ischaemic zone recorded simultaneously. In control situation, refractory period is 250 (stimuli applied close to upper cell). After 38 minutes of ischaemia, refractory period was shortened to 212 msec, and ventricular fibrillation occurs

of substrates and oxygen, but also partly to the washing out of substances that had accumulated in the extracellular space of the ischaemic compartment, otherwise the mere flushing with nitrogenated saline could not have had the effects shown in Figure 14.3. These substances have potent effects on healthy myocardium *in vitro*[8]. It is therefore possible that upon reperfusion some cells surrounding the ischaemic zone may suddenly be subjected to an increased concentration of these substances, although not as high as they are in 'ischaemic blood', with as a result temporary shortening of action potential duration.

Relation of ischaemic changes to arrhythmias
Although ventricular arrhythmias, notably ventricular fibrillation, were seen at almost any stage following coronary artery occlusion, except during the first 3 min, there were in our experiments two periods during which ventricular fibrillation was most frequently observed: (1) the period at *ca.* 5–10 min of ischaemia, at which time alternation in action potential duration and refractory period was almost always seen and (2) the period immediately following reper-

cells in border of infarct

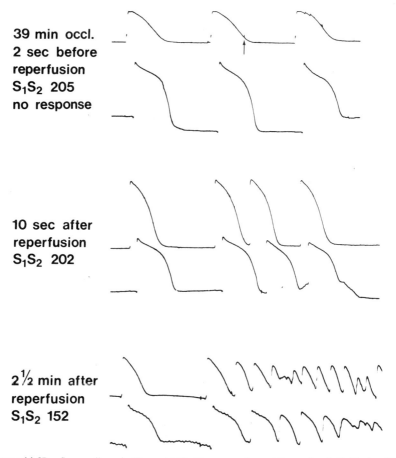

**39 min occl.
2 sec before
reperfusion
S_1S_2 205
no response**

**10 sec after
reperfusion
S_1S_2 202**

**2½ min after
reperfusion
S_1S_2 152**

Figure 14.8B   Same cells as in Figure 14.8A. Upper panel: recordings after defibrillation. Test pulse of 205 msec is unsuccessful (arrow). Action potential of upper cell shortens after reperfusion to value of 152 msec, whereas duration of action potential of lower cell does not change. Premature stimuli in lowest panel induce ventricular fibrillation

fusion, when on the one hand irresponsive cells rapidly regained their electrical activity, and on the other hand cells in the border zone showed marked shortening of the action potential. During both these periods marked dispersion in recovery of excitability was present. With our technique, in which at the most two action potentials were recorded simultaneously, it is of course impossible to prove that the arrhythmias were re-entrant in nature. Therefore, in discussing re-entry, we have to rely on circumstantial evidence, and have to examine whether factors favourable, or necessary for re-entry to occur are present in ischaemic myocardium. With regard to focal activity, we can only say that we have never observed signs of abnormal pacemaker activity – or oscillations during phase 3 or 4, such as have been reported[11] – in ischaemic myocardium. We cannot, of course, rule out the possibility of rapid pacemaker activity in the subendocardial Purkinje system. However, there are several reports in the literature suggesting that in the very first stages of ischaemia, i.e. the first 40 min, rapid pacemaker activity does not occur in the Purkinje system. Scherlag et al.[12] indicated that ventricular automaticity in the dog heart is essentially unchanged for the first two hours following coronary artery ligation. Abnormal pacemaker activity, occurring at maximal diastolic potentials of ca. – 55 mV, has been observed in excised Purkinje fibres surviving infarctions of 16–30 hours duration[4,5]. However, in Purkinje fibres that were excised after a short period of ischaemia, lasting 20–30 min, no increased automaticity was present; rather automaticity appeared depressed[6]. The possibility cannot be excluded, however, that oscillatory activity may occur in the Purkinje system, either induced by injury currents[13], or by substances diffused out of the ischaemic myocardium[14].

It is generally agreed that factors favourable for re-entry are slow conduction, short refractory periods, inhomogeneity in refractory periods in closely adjacent areas, and the occurrence of unidirectional block. As has been pointed out recently by Allessie et al.[15] the dimensions of the area of block play a key role in determining whether re-entry will occur.

Data obtained by extracellular recording have shown delayed activation and fractionation of activation in acutely ischaemic myocardium[16–18], and our data confirm that enormous delays in activation can occur. Whether this slow conduction is related to the occurrence of the so-called 'slow response'[14,19] is difficult to establish. However, the slow response seems to be blocked easily at rapid heart rates[19], and in some in vitro studies could only be evoked at stimulation rates of 1/min[20].

We have on occasion observed large action potentials with slow upstrokes when heart rate was low due to AV block. When stimulating the ventricles at a rate of 100/min, these responses disappeared and only very small responses were left (Figure 14.3). If the slow response does occur in partially depolarized ischaemic myocardium, it remains to be established that it can occur at normal heart rates.

It is well known that refractory periods shorten during ischaemia[21,22], and it has also been reported that in later stages of ischaemia, refractory periods lengthen again[22]. Increased dispersion in refractory periods has been recognized to predispose to re-entry[15,23], and our data confirm the inhomogeneity in recovery of excitability in acutely ischaemic myocardium. As already stated, the periods during which ventricular fibrillation most easily occurred, namely the phase during which post-repolarization refractoriness develops and leads to alternation, and the period following reperfusion, are the periods during which refractory periods change most rapidly and are inhomogeneous.

In the examples shown, the impulse initiating the arrhythmias was an electrically induced premature beat, whereby conduction delay and inhomogeneity in refractory periods were increased. During spontaneous sinus rhythm, there is no special initiating impulse. However, re-entry may occur in various ways, without the presence of an induced premature beat. Some cells in the ischaemic zone are activated very late, other cells close by can be activated much earlier[9]. The late activated cells may re-excite adjacent cells activated earlier, especially when these cells have short refractory periods. Slight changes in heart rate may change the response of ischaemic cells. For example, a moderate increase in heart rate can suddenly give rise to 2:1 responses in a cell that previously responded to every sinus impulse, while adjacent cells still respond in a 1:1 manner with alternation between short and long refractory periods. After the longer diastolic interval, the responses in the cell that show 2:1 block can have a much larger amplitude, and have a greater stimulating efficacy in re-exciting adjacent elements. Alternating cells in areas close to each other may get out of phase, so that at the time one cell shows a small, short action potential, the other cell exhibits a large, long response. It is easy to see how in such a situation re-entry may develop. In conclusion, therefore, we can say that the electrophysiological changes of myocardial cells in the very early stages of myocardial ischaemia strongly favour re-entry as the mechanism responsible for the arrhythmias that occur within minutes of either coronary artery occlusion, or release.

References

1. Czarnecka, M., Lewartowski, B. and Propopczuk, A. (1973). Intracellular recordings from the *in situ* working heart in physiological conditions and during acute ischaemia and fibrillation. *Acta Physiol. Pol.*, **24**, 331
2. Prinzmetal, M., Toyoshima, H., Ekmekei, A., Mizuno, Y. and Nagaya, T. (1961). Nature of ischaemic electrocardiographic patterns in the mammalian ventricles as determined by intracellular electrographic and metabolic changes. *Am. J. Cardiol.*, **8**, 493
3. Samson, W. E. and Scher, A. M. (1960). Mechanisms of ST segment alternation during acute myocardial injury. *Circ. Res.*, **8**, 780
4. Friedman, P. L., Stewart, J. R. and Wit, A. L. (1973). Spontaneous and induced cardiac arrhythmias in subendocardial Purkinje fiber surviving extensive myocardial infarction in dogs. *Circ. Res.*, **33**, 612
5. Lazzara, R., El-Sheriff, N. and Scherlag, B. J. (1973). Electrophysiological properties of canine Purkinje cells in one day old myocardial infarction. *Circ. Res.*, **33**, 722
6. Lazzara, R., El-Sherif, N. and Scherlag, B. J. (1974). Early and late effects of coronary artery occlusion in canine Purkinje fibers. *Circ. Res.*, **35**, 391
7. Woodbury, J. W. and Brady, A. L. (1956). Intracellular recording from moving tissue with a flexibly mounted ultra-microelectrode. *Science*, **123**, 100
8. Downar, E., Janse, M. J. and Durrer, D. The effect of 'ischaemic' blood on transmembrane potentials of normal porcine ventricular myocardium. Submitted to *Circulation*
9. Downar, E., Janse, M. J. and Durrer, D. The effect of acute coronary artery occlusion on epicardial transmembrane potentials in the intact porcine heart. Submitted to *Circulation*
10. Levine, H. J. (1975). In *Circulation, Suppl.* III to vols. **51** and **52**, page 145 in discussion
11. Solberg, L., Ten Eick, R. and Singer, D. (1972). Electrophysiological basis of arrhythmias in infarcted ventricle. *Circulation, Suppl.* II to vols. **45** and **46**, p. 116 (abstr.)

12. Scherlag, B. J., Hope, R. R., Williams, D. O., El-Sherif, N. and Lazzara, R. (1976). Mechanism of ectopic rhythm formation due to myocardial ischaemia: Effects of heart rate and ventricular premature beats. In: *The Conduction System of the Heart*. H. J. J. Wellens, K. I. Lie and M. J. Janse, (eds.), Lea and Febiger and Stenfert Kroese

13. Fozzard, H. (1975). Validity of myocardial infarction models. *Circulation, Suppl.* III to vols. **51** and **52**, p. 131

14. Wit, A. L. and Bigger, J. T., Jr. (1975). Possible electrophysiological mechanisms for lethal arrhythmias accompanying myocardial ischaemia and infarction. *Circulation, Suppl.* III to vols. **51** and **52**, p. 96

15. Allessie, M. A., Bonke, F. I. M. and Schopman, F. J. G. (1976). Circus movement in rabbit atrial muscle on a mechanism of tachycardia. II. The role of non-uniform recovery of excitability in the occurrence of unidirectional block on studies with multiple microelectrodes. *Circ. Res.*, **39**, 168

16. Scherlag, B. J., El-Sherif, N., Hope, R. and Lazzara, R. (1974). Characterization and localization of ventricular arrhythmias resulting from myocardial ischaemia and infarction. *Circ. Res.*, **35**, 372

17. Boineau, J. P. and Cox, J. L. Slow ventricular activation in acute myocardial infarction. A source of re-entrant premature ventricular contraction. *Circulation*, **43**, 702

18. Durrer, D., van Dam, R. Th., Freud, G. E. and Janse, M. J. (1971). Re-entry and ventricular arrhythmias in local ischaemia and infarction of the intact dog heart. *Proc. K. Ned. Akad. Wet (Biol. Med.)*, **74**, 321

19. Cranefield, P. (1975). *The Conduction of Cardiac Impulse*. (Mount Kisco, New York: Futura Publishing Company)

20. Verdonck, F., Busselen, P. and Carmeliet, E. (1972). Ca-action potentials and contraction of heart muscle in Na-free solutions. Influence of caffein. *Arch. Int. Physiol. Biochem.*, **80**, 167

21. Brooks, McC., C., Gilbert, J. L., Greenspan, M. E., Lange, G. and Mazella, H. M. (1960). Excitability and electrical response of ischaemic heart muscle. *Am. J. Physiol.*, **198**, 1143

22. Han, J., Goel, B. G. and Hanson, C. S. (1970). Re-entrant beats induced in the ventricle during coronary occlusion. *Am. Heart J.*, **80**, 778

23. Han, J. and Moe, G. K. (1964). Non-uniform recovery of excitability in ventricular muscle. *Circ. Res.*, **14**, 44

15
Cellular Electrophysiological Mechanisms for Re-entry in the Distal Purkinje System after Ischaemia or Infarction

A. L. WIT

Department of Pharmacology, College of Physicians and Surgeons, Columbia University, New York

Myocardial ischaemia resulting from coronary artery occlusion often causes ventricular arrhythmias. Such arrhythmias undoubtedly result from abnormalities in electrophysiology of the cardiac fibres deprived of their normal blood supply but in spite of all the recent advances in our knowledge of cardiac electrophysiology we cannot state with any certainty the mechanisms for myocardial ischaemic and infarction arrhythmias in humans. Recent investigations in experimental animals have provided new hypotheses concerning the mechanisms for arrhythmias after ischaemia or infarction[1]. It now seems probable that there are many different mechanisms for these arrhythmias. The mechanism of ischaemic arrhythmias may be determined by the region of the ventricles which are ischaemic, the degree of ischaemia and whether it is persistent or transient, and the time after the initiation of the ischaemic episode that the arrhythmias are occurring. Other factors are probably also important. If ischaemia occurs in a region of the ventricle abundant with specialized conducting (Purkinje) fibres, the resultant arrhythmias may have different underlying mechanisms than when ischaemia is confined to an area relatively devoid of these cells. As for the time factor, the mechanisms for cardiac arrhythmias which occur immediately after the onset of ischaemia most likely differ from the mechanisms which are important 10–24 hours after persistent ischaemia which causes infarction[1].

Ischaemic or infarction arrhythmias can probably arise in either Purkinje or ventricular muscle fibres, and like arrhythmias which occur for other reasons, are most likely due to abnormalities of impulse initiation, impulse conduction or both[2]. Abnormalities of impulse conduction cause arrhythmias by the process of re-entry and it is believed that re-entry can occur in both ventricular muscle and Purkinje fibres[3]. Although it is difficult to positively prove that re-entry is occurring in the *in situ* heart, studies on isolated tissues during the past 5 years have indicated some of the mechanisms which permit re-entry to happen[3]. The following discussion summarizes the results of some of these studies on re-entry in Purkinje fibres and relates the *in vitro* observations to the arrhythmias which occur after ischaemia or infarction in the *in situ* heart.

DISTRIBUTION OF THE VENTRICULAR SPECIALIZED CONDUCTING SYSTEM AND ITS BLOOD SUPPLY

The anatomical location of Purkinje fibres, particularly in the left ventricle, and the sources of their blood supply are among the important factors which dictate the type of electrophysiological alterations that occur in these fibres after a coronary artery occlusion. Recent detailed anatomical and electrophysiological studies on canine hearts have shown that in addition to the major fascicles the left ventricular conducting system ramifies into a network of interwoven Purkinje fibres over most of the interventricular septum, paraseptal wall and anterior and posterior papillary muscles, extending from a region level with the insertion of the free running strands into the papillary muscles to the apex[4-5]. Some of these Purkinje fibres are in free running bundles which run between the muscular trabeculae while others are subendocardial; they course beneath the endocardium although they are separated from the underlying ventricular muscle by fibrous tissue and do not seem to make contact with the muscle until they reach an area in the central septum[4]. These subendocardial fibres have some of the typical Purkinje fibre ultrastructural features which are distinct from ventricular muscle but they cannot always be identified by standard histological procedures[6]. Anatomical studies on human hearts have shown a similar network of Purkinje fibres but whether it is as extensive as in the dog is uncertain because detailed ultrastructural studies have not been done[7-9]. Alteration in the electrophysiology of both the proximal conducting system (His bundle and bundle branches) and this extensive network of peripheral Purkinje fibres can result in re-entry.

The blood supply of the His bundle in the human heart most often originates from the right coronary while the left bundle branch may receive blood from both the posterior descending branch of the right coronary and the anterior descending branch of the left. In the canine heart the His bundle is usually supplied by a branch of the left coronary but the blood supply of the left bundle branch is similar to humans[10-12]. The arteries ramify into an extensive capillary network among the Purkinje fibres in these major bundles. The His bundle and bundle branches are surrounded by a sheath of connective tissue and the Purkinje fibres toward the centre of these structures are a long distance from the endocardial surface and left ventricular cavity blood. Therefore, occlusion of the coronary arteries supplying the His bundle or bundle branches results in immediate ischaemic damage to the Purkinje fibres and subsequent necrosis if the ischaemic period is prolonged. On the other hand, the peripheral and subendocardial Purkinje systems are probably not dependent only on coronary artery blood for their nutritive requirements. Many of these fibres are very close to the endocardial surface and therefore they can probably derive at least some of their oxygen and nutritive requirements from blood in the left ventricular cavity. Subendocardial Purkinje fibres in the canine heart are also surrounded by capillaries[13] which probably receive blood from either the posterior descending, anterior descending or circumflex coronary arteries, depending on the location of the Purkinje fibres. This absence of a complete dependence on coronary artery blood for survival is an important determinant of the electrophysiological response of these Purkinje fibres to coronary artery occlusion.

EFFECTS OF ISCHAEMIA ON CELLULAR ELECTROPHYSIOLOGY OF THE VENTRICULAR SPECIALIZED CONDUCTING FIBRES

The effects of coronary artery occlusion on the cellular electrophysiology of Purkinje fibres may differ depending on whether the fibres are in the major bundles of the conducting system or are peripheral and subendocardial. When the coronary arteries supplying the His bundle or proximal bundle branches are occluded, these tissues have no alternative blood supply and the Purkinje fibres immediately begin to undergo electrophysiological changes. We must rely on *in vitro* studies on canine tissues removed from the heart after coronary artery ligation for a description of these cellular electrophysiological alterations. Lazzara *et al.*[14] ligated the septal artery in dog hearts, and removed a block of tissue containing the His bundle and bundle branches after conduction disturbances appeared *in situ*. After the His bundle and the origins of the bundle branches were exposed the electrophysiological effects of the septal artery ligation were determined by recording transmembrane action potentials from this structure during *in vitro* superfusion with Tyrode's solution. Purkinje fibres in the ischaemic His bundle had low maximum diastolic potentials (53 ± 2.8 mV as compared to a value of 72 ± 3.5 mV for fibres in non ischaemic His bundle), very slow rates of phase 0 depolarization and conduction velocities were slowed to *ca.* 0.05 m/sec from normal values of over 1.0 m/sec (Figure 15.1). In addition, refractoriness of these Purkinje fibres was largely time dependent rather than voltage dependent as in normal fibres, that is, the effective and relative refractory period outlasted complete repolarization. Accelerating the driving rate lengthened refractoriness rather than shortening it as in normal fibres. All

CL 1400

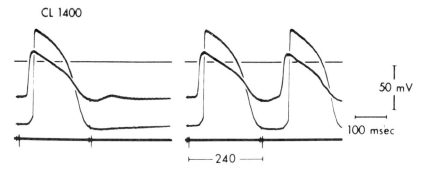

50 mV

100 msec

├── 240 ──┤

Figure 15.1 Effects of ischaemia on a His bundle action potential. Recordings were obtained from an *in vitro* preparation, previously made ischaemic *in situ* by coronary artery occlusion. The bottom trace shows an electrogram recorded from the left bundle near the stimulating electrodes. The middle trace shows an action potential recorded from the proximal right bundle which is nearly normal. The top trace was recorded from a cell in the distal His bundle which is ischaemic and has a low resting potential and action potential amplitude. The left panel shows the last of a series of action potentials driven at a cycle length of 1400 msec and a premature stimulus which excited the left bundle but did not propagate into the His bundle because of post-repolarization refractoriness. In the right panel, when the premature impulse was applied slightly later in the cycle length, it did propagate to the His bundle and right bundle. (Reproduced from Lazzara *et al.* (1975); *Circ. Res.*, **36**, 444 by permission of the American Heart Association.)

these effects of ischaemia on the Purkinje fibres in the His bundle and bundle branches may result from alterations in the cell membrane properties caused by ischaemia rather than from the acute effects of accumulated metabolites and K^+ in the extracellular space since long periods of perfusion in the Tyrode's solution did not reverse the abnormalities, although it probably washed out metabolites and excess K^+. Many of these abnormal electrophysiological properties in the His bundle fibres can cause re-entry (see later).

In contrast to this immediate direct effect of coronary artery occlusion on Purkinje fibres in the major bundles, experimental evidence suggests that the electrophysiology of peripheral subendocardial fibres is not immediately altered by a direct effect of ischaemia on the cell membrane although alterations in cellular electrophysiology may sometimes result from metabolites and electrolytes leaking into their extracellular space from the adjacent ventricular muscle cells which begin to die after a coronary occlusion. The effects of ischaemia on the electrophysiology of these peripheral Purkinje fibres have also been assessed by recording transmembrane action potentials from superfused canine left ventricular subendocardial tissue, isolated at various times after coronary artery occlusion. After superfusion *in vitro* for several hours, Purkinje fibre action potentials recorded from tissue isolated 1–3 hours after the coronary occlusion are still essentially normal though the underlying ventricular muscle is dying. The ultrastructure of these fibres is also normal, there is no evidence of ischaemic changes (unpublished observations). The lack of any immediate and direct effects on these Purkinje fibres may be attributed to their dual source of blood supply. Coronary artery occlusion completely eliminates the capillary blood flow to these subendocardial Purkinje fibres, but normal electrophysiology may be maintained for many hours because these fibres can obtain sufficient nutrients and oxygen from blood in the left ventricular cavity to meet their immediate needs[13].

The data demonstrating that subendocardial Purkinje fibre action potentials are normal after 3 hours of coronary ligation in the dog was obtained from isolated tissue which was allowed to equilibrate with the perfusing medium for 1–2 hours. Although it demonstrates that there is no direct permanent effect of this short period of ischaemia to alter membrane properties of these cells, there is also evidence to suggest that sometimes subendocardial Purkinje fibre electrophysiology may be transiently altered by K^+ and metabolites leaking from the dying adjacent ventricular muscle cells into their extracellular space. The amplitude of the electrogram recorded from subendocardial Purkinje fibres in canine hearts is sometimes markedly decreased immediately after coronary artery occlusion[15]. When the tissue was excised and action potentials recorded immediately upon superfusion *in vitro* these Purkinje fibres had low membrane potentials, slow rates of depolarization and low amplitudes[16]. Action potential duration was short and conduction velocity was slow (Figure 15.2). However, several hours of superfusion washed the substances which were responsible for

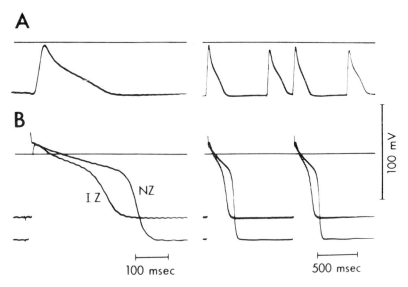

Figure 15.2 Intracellular potentials of Purkinje fibers in a preparation from a heart excised 20 min after occlusion of the left anterior descending coronary artery. (A) Potentials recorded from a cell within the ischaemic zone (IZ) 15 min after excision of the heart. (B) Potentials of the same cell recorded 20 min later and compared with those of a cell within the normal zone (NZ). (Reproduced from Lazarra *et al.* (1974); *Circ. Res.*, **35**, 391, by permission of the American Heart Association.)

these alterations out of the Purkinje fibres extracellular environment and restored nearly normal action potentials[16].

Based on this premise that there is a leakage of substances from the ischaemic ventricular muscle into the environment of subjacent subendocardial Purkinje fibres, we have studied the electrophysiological properties of Purkinje fibres isolated from normal canine hearts and superfused *in vitro* with a solution altered in composition to partially mimic the ischaemic environment[17]. The effects of elevating K^+ alone and in combination with catecholamines were investigated since it has been shown that the extracellular $[K^+]$ is markedly increased in ischaemic areas[18-19] and that ischaemia causes release of norepinephrine from sympathetic nerves in the heart[20]. However, we did not study the effects of metabolites that might be present in the ischaemic milieu. Studies were done using a three chambered tissue bath which permitted alterations to be made in the extracellular environment of a small segment of a Purkinje fibre bundle while permitting other segments to remain in a normal ionic environment, thereby mimicking a possible occurrence *in situ* where ischaemic and normal regions are adjacent to each other[17]. Elevation of the extracellular K^+ concentration to 12–16 mM from a normal value of 4 mM in the superfusate to a segment of a Purkinje fibre bundle markedly reduced resting membrane potential to between −60 and −70 mV, thereby decreasing phase 0 upstroke velocity to between 10 and 20 V/sec and markedly slowing conduction through the small segment. Besides slow conduction unidirectional block and rate dependent conduction delay also occurred in fibres depressed in this manner. The slowing of the upstroke velocity in these fibres is due to a reduction in the fast inward Na^+ current as a result of voltage dependent inactivation of the fast channel[21]. The low amplitude, slowly conducting action potentials which occur under these circumstances have depolarization phases caused by a weak inward Na current (they are highly sensentive to the fast channel blocking agent tetrodotoxin) and we have called them depressed fast responses[17]. When the K^+ in the Tyrode's solution was elevated to 16–20 mM, membrane potential declined to value < -60 mV and excitability was lost. The fast channel is inactivated at these membrane potentials and action potentials are no longer generated. Under these conditions the admission of norepinephrine to the superfusate restored excitability without increasing resting membrane potential[17,22]. The resultant action potentials arose from the low resting potentials, had extremely slow upstroke velocities and low amplitudes and as a result also conducted extraordinarily slowly. It often took the impulse 200 msec to traverse the short 10–15 mm segment of the Purkinje bundles (Figure 15.3). Unidirectional conduction block also occurred[17]. It has been suggested on the bases of a variety of experimental observations that the upstroke of these action potentials occurring in an elevated K^+ and norepinephrine environment result from a slow inward Ca^{2+} current flowing through the 'slow' membrane channel which is distinct from the fast Na^+ channel[22,23]. Although reduction of membrane potential by K^+ to < -60 mV inactivates the fast Na channel, this

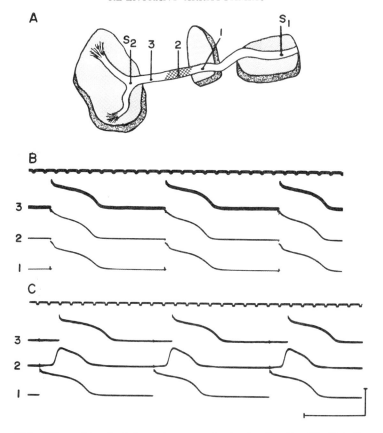

Figure 15.3   Effects of localized depression on conduction in a bundle of Purkinje fibres. (A) Diagram of the preparation with location of stimulating electrodes S_1 and S_2, and recording electrodes 1, 2 and 3. The cross-hatched area where recording electrode 2 is located has been depressed by local elevation of K^+ to 15 mM. (B) Tracing shows that conduction before depression is rapid; when the bundle is stimulated at S_1 the impulse conducted from one end of the bundle to the other in less than 5 msec. In (C) after depression of the centre segment (note the depressed action potential in trace (2) conduction between electrodes 1 and 3 required 150 msec. Conduction velocity fell in the depressed part of the bundle to *ca*. 0.07 m/sec from a normal value of *ca*. 3 m/sec. Calibrations: vertical, 100 mV, horizontal, 500 msec. (Reproduced from Cranefield *et al.* (1973); *Circulation*, **42,** 190, by permission of the American Heart Association.)

slow channel is not inactivated at membrane potentials between -60 and -20 mV. Action potentials cannot be elicited in the absence of catecholamines because of the low membrane resistance in the elevated K^+ which prevents the slow inward current from being activated and causing an action potential. Catecholamines lower the threshold for activation of the slow inward current (make threshold potential more negative) while increasing its density, thereby permitting action potentials due to the slow current to be generated[24]. We have called these action potentials slow responses[17,23].

The action potentials generated by Purkinje fibres exposed to an elevated extracellular K^+ or an elevated K^+ and catecholamines, and the action potentials generated by fibres in the ischaemic His bundle are similar in many respects. They all have low membrane potentials, slow upstroke velocities and low amplitudes and conduct very slowly. Conduction block is easily induced and unidirectional conduction may occur. Although these properties have only been demonstrated in studies conducted *in vitro*, it is reasonable to assume that Purkinje fibres in areas of ischaemia undergo similar alterations *in situ*.

MECHANISM FOR RE-ENTRY RESULTING FROM SLOW CONDUCTION AND UNIDIRECTIONAL CONDUCTION BLOCK IN PURKINJE FIBRES

The presence of slow conduction and unidirectional conduction block in Purkinje fibre bundles can lead to re-entry. We have studied re-entry in isolated bundles of canine Purkinje fibres in which the action potentials in either short segments (*ca.* 10 mm in length) or the entire bundle (15–20 mm in length) were depressed by exposure to an elevated K^+ and catecholamine environment[25,26]. Two types of re-entry were described. The first type of re-entry occurred in unbranched bundles of Purkinje fibres. The impulse travelled along the bundle into an area where conduction was depressed. After some delay, an impulse conducted retrogradely along the bundle (in the direction from which the first impulse came) as well as forward along the bundle (Figure 15.4). Slow conduction in segments as short as 6 mm generated re-entry of this type[25]. Although by mapping the spread of excitation with microelectrode recordings the sequences of excitation that led to re-entry were shown, the techniques used still did not precisely define the mechanism. We can speculate that in a segment of the conducting system showing no gross branching or loops re-entry of this type probably requires the impulse to find a circuitous re-entrant pathway within the syncytium of the depressed segment that permits the initiating impulse to enter one fibre, travel via another to a third fibre and reflect via the third fibre (Figure 15.4). This is essentially the model proposed by Schmitt and Erlanger[27]. The slow conduction is an important prerequisite for this re-entry since this is how the impulse persists while areas which it has previously excited, regain excitability. Unidirectional conduction block within part of the syncytium must be postulated to occur in order to provide the return pathway for the impulse to the region it previously excited[2,3]. An alternative mechanism involves return excitation in a single fibre where the slowly conducting action potential re-excites by an electrotonic influence a region through which it has already conducted after fibres in this area have repolarized.

Re-entry of this type does not require premature excitation for its initiation but if conduction in the depressed segment is not quite slow enough to permit re-entry or if the necessary region of unidirectional block is not present, re-entry can be initiated by a premature impulse because such impulses conduct

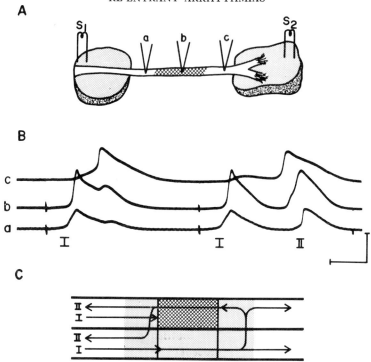

Figure 15.4 Re-entry (reflection) in a linear bundle of canine Purkinje fibres. (A) Diagram of preparation showing location of stimulating electrodes (S_1 and S_2) and recording electrodes (a, b, c). The centre segment, depressed by high K^+, is indicated by cross-hatched area. The bundle is being stimulated at S_1 only. (B) In the first group of action potentials I shows conduction of impulse originating at S_1 without re-entry; conduction from (a) to (c), through the depressed area, required 100 msec. In the second group of action potentials I shows conduction of another impulse from S_1 with marked increase in the conduction delay between recording sites (b) and (c) to 250 msec. A re-entrant impulse II returning in the opposite direction is shown at recording sites (b) and (a). (C) Diagrammatic representation of a possible pathway of impulse propagation during re-entry in two parallel fibres. Severely depressed area indicated by cross-hatches, moderately depressed area by stipples. Impulse I is completely blocked in upper fibre at area of unidirectional block but traverses the moderately depressed area in lower fibre, then re-enters upper fibre to travel in the reverse direction as impulse II. Calibrations: vertical, 100 mV for traces (a) and (c) and 50 mV for trace (b); horizontal, 250 msec. (Reproduced from Cranefield *et al.* (1973); *Circulation,* **42,** 190, by permission of the American Heart Association.)

more slowly and are more prone to conduction block[25]. The long time dependent refractory period of depressed fibres is a major cause of the additional slowing of conduction of the premature impulses.

The kind of re-entry which occurs in unbranched bundles of Purkinje fibres should be able to occur in any region of the ventricular conducting system after ischaemia, either in the His bundle and bundle branches which may be directly damaged or in the peripheral Purkinje bundles which may be exposed to an elevated K^+ and catecholamine environment.

Re-entry may also occur in Purkinje fibre bundles by a process described in the classical literature as 'circus movement'[28]. For circus movement to happen a circuitous pathway must be present and this pathway may be formed by bundles of Purkinje fibres. Many such circular arrangements exist in the peripheral conducting system. In our studies these loops of Purkinje fibre bundles were isolated from canine or bovine hearts and superfused with Tyrode's solution. Either discrete areas or the entire loop were depressed by elevated K^+ and catecholamines[26]. Under these conditions re-entry sometimes occurred when the impulse which conducted into the loop, blocked in one branch (at a site of unidirectional block) while conducting slowly around the loop in the other direction and finally returning to its point of origin (Figure 15.5). Since conduction velocity was often as slow as 0.03 m/sec in the depressed areas and the refractory periods of the Purkinje fibres were of approximately normal length (300 msec) the path length needed to permit such a circus movement was only *ca*. 100 mm[26]. Occasionally, after the re-entrant impulse returned to its site of origin it again continued to conduct around the loop and this process could be repeated many times, resulting in sustained firing at all the microelectrode recording sites. In loops in which conduction velocity was too rapid for re-entry to occur or which did not have the strategically located area of unidirectional conduction block, these necessary prerequisites for re-entry often occurred after initiation of premature impulses[26]. The premature impulses conducted more slowly than the basic impulses because they were conducting in partially refractory tissue, and they often blocked in a region of the loop. The results of these studies therefore also suggest that re-entry might occur in this manner in the peripheral conducting system of ischaemic areas in which the Purkinje fibre bundles are exposed to high concentrations of K^+ and catecholamines. To demonstrate re-entry by this mechanism in the intact heart seems like a monumental task at this time.

RE-ENTRY IN SUBENDOCARDIAL PURKINJE FIBRES SURVIVING IN AREAS OF MYOCARDIAL INFARCTION

The preceding discussion was confined mainly to events that might occur shortly after the onset of ischaemia and which may be responsible for some of the early phase arrhythmias[1]. Other electrophysiological changes have been shown to occur in Purkinje fibres in experimental studies in which ischaemia is prolonged and mycardial infarction develops. There are no studies which define what prolonged ischaemia does to electrophysiological properties of the His bundle and bundle branches but infarction of these structures which destroys the cells must eventually abolish electrical activity and when this occurs re-entry would no longer occur in these regions. Other electrophysiological changes occur in the peripheral subendocardial Purkinje system in areas of infarction which may cause the late phase of arrhythmias which develops 10–16 hours after a coronary artery occlusion in the dog[1].

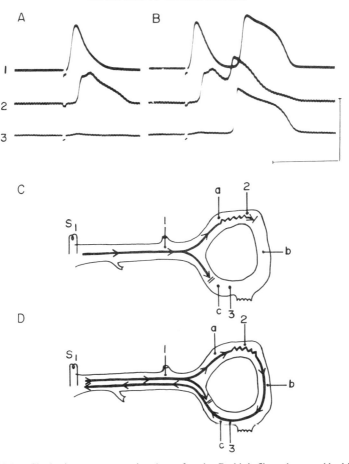

Figure 15.5 Single circus movement in a loop of canine Purkinje fibres depressed by high K⁺. (A) Action potentials recorded during conduction block in the loop, and (B) single circus movement. (C and D) Diagrams of the preparation and location of the stimulating electrode (S_1) and the recording electrodes (1, 2, 3). The branches of the loop are indicated by (a), (b) and (c). The pathway of propagation shown by arrows in C corresponds to the action potentials shown in A. Note only single depolarizations at sites 1 and 2 and the absence of depolarization at site 3 indicating block. The pathway of propagation in D corresponds to the records shown in B. In B the first depolarization at site 1 and the depolarization at 2 are followed by delayed activation at 3 (a site of unidirectional block). This is followed by the re-entrant impulse at 1 (second depolarization). Calibrations: vertical, 100mV; horizontal, 500 msec. (Reproduced from Cranefield *et al.* (1973) *Circulation*, **42**, 190, by permission of the American Heart Association.)

The documentation of the changes in transmembrane electrical activity in subendocardial Purkinje fibres in the canine heart after prolonged coronary occlusion has been accomplished by Friedman *et al.*[29], and by Lazzara *et al.*[30]. The infarcted myocardium was isolated and superfused with Tyrode's solution in a tissue chamber with the endocardial surface easily accessible for electrophysiological study. Transmembrane electrical activity of subendocardial Purkinje fibres in infarcted regions was studied in this way at times ranging from several minutes to several months after coronary artery occlusion. The technique is limited in that it does not take into account possible influences of the autonomic nervous system, blood-borne factors, or the role of hypoxia, all of which have profound effects on the *in situ* heart. However, it does provide considerable insight into the electrophysiological properties of the Purkinje fibres in the infarcted region.

Using this technique it was shown that the subendocardial Purkinje fibres in infarcted regions continued to survive and generated action potentials while the underlying ventricular muscle died[29,30]. Although these subendocardial Purkinje fibres survived, their action potential characteristics did not remain normal. Changes in the transmembrane potential were detected in preparations isolated 6 hours after coronary occlusion and these changes were more severe in preparations isolated at later times after the occlusion. Maximum diastolic potential recorded from Purkinje fibres in infarcted preparations isolated 24 hours after coronary occlusion was quite low, action potential amplitude and upstroke velocity were reduced while repolarization time was prolonged. Spontaneous diastolic depolarization was also evident which may have been a cause of some of the cardiac arrhythmias which were present in the *in situ* heart[29,30]. Action potential duration of Purkinje fibres in infarcted preparations studied 2 and 3 days after coronary artery occlusion was even longer than at 24 hours but in preparations isolated 3 days after coronary artery ligation maximum diastolic potential, action potential amplitude and V_{max} of phase 0 were not as depressed as in 24 hour old infarcts[16]. These changes in the action potentials may result from the alteration of membrane properties by the effects of ischaemia since many of the abnormalities in the action potentials even persist after long periods of superfusion with well oxygenated Tyrode's solution *in vitro*[29].

We studied the conduction of premature impulses in the subendocardial Purkinje fibres surviving in infarcts at different times after coronary artery occlusion[31]. The distribution of subendocardial Purkinje fibre action potentials with different time courses of repolarization was an important determinant of the characteristics of conduction and sites of conduction block of the premature impulses. In non-infarcted subendocardium action potential duration to 100% repolarization was longest on the false tendon at the region of the gate[32]. By recording transmembrane action potentials from subendocardial Purkinje fibres at 3–5 mm intervals distal to this site we determined that, progressing from the tip of the anterior papillary muscle to the apex of the non-infarcted heart, subendocardial Purkinje fibre action potential duration became progressively shorter (Figure 15.6). Likewise, Purkinje fibre action potential duration progressively decreased from the base of the heart to the apex in the subendocardial network of the paraseptal free wall and anterior septum. As a result of this pattern premature impulses initiated at the earliest possible time during

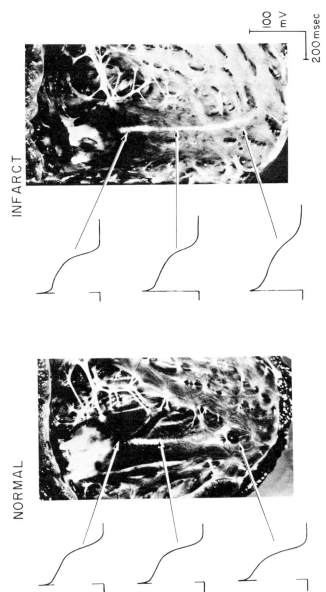

Figure 15.6 Distribution of action potential durations of subendocardial Purkinje fibres in a normal, non-infarcted preparation and an infarcted preparation. In each section, the action potentials shown were recorded from the most superficial subendocardial Purkinje fibre at sites designated on the accompanying photograph of each preparation. In the normal non-infarcted preparation (left), the action potential recorded from the tip of the papillary muscle had the longest time course of repolarization. Action potential duration to 50% repolarization $(APD_{50}) = 221$ msec and APD to 100% repolarization $(APD_{100}) = 356$ msec. Action potential duration progressively decreased from the tip of the papillary muscle and high septum toward the apex of the left ventricle. In the midregion of the anterior papillary muscle $APD_{50} = 217$ msec and $APD_{100} = 322$ msec. The shortest action potential was recorded at the apex $(APD_{50} = 179$ msec and $APD_{100} = 290$ msec). In the infarcted preparation (right), the top action potential was recorded from the non-infarcted tip of the papillary muscle; action potential duration in this region was normal $(APD_{50} = 240$ msec and $APD_{100} = 360$ msec). As the microelectrode was advanced distally across the border into the infarcted region, action potential duration progressively increased. In the midregion of the anterior papillary muscle $APD_{50} = 250$ msec and $APD_{180} = 400$ msec. Note that the action potential recorded from the apex of the left ventricle was more than 100 msec longer than the action potential recorded from the tip of the papillary muscle $(APD_{50} = 265$ msec and $APD_{100} = 500$ msec). (Reproduced from Friedman *et al.* (1973); *Circ. Res.*, **33**, 612, by permission of the American Heart Association.)

repolarization of Purkinje fibres at the tip of the papillary muscle or at the base of the paraseptal free wall or anterior septum encountered Purkinje fibres which were progressively more repolarized as they propagated towards the apex. Therefore, conduction delay and block of early premature depolarizations always occurred in Purkinje fibres in the vicinity of the stimulating electrode (Figure 15.7). Conduction block never occurred toward the apical region since action potential duration in these areas was always less than it was in the stimulated area[31].

The pattern of conduction of premature impulses and the sites of conduction block of these impulses in the subendocardial Purkinje fibre network of the 2, 3 and 4 day old infarcted preparations differed from those described for the sub-endocardial network in non-infarcted preparations[31,33]. In these infarcted preparations action potential duration of Purkinje fibres progressively increased from the base of the heart to the apex in all regions. This pattern resulted from the marked increase in action potential duration of Purkinje fibres in the infarct (Figure 15.6). As a result, premature impulses initiated either early in diastole or before complete repolarization of subendocardial Purkinje fibres in non-infarcted tissue at the tip of the papillary muscle or the base of the paraseptal free wall or anterior septum conducted extremely slowly once they propagated into the infarcted area (Figure 15.7). Such slow conduction occurred because the time course of repolarization of subendocardial Purkinje fibres in the infarcted area was 100–200 msec longer than it was in the surrounding non-infarcted areas and therefore premature impulses conducting into these suben-docardial areas encountered Purkinje fibres which were progressively less repolarized and therefore more refractory.

In addition to being prolonged, the time course of repolarization of suben-docardial Purkinje fibres in the infarcted region was strikingly inhomogeneous with action potentials in adjacent regions having markedly different durations. As a result, conduction of premature impulses through the subendocardial Purkinje fibre network of the infarct was not only slowed but was also inhomogeneous, that is, conduction of premature impulses from the base to the apex of the preparation was slower in regions with the longest action potential durations and more rapid in closely adjacent regions with shorter action potential durations. Also conduction block of early premature impulses occurred in some areas of the infarct, while conduction through other infarcted regions still proceeded slowly. This inhomogeneous conduction through the subendocardial Purkinje network often caused re-entry of the stimulated premature impulses[31]. This was documented by recording the activation sequence of up to nine recording sites in the subendocardial Purkinje network (Figure 15.8). Re-entry occurred when conduction of early stimulated premature impulses blocked in regions of the subendocardial Purkinje network with the longest action potential durations and refractory periods while conducting slowly through other regions where action potential duration and refractory periods were shorter. When conduction through these latter areas was significantly slow the impulse returned and excited regions in

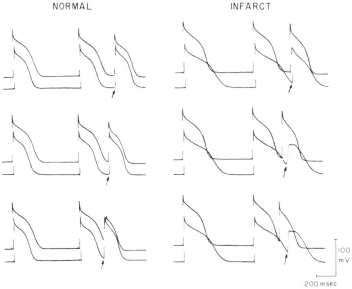

Figure 15.7 Conduction of premature impulses in the subendocardial Purkinje fibre network of a normal (left) and an infarcted (right) preparation. Premature stimuli were delivered through an intracellular microelectrode to a subendocardial Purkinje fibre on the tip of the anterior papillary muscle. In each section, the top trace is the transmembrane action potential of the prematurely stimulated fibre on the tip of the papillary muscle. The bottom trace was recorded from a subendocardial Purkinje fibre at the apex of the left ventricle. The arrows indicate the premature response at the apex. For the infarcted preparation, the apical Purkinje fibre was located in the infarcted region, but the Purkinje fibre at the tip of the papillary muscle was not. Note that the apical Purkinje fibre had a shorter action potential duration than did the fibre at the tip of the papillary muscle in the normal preparation and a longer action potential duration than did the fibre at the tip of the papillary muscle in the infarcted preparation. For the normal preparation a premature impulse initiated after complete repolarization of the proximal fibre excited the fibre in the apex after a delay of only 10 msec (top section). In the middle section, an earlier premature impulse still conducted to the apex with a delay of only 10 msec. A still earlier premature stimulus (bottom section) excited the Purkinje fibre on the tip of the papillary muscle early during repolarization, but conduction delay to the apex was still not substantial. In the infarcted preparation, a premature impulse initiated after complete repolarization of the proximal fibre (top section) conducted to the fibre in the apex with a delay of 12 msec. In the middle section, an earlier premature impulse conducted into the infarct to the apex with substantial delay; the fibre in the apex was excited nearly 50 msec after the proximal fibre. A still earlier premature stimulus (bottom section) excited the fibre on the tip of the papillary muscle and conducted to the apex with a conduction time of 88 msec. Conduction delays of this magnitude were never seen in the subendocardial Purkinje fibres of non-infarcted preparations. (Reproduced from Friedman *et al.* (1973); *Circ. Res.,* **33,** 612, by permission of the American Heart Association.)

which it initially blocked and then returned to the point of origin as a re-entrant impulse (Figures 15.8 and 15.9). This re-entry could become continuous if the Purkinje fibres over the infarcted region regained excitability by the time the reentering impulse returned to its point of origin. The impulse could once again conduct into the infarct and re-emerge as another re-entrant impulse[31]. In infarcts

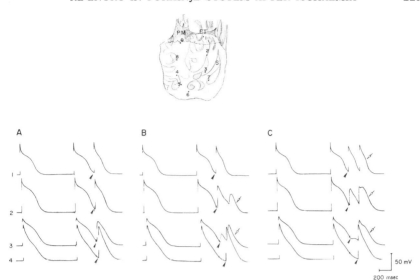

Figure 15.8   Inhomogeneous conduction of premature impulses in the subendocardial Purkinje fibre network of an infarcted preparation 24 hours after coronary occlusion. Top: Schematic representation of the preparation. Light area indicates infarcted region. PM = papillary muscle, FT = false tendon, and S = septum. The numbers in this drawing denote the locations of sites from which subendocardial Purkinje fibre action potentials were recorded during premature stimulation. Two stationary microelectrodes were utilized to record action potentials from sites 1 and 4 throughout the experiment. Premature stimuli (at variable coupling intervals with the basic stimulus) were applied through the intracellular microelectrode at site 1. The response resulting directly from this premature stimulus is indicated by the solid arrows on each trace in (A), (B) and (C). At each coupling interval a third (roving) microelectrode was utilized to record action potentials from sites 2, 3 and 5–9. These action potentials were displayed simultaneously with those recorded from sites 1 and 4. By this method, the relative sequence of activation of these nine recording sites by the premature impulse was determined. Bottom: For the records shown in (A), (B) and (C), action potentials were recorded from sites 1, 2 and 4 during premature stimulation at three given coupling intervals and then from sites 1, 3 and 4 at the same coupling intervals. The records shown are a composite of the recordings obtained at these four sites. In each of these sections the numbered traces were recorded from the correspondingly numbered sites on the accompanying diagram of the preparation. (A) Premature stimulus was applied through the microelectrode at site 1,320 msec after the basic impulse. This premature impulse conducted into the infarct to sites 2, 3 and 4 and depolarized the Purkinje fibres at these sites nearly simultaneously. (B) Coupling interval was 300 msec. This premature impulse appeared to block near recording site 3, as indicated by the low-amplitude depolarization at this site (solid arrow on trace 3). This same premature impulse, however, conducted slowly to site 4 without blocking, as indicated by the delayed depolarization at this site. Note also the additional depolarization at sites 3 and 2 (open arrows on traces 3 and 2) which followed the response at site 4. (C) Coupling interval was reduced to 280 msec. This premature impulse appeared to block before reaching site 3 (low-amplitude deflection indicated by solid arrow on trace 3) but still conducted slowly to site 4 without blocking. Now note the additional depolarizations at sites 3, 2 and 1 (open arrows on traces 3, 2 and 1) which followed the response at site 4. See discussion and Figure 15.9 for a possible interpretation of unstimulated depolarizations. (Reproduced from Friedman *et al.* (1973); *Circ. Res.*, **33,** 612, by permission of the American Heart Association.)

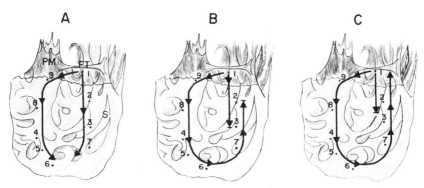

Figure 15.9 Possible conduction pathways of premature impulses in the subendocardial Purkinje fibre network of an infarcted preparation 24 hours after coronary occlusion. Experiment is the same one described in Figure 15.8. Light area on each drawing of the preparation indicates the infarcted region. PM = papillary muscle, FT = false tendon, and S = septum. Numbers denote locations of sites from which subendocardial Purkinje fibre action potentials were recorded during premature stimulation and correspond to the sites indicated in Figure 15.8. Premature stimuli were delivered through an intracellular microelectrode at site 1 at coupling intervals with the basic stimulus of 320 msec (A), 300 msec (B) and 280 msec (C). Arrows in each section indicate a possible conduction pathway for each premature impulse as determined by the relative sequence of activation of the nine recording sites. Pathways in (A), (B) and (C) are consistent with the records shown in the correspondingly lettered sections of Figure 14.8. Arrows interrupted by horizontal bars indicated sites of conduction block as determined from the records in Figure 15.8. In (A), at the long coupling interval, the premature impulse conducted along the papillary muscle and the septum to the apex. In (B), at a shorter coupling interval, conduction of the premature impulse blocked in the septum but continued slowly along the papillary muscle. The impulse then returned to the region where conduction block originally occurred in the septum before it encountered refractory tissue and died out. In (C), at a still shorter coupling interval, the same sequence of activation occurred as in (B) but conduction of the premature impulse was slower and therefore by the time it conducted retrogradely up the septum, this region had recovered excitability. Therefore the premature impulse was able to return to its site of initiation as a re-entrant impulse.

studied more than four days after coronary occlusion, the Purkinje fibre action potential durations were progressively shorter with time and nearly normal in preparations studied seven weeks after occlusion. The conduction delay of premature impulses decreased in preparations with the shorter action potential durations and a normal conduction pattern was eventually re-established. Re-entry could no longer be induced in preparations studied 10 days after the coronary occlusion. This shortening of action potential duration may be due to the re-establishment of capillary blood flow to the subendocardial Purkinje fibres, possibly through the formation of collaterals[13].

We are presently uncertain whether the mechanism for re-entry in subendocardial Purkinje fibres in infarcts demonstrated *in vitro*, occurs in the *in situ* canine or human heart. If it does it might be a mechanism for the re-entrant paroxysmal ventricular tachycardia which occurs in some cases of myocardial infarction in humans[34]. However the direct demonstration of cellular re-entrant mechanisms in the *in situ* heart after myocardial infarction in both experimental animals and in humans at the present time appears to be beyond our grasp and so for the time being we must be satisfied with attempting to extrapolate from *in vitro* observations.

Acknowledgement

Part of this work was supported by U.S. Public Health Service Grant HL-12738 and HL-14899.

References

1. Wit, A. L. and Bigger, J. T., Jr. (1975). Possible electrophysiological mechanisms for lethal arrhythmias accompanying myocardial ischemia and infarction. *Circulation,* **52,** Suppl. III, 96

2. Cranefield, P. F., Wit, A. L. and Hoffman, B. F. (1973). Genesis of cardiac arrhythmias. *Circulation,* **42,** 190

3. Wit, A. L., Rosen, M. R. and Hoffman, B. F. (1976). Electrophysiology and pharmacology of cardiac arrhythmias II. Relationship of normal and abnormal electrical activity of cardiac fibers to the genesis of arrhythmias. B. Reentry Sections 1 and 2. *Am. Heart J.,* **88,** 664, *Am. Heart J.,* **88,** 798

4. Myerburg, R. J., Nilson, K. and Gelband, H. (1972). Physiology of canine intraventricular conduction and endocardial excitation. *Circ. Res.,* **30,** 217

5. Lazzara, R., Yeh, B. K. and Samet, P. (1974). Functional anatomy of the canine left bundle branch. *Am. J. Cardiol.,* **33,** 623

6. Friedman, P. L., Fenoglio, J. J., Jr. and Wit, A. L. (1975). The time course for reversal of electrophysiological and ultrastructural abnormalities in subendocardial Purkinje fibers surviving in regions of extensive myocardial infarction. *Circ. Res.,* **36,** 127

7. Spach, M. S., Huang, S., Armstrong, S. E. and Cavent, R. V. (1963). Demonstration of peripheral conduction system in human hearts. *Circulation,* **28,** 333

8. Massing, G. H. and James, T. N. (1975). Anatomical configuration of the His bundle and bundle branches in the human heart. *Circulation,* **53,** 609

9. James, T. N., Sherf, L. and Urthaler, F. (1974). Fine structure of the bundle branches. *Br. Heart J.,* **36,** 1

10. Lev, M. (1960). The conducting system. In: *Pathology of the Heart.* S. E. Gould (ed.) (Springfield, Ill., Charles C. Thomas) 2nd ed. pp. 132–165

11. James, T. N. (1961). *Anatomy of the Coronary Arteries.* (New York, Holber.)

12. James, T. N. (1968). The coronary circulation and conduction system in acute myocardial infarction. *Prog. Cardiovasc. Dis.,* **10,** 410

13. Dangman, K. H., Albala, A., Wang, H. H. and Wit, A. L. (1976). Chronological changes in collateral blood flow to subendocardial Purkinje fibers in canine infarcts. *Fed. Proc.,* **35,** 320

14. Lazzara, R., El-Sherif, N. and Scherlag, B. J. (1975). Disorders of cellular electrophysiology produced by ischemia of the canine His bundle. *Circ. Res.,* **36,** 444

15. Scherlag, B. J., El-Sherif, N., Hope, R. and Lazzara, R. (1974). Characterization and localization of ventricular arrhythmias resulting from myocardial ischemia and infarction. *Circ. Res.,* **35,** 372

16. Lazzara, R., El-Sherif, N. and Scherlag, B. J. (1974). Early and late effects of coronary artery occlusion on canine Purkinje fibers. *Circ. Res.,* **35,** 391

17. Cranefield, P. F., Wit, A. L. and Hoffman, B. F. (1972). Conduction of the cardiac impulse. III. Characteristics of very slow conduction. *J. Gen. Physiol.,* **59,** 227

18. Harris, A. S., Bisteni, A., Russell, R. A., Brigham, J. C. and Firestone, J. E. (1954). Excitatory factors in ventricular tachycardia resulting from myocardial ischemia: Potassium: a major excitant. *Science*, **119**, 200

19. Regan, T. J., Harman, M. A., Lehan, P. H., Burke, W. M. and Odelwurtel, H. A. (1967). Ventricular arrhythmias and potassium transfer during myocardial ischemia and intervention with procaine amide, insulin or glucose solution. *J. Clin. Invest.*, **46**, 1657

20. Griffiths, J. and Leung, F. (1971). The sequential estimation of plasma catecholamines and whole blood histamine in myocardial infarction. *Am. Heart J.*, **82**, 171

21. Weidmann, S. (1970). The effect of the cardiac membrane potential on the rapid availability of the sodium carrying system. *J. Physiol. (London)*, **210**, 1041

22. Carmeliet, E. and Vereecke, J. (1972). Adrenaline and the plateau phase of the cardiac action potential. Importance of Ca^+, Na^+ and K^+ conductance. *Pfluegers Arch.*, **313**, 300

23. Cranefield, P. F. (1975). *The Conduction of the Cardiac Impulse: The Slow Response and Cardiac Arrhythmias*. (New York: Futura Press.)

24. Reuter, H. (1973). Divalent cations as charge carriers in excitable membranes. In: *Progress in Biophysics and Molecular Biology*, **26**, edited by J. A. V. Butler and D. Noble (eds.). (New York: Pergamon Press), p. 3

25. Wit, A. L., Hoffman B. F. and Cranefield, P. F. (1972). Slow conduction and re-entry in the ventricular conducting system. I. Return extrasystole in canine Purkinje fibers. *Circ. Res.*, **30**, 1

26. Wit, A. L., Cranefield, P. F. and Hoffman, B. F. (1972). Slow conduction and re-entry in the ventricular conducting system. II. Single and sustained circus movement in networks of canine and bovine Purkinje fibers. *Circ. Res.*, **30**, 11

27. Schmitt, F. O. and Erlanger, J. (1928–1929). Directional differences in the conduction of the impulse through heart muscle and their possible relation to extrasystolic and fibrillary contraction. *Am. J. Physiol.*, **87**, 326

28. Mines, G. R. (1914). On circulating excitations in heart muscles and their possible relation to tachycardia and fibrillation. *Trans. R. Soc. Can. Sec.* 4, **8**, 43

29. Friedman, P. L., Stewart, J. R., Fenoglio, J. J., Jr. and Wit, A. L. (1973). Survival of subendocardial Purkinje fibers after extensive myocardial infarction in dogs: *In vitro* and *in vivo* correlations. *Circ. Res.*, **33**, 597

30. Lazzara, R., El-Sherif, N. and Scherlag, B. J. (1973). Electrophysiological properties of canine Purkinje cells in one-day-old myocardial infarction. *Circ. Res.*, **33**, 722

31. Friedman, P. L., Stewart, J. R. and Wit, A. L. (1973). Spontaneous and induced cardiac arrhythmia in subendocardial Purkinje fibers surviving extensive myocardial infarction in dogs. *Circ. Res.*, **33**, 612

32. Myerburg, R. J., Gelband, H. and Hoffman, B. F. (1971). Functional characteristics of the gating mechanism in the canine A–V conducting system. *Circ. Res.*, **28**, 136

33. Friedman, P. L., Wit, A. L. and Hoffman, B. F. (1972). Experimental myocardial infarction: Alterations in electrophysiological properties of surviving cells. *Bull. N.Y. Acad. Med.*, **48**, 1037

34. Wellens, H. J. J., Lie, K. I. and Durrer, D. (1974). Further observations on ventricular tachycardia as studied by electrical stimulation of the heart: Chronic recurrent ventricular tachycardia and ventricular tachycardia during acute myocardial infarction. *Circulation*, **49**, 647

16
Origin of Ventricular Arrhythmias in 24-Hour-Old Septal and Anterior Infarcts Studied by Epicardial and Intramural Mapping*

E. N. MOORE and J. F. SPEAR†

Department of Medicine, Hospital of the University of Pennsylvania, Philadelphia, Pennsylvania

More than 80% of the patients who suffer an acute myocardial infarction exhibit ectopic ventricular depolarizations. These arrhythmias occur predominantly during the first few days of the acute episode. In 1950, Harris[1] described an experimental canine preparation for eliciting these early cardiac arrhythmias. He noted that two phases of ventricular arrhythmia could be induced by ligation of a major branch of the left coronary circulation. After complete acute occlusion, paroxysmal ventricular arrhythmias usually developed within 2–5 min and often degenerated to ventricular fibrillation within approximately the first 20 min thereby resulting in a very high mortality. However, Harris[1] noted that if the animals survived the initial phase of arrhythmias, the ectopic ventricular beats disappeared and again reappeared 4–8 hours after the ligation. The peak frequency of ectopic beats occurred at 15–30 hours and then decreased in frequency until at 72 hours the arrhythmias

* A report of the data from the septal artery occlusion experiments has been submitted to Circulation and was presented at the 33rd meeting of the American Federation for Clinical Research (E. L. Michelson *et al.* 1976, *Clin. Res.* 24:231A). The data from the left anterior descending coronary artery occlusion experiments have also been previously published (Horowitz *et al.* 1975, *Circ.* 53:56).

† Dr. Spear is an established investigator of the American Heart Association.

usually disappeared. After left anterior descending coronary (LAD) occlusion, the infarcted region involves the anterior left ventricular free wall as well as the anterior inferior aspect of the left side of the ventricular septum. In contrast, acute ligation of the anterior septal artery results in infarction of only the septum and extends variably to the right and left surfaces. The experimental septal occlusion model also differs from the LAD occlusion model in that the specialized conduction system consisting of the bundle of His, bundle branches and parts of the peripheral Purkinje system are located over the infarcted septal myocardial tissue. Previous studies in our laboratory as well as work by other investigators, suggests that following LAD occlusion and septal artery occlusion, the ventricular arrhythmias originate in surviving Purkinje tissues within the infarcted region[2-8]. This paper describes the origin and characteristics of the ventricular arrhythmias which occur 24 hours after anterior septal artery ligation and following LAD ligation.

METHOD

Twenty-four healthy mongrel dogs weighing 10–18 kg were anaesthetized with sodium pentobarbital (30 mg/kg i.v.). Two different procedures were used in these experiments. In one series, after the animals were anaesthetized their chests were opened through a small left lateral thoracotomy, the left anterior descending coronary artery (LAD) was occluded by the two stage procedure described by Harris[1]. The ligation was located *ca.* 1 cm from the origin of the main left coronary artery and did not involve the anterior septal or circumflex arteries. After the ligation, the animals' chests were closed, antibiotics administered, and the animals allowed to recover for 18–24 hours before being restudied. The second group of animals underwent anterior septal coronary artery ligation. The artery was located by blunt dissection and a one-stage acute ligation of the septal artery was performed. These animals also were allowed to recover.

Twenty-four hours after the coronary ligation the animals were re-anaesthetized with diazepam (1.0 mg/kg) and sodium pentobarbital (10 mg/kg). The animals were ventilated using a positive pressure Harvard pump and the chests re-opened in the fifth left intercostal space. Standard electrocardiographic leads were monitored continuously, and the arrhythmias studied initially using epicardial surface mapping techniques as previously described[5,8]. The technique involves placing a reference electrode at a site distant from the infarct. A plunge-type electrode was inserted into viable myocardium and was used as a reference point for all mapping procedures. A hand-held bipolar roving electrode was then placed at 40 or more predetermined points along the epicardial surfaces of both the right and left ventricular epicardium. Time of activation at these epicardial points relative to the time of activation of the fixed reference electrogram allowed construction of an epicardial activation map defining the sequence and direction of epicardial activation. A custom-made digital timing module permitted the immediate registration of the time of activation at each recording site thereby permitting rapid location of the earliest epicardial activity. Also, plunge electrodes and multi-polar intramural electrodes were utilized to record from the bundle of His, bundle branches and peripheral Purkinje system. Plunge electrodes also were used to record from different regions of the septal myocardium in order to define the sequence of activation of both the specialized A–V conduction system and septal muscle during these ectopic ventricular depolarizations. The endocardial electrodes were left in place and their anatomical location verified at post-mortem. The conduction system was stained using 2% Lugol's solution. The region of myocardial septal infarction was defined using the vital stain nitroblue tetrazoleum according to the technique of Nachlas and Schnitka[9].

RESULTS

Ventricular tachyarrhythmias were observed in all animals 24 hours after either left anterior descending coronary artery ligation or anterior septal coronary artery ligation. In some animals, two competing foci were observed. Since it is impossible to construct an activation sequence map in the presence of two different rhythms, several procedures were utilized to ensure a unifocal ventricular tachycardia. First, the sinus node was crushed to eliminate supraventricular competition with the ventricular tachycardia. In the few animals with competing ventricular foci, it was necessary to overdrive the ventricular tachycardia by pacing the atrium at a rate more rapid than the rate of the ventricular tachycardia. A pause in the supraventricular stimulus sequence was provided which allowed a monofocal ventricular ectopic beat to manifest itself.

Table 16.1 shows the average spontaneous rates of escape rhythms in anaesthetized dogs during junctional rhythms, during A–V dissociation

Table 16.1   Spontaneous Rates of Ectopic Rhythms

Junctional	A–V Dissociation	LAD Occlusion	Anterior septal occlusion
(beats/min)	(beats/min)	(beats/min)	(beats/min)
100.6 ± 33.0	49.2 ± 8.4	196 ± 19.5	133 ± 35.9

produced by interruption of the bundle of His by electrocautery[10], and during the ventricular rhythms following LAD occlusion and following anterior septal artery occlusion. The ectopic rhythm following anterior septal occlusion (13 animals) was somewhat slower than that associated with LAD occlusion (133 v. 196 beats/min). However, the ventricular rhythms following coronary occlusion are far more rapid than the normal escape ventricular rhythms observed in animals without myocardial ischaemia (49.2 ± 8.4 beats/min).

VENTRICULAR ACTIVATION DURING RHYTHMS INDUCED BY LAD OCCLUSION

In five of twelve animals which underwent LAD occlusion, multifocal tachycardias were observed. The other seven animals developed stable unifocal tachyarrhythmias. In the animals with multifocal tachyarrhythmias programmed pacing was used to establish a stable pattern of escape depolarization. Figure 16.1 presents an example of an epicardial activation map together with an inscribed electrocardiogram. The electrocardiogram shows ectopic ventricular depolarizations exhibiting predominantly a rS pattern. In this instance, the monofocal rhythm was brought out by driving the atrium for three beats followed by a pause to permit the ventricular escape. Only the ventricular escape beat was mapped. The calibration grid located between the epicardial map and electrocardiogram indicates the time of activation for the various ventricular epicardial regions. The earliest area of epicardial activity began inferiorly (solid black area) near the apex along the left border of the infarct (diagonal broken lines) and spread concentrically to excite the entire left ventricle. Total time for overall epicardial activation was 51 msec with the right ventricle being activated 32 msec after the earliest left ventricular epicardial site. This suggests that there may have been sufficient time for the right ventricle to have been activated in part by retrograde conduction through the His and antegrade conduction over the right bundle branch–Purkinje system.

In Figure 16.2, analog records are presented. These were recorded from various regions of the specialized conduction system simultaneously with a lead II electrocardiogram. The animal was in a monofocal ventricular tachyarrhythmia and the ECG showed a ventricular complex with a predominant rS pattern. HBE is a recording from the bundle of His, LBE a bipolar recording from the left bundle branch, PF_i an electrogram from the endocardial surface 1 cm within the infarct, PF_b is a recording from a Purkinje fibre on the endocardial surface at the border of the infarcted region, REF is the reference electrogram utilized for constructing the epicardial activation map, and ECG is the lead II electrocardiogram. Time lines denote 100 msec intervals. It can be noted in this figure that the earliest recordable activity in any of the analog records occurred in the Purkinje fibre (p) located within the zone of infarction (PF_i). This Purkinje spike was the earliest recordable activity from the heart. Activation from this Purkinje region gave retrograde conduction back through the left bundle to the bundle of His. These analog records are typical for all of the dogs studied with LAD ligation in that Purkinje activity preceded recordable activity within any other part of the ventricles. Further verification that the arrhythmia was originating within this region was accomplished by pacing at a rate slightly exceeding the spontaneous ectopic rate through the recording electrode which measured this early activation. When this was done, the activation sequence of the conduction system, as well as the surface electrocardiogram configuration and epicardial activation sequence, was identical with

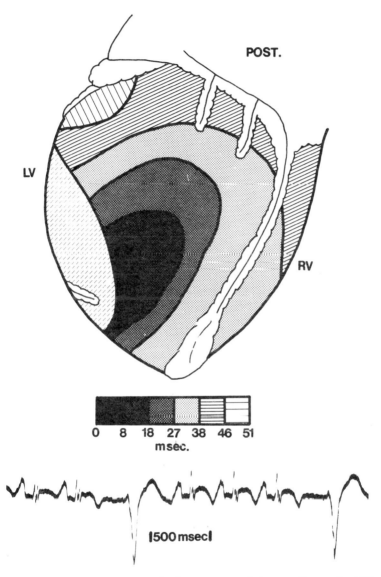

Figure 16.1 Ventricular epicardial activation sequence and electrocardiogram (lead II) of ectopic ventricular depolarizations originating on the posterolateral surface of the dog heart 24 hours following acute myocardial infarction. The infarcted myocardium is indicated by the broken diagonal lines. The concentric isochronic lines indicate activation times and the scale is shown below. Note that the earliest site of epicardial depolarization is along the border of the infarct in the left ventricle near the apex. (From Horowitz *et al.* (1975). *Circulation,* **53,** 56, reproduced by permission of the American Heart Association.)

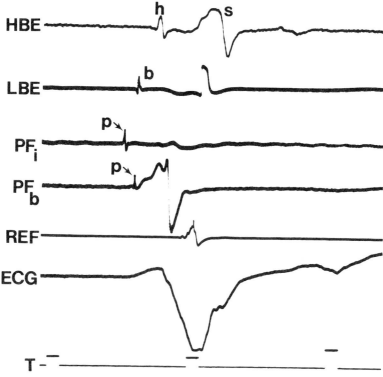

Figure 16.2 Depolarization of the ventricular specialized conducting system during spontaneous ventricular tachycardia 24 hours following left anterior descending coronary artery occlusion. The records are bipolar recordings from the His bundle (HBE), the left bundle branch (LBE), a Purkinje fibre within the infarct (PF$_i$), a Purkinje fibre in the border zone of the infarct (PF$_b$), non-infarcted myocardium (REF) and a lead II electrocardiogram (ECG). In the HBE record, h indicates the retrograde His deflection and s indicates the underlying ventricular septal activation. The time signal (T) indicates 100 msec intervals. The records were obtained during spontaneous ventricular tachycardia originating in the inferior–posterior margin of the infarct. PF$_i$ precedes activation of the proximal conducting system as well as the distal ventricular conducting system and ventricular muscle. (From Horowitz *et al.* (1976). *Circulation*, **53**, 56; reproduced by permission of the American Heart Association.)

the spontaneous ventricular rhythm. This is strong supportive evidence that the ventricular tachyarrhythmia was originating very near this Purkinje site.

In Figure 16.3 data from the same experiment as Figure 16.2 are plotted showing the relationship of the early epicardial activation site to the activation sequence within the conduction system. In Figure 16.3 (A) the anterior and posterior surfaces of the heart are shown schematically. The circumscribed dark area at the infero-posterior region of the heart locates the earliest site of epicardial activation. The region of infarction is indicated by the cross-hatched area. In Figure 16.3 (B), the time of activation of Purkinje fibres, left bundle branch, bundle of His and left and right ventricular epicardial sites are indicated. The time bar below the schematic lead II ECG indicates time in msec. Time = 0 of this axis is the occurrence of the earliest recorded Purkinje fibre activity. This was obtained from the subendocardium within the region of infarction. It can be noted that Purkinje activity preceded activation of the bundle branch (B) and His bundle (H). Also, the circles denote the fact that most of the left ventricular epicardium was activated prior to activation of the right ventricular epicardium. In all twelve ectopic ventricular rhythms investigated 24 hours after LAD occlusion, the left ventricular depolarization always occurred earlier than activation of the right ventricle. In none of the LAD occlusions was an early site found on the right ventricular epicardium.

In Figure 16.3, the right ventricular epicardium was activated 32 msec later than left ventricular epicardial breakthrough. To determine if part of the right ventricular epicardium was being activated due to retrograde conduction over the left bundle to the right bundle of His and then via normal antegrade conduction over the right bundle conduction system, the bundle of His was stimulated 2, 4 and 6 msec earlier than the anticipated retrograde His bundle activation during the monofocal ventricular tachyarrhythmia. Interestingly, it was noted that the right ventricular epicardial sites were similarly pre-excited 2, 4 and 6 msec earlier and in nearly the identically time sequence of activation, i.e. the whole right ventricular epicardial activation sequence was similarly stepped 2, 4 and 6 msec earlier. This strongly suggests that indeed the right ventricle was being activated via antegrade conduction over the right specialized conduction system.

VENTRICULAR ACTIVATION DURING RHYTHMS INDUCED BY SEPTAL ARTERY OCCLUSION

Sixteen healthy mongrel dogs underwent anterior septal artery occlusion. At 24 hours following the occlusion, the animals had developed spontaneous ventricular ectopic rhythms competing with normal sinus rhythm. Following re-anaesthesia and crushing the sinus node, the animals exhibited stable ventricular rhythms, which by electrocardiographic criteria, appeared to be originating in one or two competing foci. Utilizing ventricular mapping techniques, the earliest area of epicardial activation was determined to be on the right ventricle in eight of 13 rhythms, and on the left ventricle in five of 13 rhythms. These early epicardial activation sites all occurred near the interventricular septum.

Figure 16.4 presents analog records recorded from different sites of the ventricular septum in an animal following anterior septal artery ligation. At the top of the figure are shown schematically an anterior view of the heart as well as right and left septal views. The bundle of His and right bundle branch are shown on the right septal schematic drawing and the divisions of the left bundle are shown on the drawing of the left septal surface. The analog records located immediately below the schematic drawings were recorded during a

L.A.D. OCCLUSION

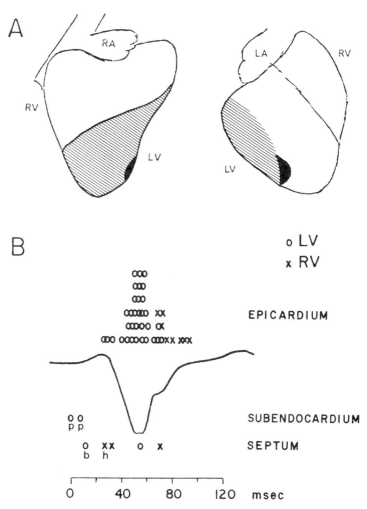

Figure 16.3 A comparison of early epicardial activation and subendocardial Purkinje and septal activation during a ventricular tachycardia following left anterior descending coronary artery occlusion. In (A) the cross-hatched areas indicate the approximate extent of the infarcted myocardium. The dark crescent area indicates earliest epicardial activation. In (B) the electrocardiographic lead II wave form and epicardial, subendocardial and septal activation times are plotted on the common time axis. The open circles are left ventricular sites, the x's are right ventricular sites. Epicardial activation times are shown above the ventricular complex, subendocardial and septal activation times are shown below the electrocardiographic complex. The p below the open circles indicate that these represent peripheral Purkinje fibre activations. The b below the open circle indicates that this represents a left bundle activation time and the h below the x indicates that this represents His bundle activation. From *Pathophysiology and Therapeutics of Myocardial Ischemia* (1976). (Reproduced by permission of Spectrum Publications, Inc.)

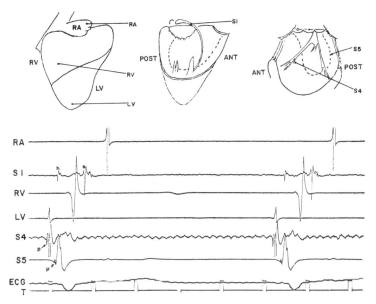

Figure 16.4   Analog records obtained during spontaneous ventricular tachycardia 24 hours following anterior septal artery occlusion. The schematic drawing above indicates the approximate recording sites for the analog records displayed below. Records were obtained from the right atrium (RA) and right ventricle (RV) as well as from the earliest left ventricular activation site LV, S1, S4 and S5 indicate septal recording sites. A lead II electrocardiogram (ECG) was recorded simultaneously. The h, and s in the S_1 record indicate His bundle and underlying ventricular septal muscle activation. The p's indicate Purkinje fibre spikes. The timing signal (T) represent 100 msec. (Reproduced by permission of the author and the publisher. From Spear, J. F. *Pathology and Therapeutics of Myocardial Ischemia*. Spectrum Publications, Inc. (1976).)

monofocal ventricular tachycardia. The electrograms were recorded from the right atrium (RA), bundle of His (S_1), right ventricle (RV), left ventricle (LV), and left septal surface (S_4, S_5). The ECG is a lead II electrocardiogram showing the characteristic configuration of the ectopic focus. Time lines denote 100 msec intervals. Earliest activity originated in the Purkinje fibre located at site S_4 near the anterior division of the left bundle. Activity in this region preceded retrograde bundle of His activation by 25 msec. Electrogram LV indicates that the earliest left ventricular epicardial site of activation was located at the left ventricular apex. Left ventricular epicardial activity followed the earliest recordable Purkinje activation by only 7 msec. This resulted from the fact that epicardial breakthrough was directly overlying the early septal activation site.

Figure 16.5 shows schematic drawings of the anterior and left lateral views of the heart with the earliest epicardial activation being indicated by the black area on the left ventricular apex. In Figure 16.5 (B), the onset of activation of the left and right ventricular epicardium and septal sites is indicated

SEPTAL OCCLUSION

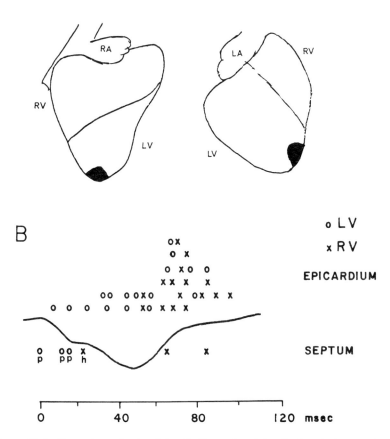

Figure 16.5 Comparison of epicardial activation and septal activation during spontaneous ventricular tachycardia following anterior septal artery occlusion. In (a) the dark crescent indicates earliest epicardial activation occurring in the left ventricle. Below are shown the electrocardiographic wave form, left and right epicardial and septal activation times plotted on a common time axis. The open circles are left ventricular sites, the x's are right ventricular sites. Epicardial activation is shown above the electrocardiographic waveform, septal activation is shown below. The p indicates Purkinje fibre activation. The h indicates His bundle activation. (Reproduced by permission of the author and the publishers. From Spear, J. F., *Pathophysiology and Therapeutics of Myocardial Ischemia.* Spectrum Publications, Inc. (1976).)

simultaneously with the lead II electrocardiogram. P denotes Purkinje activation and h denotes bundle of His depolarization. It can be noted again that Purkinje activity preceded any activation of the ventricular epicardium and that the right ventricle was activated considerably later than the left ventricular epicardium. Again, pre-excitation of the bundle of His demonstrated that the right ventricular epicardium was being activated by retrograde conduction over

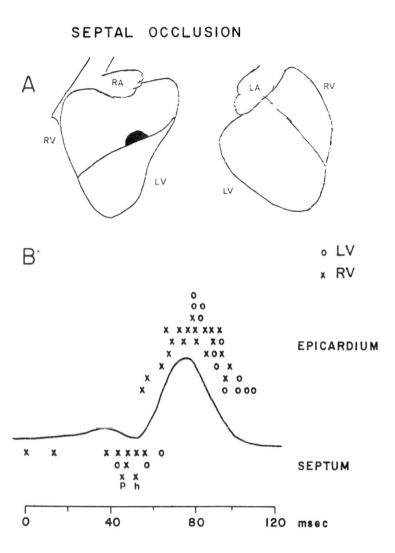

Figure 16.6 The relationship between epicardial activation, septal and ventricular conducting system activation during a ventricular tachycardia following occlusion of the anterior septal coronary artery. The dark crescent overlying the right ventricle in the schematic diagram in (A) indicates earliest epicardial breakthrough during the ectopic rhythm. In (B) are shown the electrocardiographic configurations as well as the relative times of activation of right and left epicardial and septal sites plotted on a common time axis. The open circles are left ventricular activation sites, the x's are right ventricular activation sites. Epicardial activation is shown above the electrocardiographic complex and septal activation is shown below. The p indicates Purkinje fibre activation; h indicates bundle of His activation. (Reproduced by permission of the authors and the publishers. From Spear, J. F. *Pathophysiology and Therapeutics of Myocardial Ischemia.* Spectrum Publications, Inc. (1976).)

the left bundle to the bundle of His and antegrade conduction down the right conduction system.

Figure 16.6 is similar to Figures 16.3 and 16.5. In this animal after anterior septal artery occlusion, the ectopic focus produced early activity on the right epicardium rather than on the left epicardium. Above are shown schematic drawings of the right septal surface and left septal surface. As in Figure 16.5 the analog recordings shown below were recorded at the sites indicated on the drawings. In this experiment, the earliest activity recorded was from the right septal surface (site S4, in Figure 16.4) and preceded right epicardial breakthrough by 55 msec and retrograde His bundle activation by 51 msec.

Discussion

Twenty-four hours after either left anterior descending or anterior septal artery occlusion our experiments demonstrate that the origin of the ectopic ventricular rhythms is from the peripheral Purkinje system within the region of infarction. These ectopic rhythms exhibit characteristics which suggest they are due to enhanced automaticity. The rhythms can be readily overdriven by supraventricular and ventricular pacing. They manifest warm-up phenomena following cessation of pacing, and they are suppressed by lidocaine.

Table 16.1 demonstrates that the ventricular rhythms associated with the experimental infarction have rates which are three or four times the rate of normal ventricular automaticity during experimentally induced atrioventricular dissociation. In the case of the septal infarction, the bundle of His and right and left bundle branches, as well as peripheral Purkinje fibres lie within the region of infarction, yet it is the peripheral Purkinje system whose automaticity is selectively enhanced in this model. It is possible that the automaticity of the junctional tissue is also enhanced, but it is not able to be manifest due to its suppression by the more rapid ventricular rhythm. However, if this were the case, our experiments still demonstrate a preferential enhancement of automaticity of the peripheral Purkinje system. Table 16.1 shows that the rate of the normal junctional rhythm which occurs following experimental sinus node ablation averages 100.6 ± 33.0 beats/min. If automaticity of the junction were enhanced by the septal infarction to a proportional degree as measured for Purkinje fibre automaticity, it would be reasonable to expect accelerated junctional or fascicular rhythms at rates of 300–400 beats/p min. We did not observe junctional or fascicular rhythms in our 24 hour infarction model.

In our experiments we observed that the true origin of the ectopic rhythm occurred in the Purkinje system associated with the infarct, but at some distance from the site of its earliest epicardial breakthrough. In the case of the LAD occlusion, the activity originated from the subendocardial Purkinje system within the infarcted area. Epicardial activation was by way of Purkinje conduction from this site to the border where viable muscle was then activated. In the case of the septal occlusion, the time from the earliest septal Purkinje fibre activation to the ultimate epicardial breakthrough could be as much as 52 msec (Figure 16.6) and the distance could be as great as 4 cm. These experiments imply that the epicardial mapping technique alone is limited in its ability to locate the origin of ventricular activity. In situations where it is desirable to locate the source of an ectopic ventricular rhythm for possible surgical resection, epicardial mapping may not in itself provide sufficient information, and transmural recordings may be necessary to exactly locate the source of the rhythm.

Acknowledgement

These studies were supported in part by grants HL 16076-03 and HL 19045-01 from the National Heart and Lung Institute and by grant 75-733 from the American Heart Association.

References

1. Harris, A. S. (1950). Delayed development of ventricular ectopic rhythms following experimental coronary occlusion. *Circulation*, **1**, 1318
2. Friedman, P. L., Steward, J. R., Fenoglio, J. J. and Wit, A. L. (1973). Survival of subendocardial Purkinje fibers after extensive myocardial infarction in dogs. *Circ. Res.*, **33**, 597
3. Scherlag, B. J., El-Sherif, N., Hope, R. and Lazzara, R. (1974). Characterization and localization of ventricular arrhythmias resulting from myocardial ischemia and infarction. *Circ. Res.*, **35**, 372
4. Friedman, P. F., Fenoglio, J. J. and Wit, A. L. (1975). Time course of reversal of electrophysiological and ultrastructural abnormalities in subendocardial Purkinje fibers surviving extensive myocardial infarction in dogs. *Circ. Res.*, **36**, 127
5. Horowitz, L. N., Spear, J. F. and Moore, E. N. (1975). Subendocardial origin of ventricular arrhythmias in 24-hour-old experimental myocardial infarction. *Circulation*, **53**, 56
6. Lazzara, R., El-Sherif, N. and Scherlag, B. J. (1973). Electrophysiological properties of canine Purkinje cells in one-day-old myocardial infarction. *Circ. Res.*, **33**, 722
7. Michelson, E. L., Spielman, S. R., Spear, J. F. and Moore, E. N. (1976). The origins of late ventricular rhythms and their activation patterns in experimental septal infarction in dogs. *Clin. Res.*, **24**, 232A
8. Spear, J. F., Michelson, E. L., Spielman, S. R. and Moore, E. N. (1977). The origin of ventricular arrhythmias following experimental anterior septal coronary artery occlusion. *Circulation*. In press
9. Nachlas, M. M. and Shnitka, T. K. (1963). Macroscopic identification of early myocardial infarcts by alterations in dehydrogenase activity. *Am. J. Pathol.*, **42**, 379
10. Spear, J. F. and Moore, E. N. (1973). Influence of brief vagal and stellate nerve stimulation on pacemaker activity and conduction within the atrioventricular conduction system of the dog. *Circ. Res.*, **32**, 27

17
Electrophysiology Following Healed Experimental Myocardial Infarction

A. L. BASSETT, H. GELBAND, K. NILSSON
A. R. MORALES and R. J. MYERBURG

Departments of Medicine, Pharmacology, Pediatrics, Pathology, and Physiology,
University of Miami School of Medicine;
and the Miami Veteran's Administration Hospital, Miami, Florida

Clinical and epidemiologic data in man suggest the persistence of cardiac electrophysiological instability for at least 6 months following *acute* myocardial infarction, and further that the manifestations of electrophysiological instability are unpredictable in the setting of *chronic* ischaemic heart disease[1-3]. Most efforts to develop experimental animal models of electrophysiological instability in the setting of ischaemia have emphasized arrhythmogenesis in acute myocardial infarctions in dogs[4-11], and the majority of the studies have been oriented to the electrophysiological events occurring soon after coronary occlusion through the first 72 hours. More limited investigations have been carried out in longer-term canine preparations to determine whether chronic electrophysiological abnormalities persist after acute coronary occlusion in this species. In studies reported to date, the canine model has demonstrated neither chronic rhythm disturbances nor long-term cellular electrophysiological abnormalities[9,12], in studies up to three months after the acute coronary occlusion. Thus, in contrast to its value as a model of electrophysiological instability during the first few days following acute myocardial infarction, the canine heart has not been reported to provide a suitable model for study of chronic electrophysiological instability.

Because of the limitations of the canine model in respect to chronic electrophysiological abnormalities as a consequence of experimental myocardial infarction, and the desirability of devising a model which demonstrated these characteristics, a group of investigators in our laboratory embarked upon efforts to devise a new myocardial infarction model[13]. During the course of other studies using a cat heart model, we carried out a series of experiments to determine the long-term electrophysiological effects of myocardial infarction in that species. The infarcted cats were studied up to six months following experimental myocardial infarction. Spontaneous ventricular arrhythmias were recorded immediately prior to terminal studies in 25% of the chronic cats; electrophysiological evidence for a propensity to ventricular arrhythmogenesis was observed in a total of 50% of the long-term survivors; and cellular electrophysiological abnormalities were recorded from surviving subendocardial Purkinje fibre and ventricular muscle cells coursing over the surface of the myocardial infarction in 91% of the cat hearts studied in tissue bath after sacrifice. Pathologic correlations demonstrated survival of bands of subendocardial fibres two to ten cell layers in depth, composed of both Purkinje fibres and ventricular muscle cells.

THE CAT MYOCARDIAL INFARCTION MODEL

Acute myocardial infarctions were created in cats anaesthetized with sodium pentobarbital, 30 mg/kg intraperitoneally, by single stage ligation of two or three distal vessels of the left coronary system through a left thoracotomy incision. Electrocardiographic documentation of acute myocardial infarction was acquired by standard six-lead electrocardiography. The vessels ligated were located in an area which produced an anterior and apical infarction of the left ventricle which, on the endocardial surface, uniformly involved the base of the anterior papillary muscle and adjacent free wall and apex. In some preparations, the infarction extended on to the base of the posterior papillary muscle and lower septum. In the initial series, myocardial infarctions were created in 48 cats, of which 42 (87.5%) survived the first day. Ten more spontaneous deaths among the 42 initial survivors occurred predominantly during the first week after infarction. Thus, a colony of 32 long-term survivors was available for long-term electrophysiological studies. Terminal studies were carried out seven days to six months after the acute infarction, using a 30-min period of rhythm monitoring by ECG to identify spontaneous ventricular arrhythmias, and vagal stimulation to unmask increased ventricular automaticity, immediately prior to sacrifice. Following sacrifice, the left ventricles were immediately studied in isolated tissue bath by surface electrogram and transmembrane action potential recording techniques. In addition, eleven control cats were studied, using the same protocol.

ANATOMY AND HISTOPATHOLOGY OF THE INFARCTED CAT HEARTS

Discrete scars were seen on the epicardial and endocardial surfaces of the left ventricle in locations generally predictable by the distribution of coronary artery ligations. The surface area of the scar on the epicardium was not easily measured because of dense adhesions between the epicardium and pericardium over the site of the infarction partially obscuring the borders of the scar. A corresponding scar on the endocardial surface was seen in nearly all preparations, the gross appearance of which depended upon the age of the infarction. In studies carried out two weeks or less after the myocardial infarction, a dark red patch was seen on the endocardium, while in later preparations (especially beyond two months after the myocardial infarction), a pale retracted scar was seen. On histopathological studies, transmural myocardial infarctions were demonstrated in 13 of the preparations (Figure 17.1), and non-transmural infarctions involving more than one-half of the ventricular wall were present in an additional 13 (Figure 17.2). In 6 preparations, subendocardial infarctions involved less than one-third of the wall thickness. In all preparations, multiple layers of surviving subendocardial cells were observed overlying the infarction area. The width of this band of surviving cells was usually $100\,\mu$m or less, but occasionally in the range $100-200\,\mu$m (Figures 17.3, 17.4 and 17.5). Surviving fibres demonstrating features of both specialized conducting tissue and or-

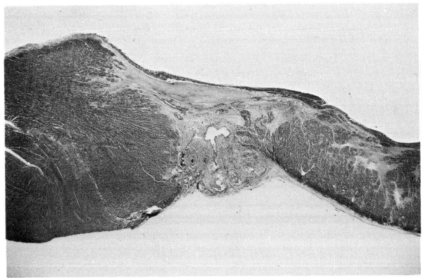

Figure 17.1 Transmural myocardial infarction. A dense scar has formed at the base of an anterior papillary muscle $3\frac{1}{2}$ months after coronary ligation. Note the layer of surviving subendocardial cells overlying the scar

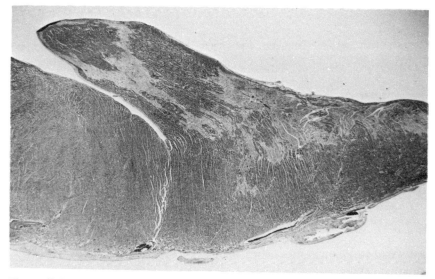

Figure 17.2 Non-transmural myocardial infarction. The preparation was obtained one week after coronary artery ligation. Most of the papillary muscle is infarcted, and about one-half of the thickness of the ventricular free wall demonstrates changes of myocardial infarction. Note the thin band of surviving cells on the endocardial surface overlying the infarcted tissue

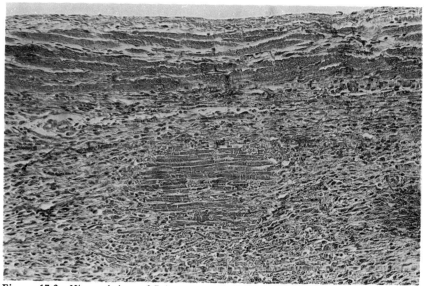

Figure 17.3 Histopathology of 7-day myocardial infarction. The section demonstrates surviving subendocardial cells of the one-week myocardial infarction shown in Figure 17.2. Note the intercellular edema from the endocardial surface through the subendocardial layer of cells, the irregular cell borders, and small areas of cytoplasmic vacuolization. The deeper tissues demonstrate fibroblastic and vascular proliferation, and a sequestrum of infarcted cells which retain cross-striations, but are fragmented and anuclear

dinary ventricular muscle were identified. In addition, islands of viable appearing muscle cells were present within the depths of the myocardial infarction. These became smaller and more fragmented in the longer-term preparations. The histopathologic studies were analyzed in two categories: (1) the features of the healing myocardial infarction process and (2) the details of the surviving subendocardial cells.

The general healing process took place primarily by fibroblastic proliferation, with no apparent inflammatory reaction. The one-week old myocardial infarctions were characterized by intense proliferation of fibroblasts with early collagen deposition (Figure 17.3). Since no infarctions were studied before one week after coronary artery ligation, the possibility of early resolution of an inflammatory reaction, which had subsided by seven days, could not be excluded. Examination of longer term infarctions revealed a decrease in the fibroblastic cellular component as the collagen component became more abundant (Figure 17.4—1 month infarction). By three months after the infarction (Figure 17.5), a dense scar was formed with only a few remaining fibroblasts. There was no apparent progression in the density of scar tissue beyond this stage. Vascular proliferation accompanied the fibroblastic proliferation. In the one week infarctions, many small capillaries were present throughout the infarcted field, these vessels becoming larger, thin-walled, and more numerous at the periphery of the scar tissue in infarcts studied one month or longer after myocardial infarction (see Figures 17.4 and 17.5). Necrotic myocardial fibres usually appeared as an irregular nest of muscle cells in the midst of the healing process described above (Figure 17.3). In 7-day-old myocardial infarctions, the myocardial cells in these nests retained their cross-striations, but contained no nuclei and the cytoplasm had a basophilic hue with trichrome stain, distinct from the bright red stain of the normal myocardium (Figure 17.3). A number of infarcted fibres, particularly at the infarction–fibroblastic interface, demonstrated marked irregular clumping of the cytoplasm. In one-month-old infarcts, the basophilic hue of the necrotic fibres was more intense, and the anuclear infarcted group of myocardial fibres appeared as a more distinct sequestered island surrounded by the healing process. Some cross-striations were still present at this stage, but the borders of the necrotic group of fibres were irregular, with evidence of dissolution of the cytoplasm. Van Kosse's stain demonstrated precipitation of calcium in these necrotic fibres. In most of the two-month-old infarcts, and all of the infarcts three months or beyond, all of the infarcted fibres had been replaced by scar tissue. Sparse nests of sequestered normal-appearing myocardial cells were sometimes seen within the dense scar[14].

The second phase of histopathologic analysis involved the surviving band of subendocardial fibres which remained over the infarcted portion of the left ventricle. These fibres had histologic criteria for viability, although they appeared structurally abnormal in the earlier post-myocardial infarction stages. Criteria for both surviving Purkinje fibres and ventricular muscle cells were evident. In the one-week preparations (Figures 17.3), the surviving subendocardial cells

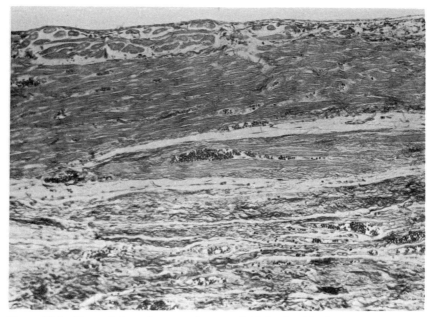

Figure 17.4   Histopathology of one-month myocardial infarction. The intercellular edema and cytopathology of the band of subendocardial surviving cells are less pronounced, although regional areas of abnormalities persist. In addition, the fibroblastic infiltration is less pronounced, and collagen deposition is more evident

demonstrated varying degrees of myofibrillar disorganization, irregular vacuolization of some cells, and irregular cell outlines. Many of these changes may have resulted from loss or disruption of sarcoplasmic myofibrils as a result of cellular injury. Evidence of some degree of cytopathology was relatively uniform in these early preparations, and was accompanied by widening of interstitial spaces and of the endocardial fibrous tissue layer, suggesting endocardial and interstitial edema. During later stages of healing, such as the one-month myocardial infarction, cellular abnormalities were less uniform. Areas of normal-appearing fibres having good cross-striations, euchromic nuclei, and no abnormal vacuolization of cytoplasm, were interspersed with areas of cellular disruption and with intermediate areas in which cross-striations were maintained, but minor degrees of vacuolization persisted. Interstitial edema was somewhat more variable at this time, remaining a prominent component in some preparations, and much less so in others. Finally, the encroachment of fibroblasts into the layers of surviving cells was seen, and was accompanied by focal fibrous disruption of the subendocardial bands of fibres beginning one month after myocardial infarction. The cellular abnormalities continued to become less apparent in the older infarctions, and the surviving fibres in the subendocardium overlying infarctions over three months of age often showed no cellular abnormalities (Figure 17.5). The absence of interstitial edema in

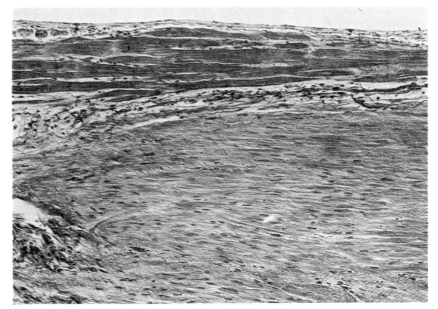

Figure 17.5   Histopathology of 3½-month myocardial infarction. At this stage there is essentially complete resolution of intercellular edema, and very limited evidence of cellular abnormalities
in the surviving band of subendocardial fibres. The endocardial surface is thickened with fibrous
tissue. Under the discrete layer of surviving cells, there is a dense scar with little or no
fibroblastic infiltration. This preparation is from the endocardial surface of the preparation
shown in Figure 17.1

these preparations was accompanied by the presence of some encroachment of
fibrous tissue in the interstitial area between surviving cells; but the cells
themselves showed good cross-striations, euchromic nuclei, and nearly complete disappearance of the myocytoplasmic abnormalities seen in earlier
specimens.

LONG-TERM ELECTROPHYSIOLOGICAL INSTABILITY

Cardiac rhythm was monitored for 30 min under anaesthesia immediately prior
to terminal studies of each animal. The eleven control cats included in the
study demonstrated no rhythm disturbances during the monitoring period, but
ventricular ectopic activity was observed in eight of the 32 long-term
experimental cats (25%). All eight had premature ventricular contractions,
while several also had more complex ventricular arrhythmias, including
recurrent ventricular tachycardia and ventricular bigeminy. Examples of ventricular ectopic activity are shown in Figure 17.6. The recordings were obtained in cats studied 1 week, 1 month, 3 months and 6 months after myocardial infarction. The ventricular rhythm disturbances in the eight cats were dis-

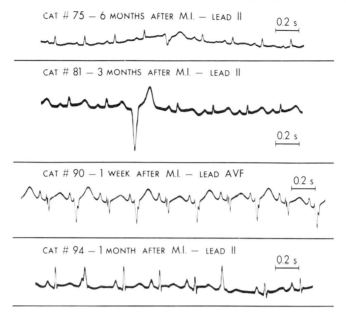

Figure 17.6 Spontaneous ventricular ectopic activity in cats surviving myocardial infarction. Short rhythm strips, selected from four cats studied at 1 week, 1 month, 3 months and 6 months after myocardial infarction, demonstrate ventricular ectopic activity

tributed among chronic animals of various post-myocardial infarction durations. Finally, the limited sampling technique of 30 min of monitoring immediately prior to sacrifice almost certainly precluded the identification of rhythm disturbances in other infarcted cats.

A second method used to establish the presence of a propensity to ventricular ectopic activity involved studies during vagal stimulation. These were carried out in 21 of the 32 experimental cats, and in ten of the eleven controls. The response to vagal stimulation was analyzed with regard to the occurrence and rate of ventricular escape mechanisms. Sinus node slowing, without escape mechanisms, was observed in ten of the 21 infarction cats, and in seven of the ten controls. However, accelerated ventricular escape rhythms, having escape cycle lengths ranging from 500 to 700msec, were recorded in seven of the myocardial infarction cats, and in none of the controls. Thus, 33% of the infarcted cats studied by this technique (seven of 21) had accelerated ventricular foci which were suppressed by a faster sinus rate during anaesthesia.

The third technique for evaluating propensity to arrhythmias involved observation of the behaviour of the isolated left ventricular preparations in tissue baths after removal of the heart from the chest. Automatic activity in preparations from the control cats was always suppressed by overdriving at cycle lengths of 800 msec or more. However, eleven of the 32 myocardial infarction preparations required overdrive cycle lengths of 630msec or less, dis-tributed uniformly among infarction preparations of various ages, up to six months.

When the three criteria for study of long-term electrophysiological instability were cross-correlated, it was determined that a total of 16 of the 32 myocardial infarction cats (50%) had one or more manifestations of electrophysiologic instability; three demonstrated all three criteria; four demonstrated two of the three criteria; five demonstrated one of the three criteria; and four demonstrated one of only two criteria in which they were tested. From these observations it appears that the cat surviving an acute experimental ischaemic event provides a model for chronic ventricular arrhythmias and is appropriate for further electrophysiological studies.

ISOLATED TISSUE STUDIES

Surface electrogram recordings and transmembrane action potential recordings were used to determine the electrophysiologic properties of the isolated left ventricle of cats having survived long-term infarctions. The surface electrograms were used to map the sequence of excitation and to identify areas of abnormalities. Areas over myocardial infarction scars demonstrated regions of decreased surface electrogram voltage interspersed between areas of normal voltage and configuration (Figure 17.7). In many preparations, areas in the centre of the endocardial surface overlying the myocardial infarction scars demonstrated extremely low voltage electrogram activity or even total quiescence. In these areas, transmembrane action potential recordings were difficult and only scattered cellular responses were recorded.

Transmembrane action potential recordings in grids 1 cm² or less from viable areas overlying the myocardial infarction demonstrated three distinct types of transmembrane action potential abnormalities and a number of mixed forms. Early myocardial infarctions (less than two weeks) usually demonstrated a fairly uniform pattern of transmembrane action potential abnormalities characterized by action potential prolongation with slurring of phases 2 and 3 (see Figure 17.8 (A-2)). This 'Type 1' abnormality was seen most commonly in early infarctions, and decreased in frequency in infarctions over one month. It was rarely seen beyond two months after myocardial infarction. A second characteristic waveform, the 'Type 2' abnormality, was characterized by a very short transmembrane action potential duration resulting from a nearly absent phase 2 and a normal phase 3. These patterns appeared at approximately two months after myocardial infarction, and were commonly recorded in preparations over three months after infarction. In Figure 17.8, action potential (B-4) demonstrates a transmembrane potential similar to the 'Type 2' abnormality with the exception of the co-existent presence of slight slurring of terminal repolarization during phase 3. The 'Type 3' abnormality was identified as those potentials having the characteristics of a slowly rising, low-amplitude potential, arising from partially depolarized tissue.

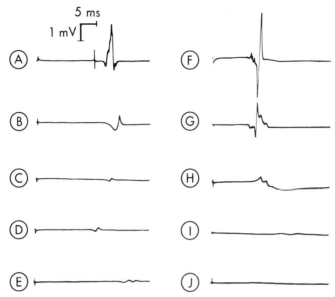

Firgure 17.7 Surface electrogram recordings from multiple areas on the endocardium overlying a healed myocardial infarction. Ten surface electrogram recordings are demonstrated. Tracing A demonstrates a normal waveform including a sharp Purkinje fibre spike followed by a broader ventricular muscle spike. Recordings B, C, D and E are obtained from sites progressively further into the centre of the endocardial surface of the infarction. Electrograms F–J are recorded on a line perpendicular to A–E, F and G are recorded on the border of the infarct and 1 mm toward the centre of the infarct. Electrograms H, I and J are recorded each at 1 mm intervals further toward the centre. Note that no recordable activity is evident on electrogram J and extremely low voltage on electrogram C, D, E, H and I

The transmembrane potentials in Figure 17.8 were recorded from a grid, having interelectrode distances of 0.2 mm, and recording from the first cell layer impaled over the surface in the centre of a myocardial infarction studied two months after acute coronary occlusion. The transmembrane potentials have characteristics found predominantly in earlier infarctions (e.g. A-2), as well as those seen in later infarctions (e.g. B-4, and C-1). The 'Type 3' abnormalities have been found in myocardial infarction preparations of all ages, although they were somewhat more common in the older infarctions.

The transmembrane action potential characteristics demonstrated an evolution which temporally paralleled changes in the histology of the surviving band of subendocardial fibres overlying the myocardial infarction area. Specifically, the early period, characterized by prolonged action potential durations, was accompanied by histologic abnormalities of the surviving cells and prominent intercellular edema in this region. As 'Type 1' action potentials disappeared and 'Type 2' action potentials became more dominant, the cellular abnormalities and intercellular edema were no longer seen. It was not technically possible to determine the specific histologic characteristics of cells from

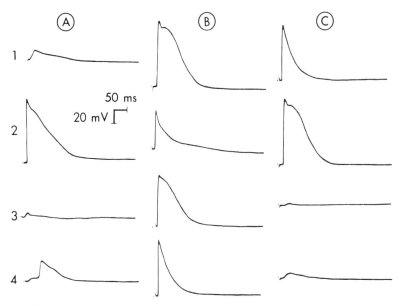

Figure 17.8 Transmembrane action potentials recorded from a 2-month myocardial infarction. A grid constructed of equidistant points between microelectrode recordings demonstrates variability of transmembrane action potential abnormalities recorded from a surviving band of subendocardial cells overlying a healed myocardial infarction. There are normal cells (B-1 and C-2), in addition to various forms of abnormal cells. Cells similar to A-2 are more commonly seen in infarcts from 1 week to 1 month after coronary occlusion, while cells similar to B-4 and C-1 are more common in infarcts studied beyond two months after coronary occlusion. Abnormalities such as A-4 may be recorded any time after myocardial infarction, but are somewhat more common after 2–3 months

which 'Type 2' abnormalities were recorded; and so we can only make a hypothesis that electrophysiological abnormalities, of a variety different from those seen in the acute infarction, persisted in cells which had regained cytological normalcy after a period of healing. Such an hypothesis would invoke the occurrence of a cellular membrane injury as a result of acute myocardial ischaemia with subsequent survival of the cell in an altered state of electrophysiological function. Further data are required to establish this hypothesis.

MECHANISMS OF ARRHYTHMIAS

The long-term goal of our studies of a myocardial infarction preparation demonstrating chronic arrhythmias is oriented to a determination of the mechanism(s) of the *chronic* arrhythmias recorded. Studies carried out to date suggest that re-entry, automaticity, and a combination of both, play a role in the various ventricular arrhythmias. Figure 17.9 demonstrates a transmembrane action potential study carried out in an isolated left ventricular preparation from a cat studied $2\frac{1}{2}$ months after myocardial infarction. The cat had

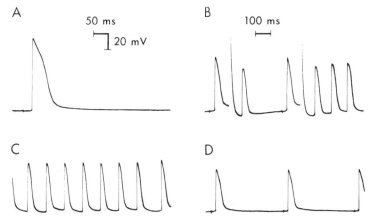

Figure 17.9 Arrhythmia triggered in isolated preparations by premature stimulation in the infarct zone. The preparation consists of the entire left ventricle isolated in tissue bath and stimulated by surface electrodes on the left bundle branch. The cat was studied $2\frac{1}{2}$ months after myocardial infarction. Driving stimulation was at a cycle length of 500 msec, and premature impulses were delivered intracellularly to an abnormal cell in the surviving band over the infarct zone. Panel A demonstrates the transmembrane action potential recorded from a cell which is to be stimulated prematurely. The sweep speed of the oscilloscope for this recording was 50 msec/division. Panel B demonstrates intracellular stimulation, followed by a single premature impulse, and another followed by a burst of repetitive impulses, recorded at a sweep speed of 100 msec/division. Panel C demonstrates a continuing burst of unstimulated activity 30 sec after Panel B. Panel D demonstrates return to a driven rhythm after spontaneous cessation of the repetitive ventricular activity. This phenomenon was reproducibly triggered at appropriately premature coupling intervals between the driving stimulus and premature intracellular stimulation

demonstrated premature ventricular contractions on ECG monitoring prior to sacrifice. Transmembrane action potential recordings demonstrated 'Type 2' and 'Type 3' action potential abnormalities. Figure 17.9 demonstrates studies of premature stimulation carried out at a driving cycle length of 500 msec. When a premature impulse was delivered during late repolarization to the same Type 2 cell from which the recording is obtained, repetitive ventricular responses were triggered. At appropriate cycle lengths, bursts of sustained ventricular ectopic activity occurred, and abruptly terminated after periods ranging from 2 to 30 sec. Automaticity in the isolated preparation could be overdriven at a cycle length of 800 msec. This appears to be an instance of a re-entrant tachycardia triggered by premature excitation of a cell having residual electrophysiological abnormalities more than two months after myocardial infarction. In contrast, Figure 17.10 demonstrates automatic activity within an infarct zone, associated with exit block. The first, third and fifth action potentials on the top tracing are preceded by a prepotential, while the simultaneous tracing recorded from a cell outside the infarct zone follows every fourth impulse in the infarct zone. The cat from which this preparation was obtained had spontaneous bursts of ven-

INFARCT ENDOCARDIUM

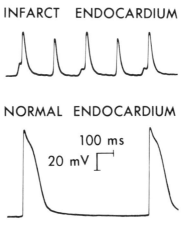

NORMAL ENDOCARDIUM

Figure 17.10 Automatic activity in cells overlying a 'healed' infarction showing exit block and 4:1 conduction into the remainder of the ventricle. In the upper tracing, recorded from the infarct subendocardium, prepotentials precede the upstrokes of action potentials of the first, third and fifth (spontaneous) impulses. In a recording from normal muscle simultaneously in the same preparation, ventricular excitation follows only the first and fifth automatic impulses. The preparation sporadically alternated between 2:1 and 4:1 conduction from the infarct into the remaining ventricle. The cat from which this preparation was obtained had manifested bursts of ventricular tachycardia during terminal studies. These studies were carried out three months after myocardial infarction

tricular tachycardia recorded on ECG at a rate nearly identical to that of the rate of maturity outside the infarction zone. Thus, the mechanism of the arrhythmia in this instance appears to be automaticity within the infarct zone at a rate more rapid than the manifest ventricular rhythm.

The cellular electrophysiological abnormalities recorded from the experimental preparations lead us to make the hypothesis that mechanisms of ventricular arrhythmias involve re-entry, automaticity, and/or exit block all three of which are supported, in part, by Figures 17.9 and 17.10. However, further direct demonstration of these mechanisms is required to confirm these hypotheses.

Acknowledgement

This work was supported in part by funds from NIH (NHLI) Grant No. HL–19044–01, from NIH (NHLI) Contract No. NHLI–72–2975–M, from Veterans Administration Institutional Research Funds, and from Grants-in-Aid of the Heart Association of Greater Miami, Heart Association of Broward County, Florida Heart Association, and the National Foundation March of Dimes.

References

1. Coronary Drug Project Research Group (1973). The prognostic importance of premature beats following myocardial infarction: experience in the coronary drug project. *J. Am. Med. Ass.*, **223**, 1116

2. Doyle, J. T. (1975). Profile and risk of sudden death in apparently healthy people. *Circulation,* **52** (suppl. III), 176

3. Moss, A. J., De Camilla, J., Mietlowski, W., Green, W. A., Goldstein, S. and Locksley, R. (1975). Prognostic grading and significance of ventricular premature beats after recovery from myocardial infarction. *Circulation,* **52** (suppl. III), 204

4. Friedman, P. L., Fenoglio, J. J. and Wit, A. L. (1975). Time course for reversal of electrophysiological and ultrastructural abnormalities in subendocardial Purkinje fibers surviving extensive myocardial infarction in dogs. *Circ. Res.,* **36,** 127

5. Friedman, P. L., Stewart, J. R., Fenoglio, J. J. and Wit, A. L. (1973). Survival of subendocardial Purkinje fibres after extensive myocardial infarction in dogs. *Cir. Res.,* **33,** 597

6. Friedman, P. L., Stewart, J. R. and Wit, A. L. (1973). Spontaneous and induced cardiac arrhythmias in subendocardial Purkinje fibers surviving extensive myocardial infarction in dogs. *Circ. Res.,* **33,** 612

7. Lazzara, R., El-Sherif, N. and Scherlag, B. (1973). Electrophysiological properties of Purkinje cells in one-day old myocardial infarction. *Circ. Res.,* **33,** 722

8. Lazzara, R., El-Sherif, N. and Scherlag, B. J. (1974). Early and late effects of coronary occlusion on canine Purkinje fibers. *Circ. Res.,* **35,** 391

9. Scherlag, B. J., Helfant, R. H., Haft, J. I. and Damato, A. N. (1970). Electrophysiology underlying ventricular arrhythmias due to coronary ligation. *Am. J. Physiol.,* **219,** 1665

10. Scherlag, B. J., El-Sherif, N., Hope, R. and Lazzara, R. (1974). Characterization and localization of ventricular arrhythmias resulting from myocardial ischemia and infarction. *Circ. Res.,* **35,** 373

11. William, D. O., Scherlag, B. J., Hope, R., El-Sherif, N. and Lazzara, R. (1974). The pathophysiology of malignant ventricular arrhythmias during acute myocardial ischemia. *Circulation,* **50,** 1163

12. Fenoglio, J. J. Jr., Albala, A., Silva, F. G., Friedman, P. L. and Wit, A. L. (1977). Structural basis of ventricular arrhythmias in human myocardial infarction: An hypothesis. *Hum. Pathol.* (in press)

13. Myerburg, R. J., Gelband, H., Nilsson, K., Sung, R. J., Thurer, R. J., Morales, A. R. and Bassett, A. L. (1977). Long-term electrophysiologic abnormalities resulting from experimental myocardial infarction (abstract). *Circulation* (in press)

14. Durrer, D., Van Lier, A. A. W. and Büller, J. (1964). Epicardial and intramural excitation in chronic myocardial infarction. *Am. Heart J.,* **68,** 765

18
Evidence for Re-entry within the His-Purkinje System in Man during Extrasystolic Stimulation of the Right Ventricle: Macro- versus Micro-re-entry*

D. W. FLEISCHMANN, T. POP AND J. M. T. de BAKKER

Department of Internal Medicine I and Helmholtz Institute, Rhein.-Westf. Technische Hochschule, Aachen, West Germany

INTRODUCTION

The recent development of intracardiac recording and stimulation techniques of the human heart makes it possible to test directly in the human the validity and applicability of theories on the genesis of cardiac arrhythmias which are based on electrophysiological studies from *in vitro* or *in situ* animal heart preparations. However, clinical electrophysiological investigations, although sophisticated, will be crude as compared with animal research work. At best, they can supply indirect evidence in favour of a certain hypothesis. This especially applies to studies like our own, which are concerned with the re-entry mechanism as a cause of cardiac arrhythmias[1,2].

Several authors[3-9] have reported the occurrence of non-stimulated ventricular extrasystoles in the human heart after one prematurely stimulated ventricular extra beat during constant right ventricular pacing rhythm. It is interesting to note that neither in the dog nor in the rabbit heart has it been possible so far to reproduce this artificially induced, possibly intraventricular, echo beat by one premature beat alone either stimulating myocardial fibres[10-12] or fibres of the peripheral Purkinje system[13]. In animal studies two stimulated early extrasystoles in succession were always needed to produce the non-stimulated extrasystole.

In this chapter we shall summarize our experience on extrasystolic stimulation of the right ventricle in 93 cases. We think from the results of our studies that the observed non-stimulated ventricular extrasystoles are re-entrant in origin, the re-entrant circuit being localized near the site of stimulation in the majority of cases. In some cases, there occurs probably a macro-re-entry circuit including structures of the contralateral ventricle. Additionally, indirect evidence suggests that the main conduction delay of the prematurely stimulated right ventricular impulse is confined to the peripheral Purkinje network in close proximity to the stimulation site which would correspond with the local re-entry hypothesis of the non-stimulated extrasystoles.

METHODS

During clinical electrophysiological studies for various rhythm disorders premature right ventricular (RV) stimulation was performed in 93 patients without evidence for an acute myocardial infarction. Utilizing the single test stimulus method, the premature impulses were elicited during a constant RV drive rhythm after every tenth beat until the effective refractory period of the right ventricle was reached. This procedure was performed in all cases at several different driving rates. In at least 30 unselected cases premature RV stimulation was repeated during a constant right atrial drive rhythm at rates identical to those during the RV drive.

Initially we used a bipolar stimulation technique[6,7] for the right atrium as well as for the right ventricle. Lately, for the last 50 cases, we used unipolar cathodal rectangular impulses of 1 msec duration and double diastolic threshold to stimulate the right ventricular apex both for driving and testing. The mean diastolic threshold for the RV was 0.44 ± 0.14 V ($n = 64$). A programmable stimulator adjustable to select two different basic driving rates and to deliver three additional, independent test stimuli was used for atrial and ventricular pacing[14]. Several surface ECG leads, a bipolar electrogram of the high lateral wall of the right atrium, the bundle of His and a unipolar electrogram recorded 1 or 10 mm proximal to the RV unipolar stimulating electrode were registered simultaneously on an eight-channel direct-writing recorder at a paper speed of 100 mm/sec[6,7].

RESULTS

Retrograde intraventricular conduction of premature right ventricular stimuli

A premature test impulse (S_2) elicited at the same right ventricular myocardial site as the basic driving impulse (S_1) will be conducted retrogradely to the bundle of His with increasing delay (S_2–H_2 interval) as the premature beat interval—S_1–S_2 interval— is shortened. This has been reported previously[3,6,7]. An increase of the basic driving rate leads to shorter retrograde interventricular conduction times (S_2–H_2 interval) at the same coupling interval of the premature test impulse[7] suggesting a rate dependency of the action potential duration of the structures participating in retrograde conduction from the site of stimulation to the bundle of His. These structures are the right ventricular myocardium at the site of the stimulating electrode, the peripheral Purkinje fibres which are activated either directly by the electrode or by way of myocardial fibres and finally, the proximal Purkinje network, the bundle branch system and the bundle of His.

The retrograde intraventricular conduction time S_2–H_2 measured as long as 350 msec in several cases. The main conduction delay is not located within the myocardial fibres but within the His–Purkinje system. This can be deduced from Figures 18.1 and 18.2. While the S_2–H_2 interval was 200 msec at a coupling interval S_1–S_2 of 340 msec there was no increase of the V_1–V_2 interval

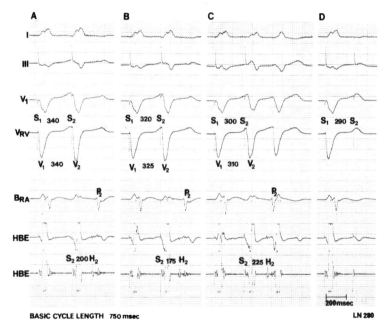

Figure 18.1 Occurrence of a non-stimulated ventricular extrasystole during premature right ventricular stimulation at a constant right ventricular pacing rhythm. Simultaneous recording of ECG leads, I, III, V_1, a unipolar right ventricular electrogram (v_{RV}) registered 10 mm from the stimulation site, a bipolar atrial electrogram (B_{RA}) and two His bundle leads (HBE) recorded from the same site with different band pass-filters. From A to D: S_1 is the last of a series of ten driving impulses, S_2 is delivered with decreasing prematurity at the same site of stimulation. Note that the QRS morphology of the spontaneous ventricular beat (part C of the figure) is almost identical to the beat V_1 and V_2.

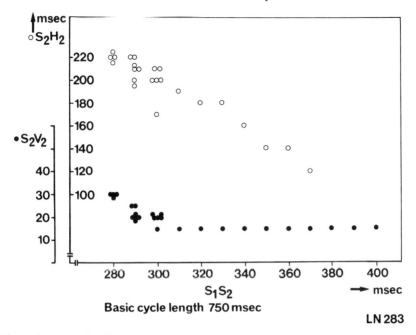

Figure 18.2 Relationship between the right ventricular test beat interval S_1–S_2 (abscissa) and the retrograde intraventricular conduction time S_2–H_2 (ordinate) and the myocardial conduction time S_2–V_2 (ordinate). The S_2–V_2 interval was measured from the stimulus S_2 to the intrinsic deflection of the unipolar ventricular electrogram recorded 10 mm from the site of stimulation

in the ventricular electrogram or any increase of the latency between the stimulus impulse S_2 and the unipolar ventricular electrogram V_2 which was recorded 10 mm from the electrode site (the S_2–V_2 interval, Figure 18.1). The myocardial conduction velocity started to decrease only 30 msec before the effective refractory period of the right ventricle was reached. At these very short coupling intervals of the test impulse S_2 an initial slurring of the first rapid deflection of the ventricular electrogram was seen. Figure 18.2 shows graphically the disparity between the early increase of the retrograde intraventricular conduction time S_2–H_2 and the late increase of the myocardial conduction time S_2–V_2 upon premature stimulation of the right ventricle. From this graph and Figure 18.1, it becomes evident that the conduction delay within the myocardial fibres near the stimulation site plays a rather minor role as compared to the major and essential retrograde conduction delay in the subsequently activated His–Purkinje system.

There was a striking difference between the retrograde conduction delay during a RV drive rhythm and the retrograde conduction delay during a supraventricular, atrial drive rhythm as premature RV stimulation was performed. Retrograde conduction of the premature RV impulse S_2 was significantly faster and less impaired during right atrial driving rhythm (Figure

18.3, Table 18.1) than during ventricular driving provided the driving and testing impulse during the ventricular drive was delivered at the same stimulation site. We could identify a retrograde His potential in only two of 20 cases in whom a right atrial drive was maintained (Table 18.1), the maximal retrograde intraventricular conduction time S_2-H_2 being 140 and 90 msec, respectively as compared to the mean S_2-H_2 value of 250 msec which was seen during a RV drive rhythm in 17 of 20 cases. The fast retrograde conduction velocity of the S_2 impulse during the supraventricular driving rhythm is explained by the

Table 18.1   Effect of premature right ventricular stimulation upon retrograde intraventricular conduction. Comparison of electrophysiological data during right ventricular versus right atrial drive rhythm at identical rates (basic cycle length 750 msec)

	Premature right ventricular stimulation ($n = 20$)	
	Right ventric. drive rhythm	*Right atrial drive rhythm*
Retrograde His potential visible	17 (85%)	2 (10%)
Maximal retrograde intraventric. conduction time	$n = 17$ 250 msec ± 50 msec	$n = 2$ 140 msec 90 msec
Intermittent failure of retrograde intraventricular conduction	12 (60%)	0 (0%)
Intraventricular echo beats	12 (60%)	0 (0%)

rapidly advancing recovery of excitability of the His–Purkinje system as the premature beat S_2 travels retrogradely. During this rhythm, the ventricles were activated in an antegrade direction; the S_2 impulse, however, was propagated in the opposite direction thereby reaching structures almost completely recovered from previous excitation. On the other hand, when the driving and testing impulses take the same way there will be a slow retrogradely progressing recovery of conduction within the His–Purkinje system from the driving impulse, in this way retarding the spread of the premature test impulse S_2 (Figure 18.5).

It is obvious that the intramyocardial conduction delay of the S_2 impulse is of minor importance as compared to the delay of conduction within the His–Purkinje system. Additionally, the marked differences between the retrograde conduction times of the S_2 impulse during right atrial versus RV drive imply that the main delay of retrograde His–Purkinje conduction is confined to the peripheral Purkinje system rather than located in the proximal bundle branches. Otherwise, the differences in conduction times should be small. This hypothesis is supported by the effect of premature RV stimulation upon the retrograde intraventricular conduction time S_2-H_2 during a ventricular rhythm showing supraventricular and ventricular fusion characteristics. In Figure 18.4B the configuration of the S_1 impulse shows a slight fusion as the right atrium was activated 125 msec before the right ventricle. It is reasonable to assume that at least the bundle of His and the proximal His–Purkinje system are activated antegradely whereas the myocardium near the ventricular stimulation site and the peripheral Purkinje system are activated retrogradely by the ventricular stimulus. Figure 18.4B shows that the retrograde conduction time S_2–H_2 of the prematurely elicited impulse S_2—having the same S_1–S_2 interval as in Figure 18.4A—is only 35 msec less than the retrograde conduction time of S_2 during the purely ventricular drive rhythm. This strongly suggests that the proximal His–Purkinje system contributes little to the overall

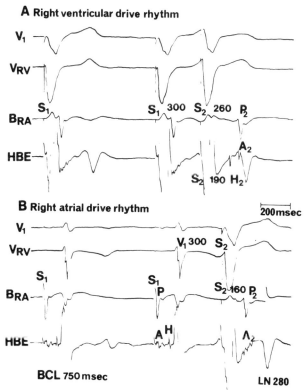

Figure 18.3 Different retrograde conduction pattern of a premature right ventricular stimulus S_2 delivered at the same site of stimulation, in A during a constant right ventricular drive rhythm, in B during a constant right atrial drive rhythm. The premature beat interval is the same in part A and B, of the figure, measured in B from the first rapid deflection of the unipolar right ventricular electrogram (V_{RV}) to the S_2 impulse. A retrograde His deflection can only be delineated during ventricular pacing rhythm, the retrograde intraventricular conduction time S_2–H_2 is 190 msec

retrograde conduction time of the premature impulse S_2 while the structures with the longest action potential duration in the periphery of the His–Purkinje system will cause the main delay of retrograde conduction. A modified ladder diagram (Figure 18.5) illustrates the conduction pathway of the premature RV impulse S_2 elicited during the above described three different types of driving rhythms thereby taking into consideration the change of action potential duration along the course of the His–Purkinje system[15–21].

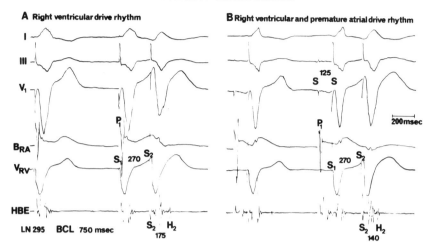

Figure 18.4 Effect of premature right ventricular stimulation upon the retrograde intraventricular conduction time S_2-H_2 during a pure right ventricular drive rhythm (part A) versus a ventricular rhythm showing ventricular and supraventricular fusion characteristics (part B). In part B of the figure: the right atrium was stimulated 125 msec before the right ventricular driving impulse S_1 was delivered. The premature beat interval S_1-S_2 and the driving rate are identical in A and B. Notations as in Figure 18.1

Intraventricular echo beats during premature right ventricular stimulation

In 59 of 93 cases we observed spontaneous, non-stimulated ventricular extrasystoles (Figures 18.1 and 18.9) after premature ventricular stimulation during a right ventricular pacing rhythm. In the vast majority of cases there was only one spontaneous ventricular beat after the artificially induced, stimulated extrasystole, in some cases two or three spontaneous ventricular contractions occurred in succession. We never observed sustained ventricular tachycardias, ventricular flutter or fibrillation although in all patients extrasystolic stimulation of the right ventricle was performed with decreasing coupling intervals of the test impulse until the effective refractory period of the right ventricle was reached.

The non-stimulated ventricular extrasystoles occurred when the retrograde intraventricular conduction time S_2-H_2 of the premature test beat S_2 was critically prolonged[3,6,7]. This is clearly shown in Figure 18.6. As can be seen from the same Figure, the non-stimulated extrasystoles appeared at coupling intervals of the test impulse outside the relative refractory period of the right ventricle. They were evoked when there was a step-like increase of the retrograde conduction time S_2-H_2. A correlation between the delayed retrograde intraventricular conduction time S_2-H_2 and the occurrence of spontaneous ventricular extrasystoles could be demonstrated for all driving frequencies tested (Figure 18.7). Additionally, the spontaneous extrasystoles were ab-

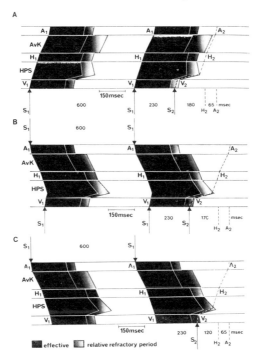

Figure 18.5 Hypothetical retrograde conduction pathway of a premature right ventricular test impulse S_2 elicited during a constant right ventricular drive (part A), during a constant right atrial drive rhythm (part C) and during a ventricular rhythm showing fusion characteristics (part B of the figure). In B the myocardium and the peripheral Purkinje system are activated retrogradely by a ventricular driving stimulus whereas the proximal His–Purkinje system is activated antegradely by a right atrial driving stimulus. There is a change of the refractory periods along the course of the His–Purkinje system, the longest refractory period being located in the periphery of this system (gate). Note the different state of recovery of excitability of the driving impulse S_1 in part A, B and C as the testing impulse S_2 travels retrogradely. Note further the significant difference in the retrograde intraventricular conduction time S_2–H_2 between part A and C and the slight difference between A and B

sent during intermittent failure of retrograde conduction of the test beat S_2[3,7,8] a phenomenon which was observed in 50% of the cases studied (Figure 18.9, Tables 18.1 and 18.2). As there was a marked difference between the retrograde conduction time of the premature beat S_2 during a right ventricular versus a right atrial drive rhythm there was a significant difference between the frequency with which spontaneous ventricular extrasystoles could be generated during both stimulation procedures (Table 18.1). Tested in 20 cases we found no vulnerability of the right ventricule during a right atrial drive rhythm in contrast to the frequency of 60–64% vulnerability during a RV drive rhythm.

The obvious dependency of the ventricular vulnerability just described on the degree of the retrograde intraventricular conduction delay of the premature

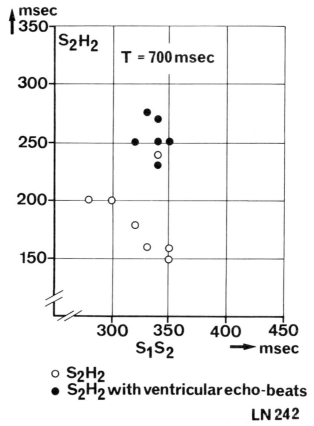

Figure 18.6 Step-like increase of the retrograde intraventricular conduction time S_2–H_2 (ordinate) coinciding with the occurrence of non-stimulated ventricular extrasystoles (echo beats). Premature test beat interval S_1–S_2 on the abscissa. Basic cycle length (T) 700 msec

test beat S_2 suggested a re-entry mechanism within the ventricular chambers underlying the occurrence of the non-stimulated ventricular extra-systoles[2,3,6,7,22,23]. As the spontaneous ventricular extrasystoles were observed independent of the AV nodal conduction time of the premature beat S_2 as well as during atrial fibrillation the hypothesis of an AV nodal echo phenomenon seemed remote. In 73% of all cases (Table 18.2) the QRS morphology of the non-stimulated extrasystoles showed a left bundle branch block pattern similar to the basic right ventricular driving beat S_1 (Figures 18.1 and 18.9). This clearly means that the extrasystoles originated in the right ventricle. The presumably re-entrant activation probably started near the site of the right ventricular stimulation electrode.

The left bundle branch block pattern of the spontaneous extrasystoles may be explained by a re-entrant circuit within the peripheral Purkinje network of the right ventricle at or near the site of stimulation—a micro-re-entry—or by a

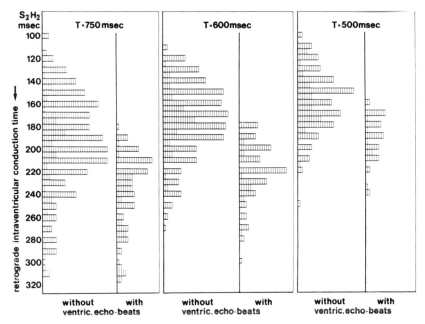

Figure 18.7 Relationship between retrograde intraventricular conduction time S_2–H_2 (ordinate) during premature right ventricular stimulation at three different driving rates and the genesis of intraventricular echo beats. The S_2–H_2 intervals of all cases tested at the three different driving rates 80, 100 and 120/min were plotted as single dashes adding up to bars on the ordinate. The S_2–H_2 intervals occurring without spontaneous ventricular extrasystoles were plotted on the left of each panel, the S_2–H_2 intervals preceding spontaneous extrabeats were plotted on the right. The ventricular echo beats occurred only at delayed retrograde conduction times S_2–H_2 of the test beat S_2

macro-re-entry pathway[3,6] including the ventricular septum and the left bundle branch system during unidirectional block of the right bundle branch. A support of the last hypothesis would include an unchanged QRS configuration of the spontaneous extrasystoles as the right ventricular pacing site is altered. On the other hand, however, an analogous change of the left bundle branch block pattern of the non-stimulated extrasystoles as the site of stimulation varies within the right ventricular chamber would be in favour of a local re-entry mechanism. Figure 18.8 shows the occurrence of spontaneous ventricular extrasystoles during stimulation of the right ventricular apex and the right ventricular septum in the same patient. The QRS morphology of the non-stimulated extrasystoles resembled closely the left bundle branch block configuration of the basic driving beat S_1 at both stimulation sites. The spontaneous extrasystoles must be generated near the site of stimulation by way of a local re-entry phenomenon within the network of the peripheral Purkinje fibres where we have confined the main delay of conduction of the premature ventricular impulse S_2.

Table 18.2 Frequency of intraventricular echo – beats and intermittent failure of retrograde intraventricular condition during premature right ventricular stimulation at constant ventricular pacing in 93 cases. The bundle branch block (BBB) pattern of the echo – beats showed a left bundle branch block (LBBB) configuration in the majority of cases

| | Intraventricular echo beats | BBB – pattern of echo beats | | | Intermittent failure of retrograde intraventricular conduction |
| | | LBBB | RBBB | LBBB + RBBB | |
	n (%)	n (%)	n (%)	n (%)	n (%)
normal QRS, $n = 73$	51 (70)	39 (76.5)	3 (5.9)	9 (17.6)	40 (55)
LBBB (QRS ⩾ 0.12 sec) $n = 7$	4 (57)	3 (75)	1	—	3 (43)
RBBB (QRS ⩾ 0.11 sec) $n = 13$	4 (30.5)	1	2 (50)	1	7 (54)
all cases, $n = 93$	59 (63.5)	43 (73)	6 (10)	10 (17)	50 (54)

In some patients we observed a right bundle branch morphology of the spontaneous extrasystoles (Figure 18.9). It implies that the reactivation of the cardiac chambers started within the left ventricle. As is shown in Figures 18.9 and 18.10 the non-stimulated extrasystoles with a right bundle branch block pattern occurred with another step-like increase of the retrograde intraventricular conduction time S_2–H_2 compared with the S_2–H_2 intervals preceding the spon-

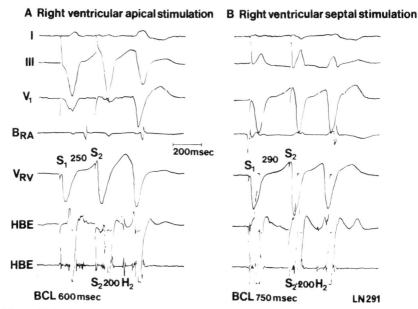

A Right ventricular apical stimulation   B Right ventricular septal stimulation

Figure 18.8 Spontaneous ventricular extrasystoles during premature right ventricular stimulation at two different pacing sites within the right ventricular chamber. Driving and testing impulses were delivered at the right ventricular apex (part A) or the upper part of the right ventricular septum (part B). Notations as in Figure 18.1. S_1: the last of a series of ten driving impulses

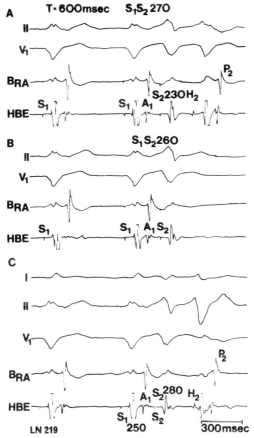

Figure 18.9 Occurrence of spontaneous ventricular extrasystoles with a left bundle branch block pattern (part A) at a test beat interval S_1–S_2 of 270 msec. Part B retrograde conduction failure at a test beat interval of 260 msec. Part C: as the test beat interval was shortened to 250 msec there was a step-like increase of the S_2–H_2 interval, the non-stimulated ventricular extrasystole showing a right bundle branch block pattern

taneous extrasystoles originating in the right ventricle. We speculate that in these instances retrograde conduction of the S_2-impulse into the right bundle branch Purkinje system was blocked with additional asymmetrical conduction and local block within the peripheral Purkinje network of the left bundle branch leading to a re-entry circuit which resulted in an early re-excitation of the left ventricle.

CONCLUSIONS

Direct recordings from the endocardial surface of the right ventricle, from the bundle of His and the right atrium combined with various stimulation

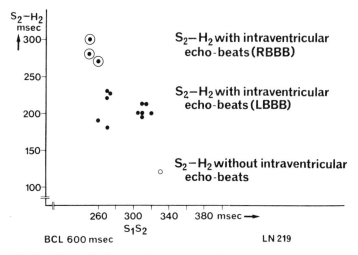

Figure 18.10   Relationship between the occurrence of intraventricular echo beats of different QRS configuration and delayed retrograde intraventricular conduction time S_2–H_2 after premature right ventricular stimulation. Same patient as in Figure 18.9

techniques allow a detailed analysis of the retrograde intraventricular conduction pattern of premature right ventricular impulses in the human heart. It was found that the delay of the retrograde intraventricular conduction time is not only dependent upon the prematurity of the test beat but also on the local activation sequence at the time of premature stimulation[24]. Extrasystolic stimulation of the right ventricle during a supraventricular drive rhythm leads to fast retrograde intraventricular conduction. On the other hand premature right ventricular stimulation during a ventricular drive rhythm when the sites of stimulation during testing and driving are identical is characterized by a prominent delay of retrograde intraventricular conduction.

As we localized the main delay of retrograde intraventricular conduction of premature right ventricular test impulses within the peripheral His–Purkinje system of the right ventricle, we assume a local re-entry mechanism near the site of stimulation underlying the genesis of non-stimulated ventricular extrasystoles occurring after one artificially induced premature right ventricular beat. This type of intraventricular echo beat occurs in the majority of cases; in some cases an echo phenomenon may be observed including structures of the left ventricle.

The relevance of the described results to clinically observed arrhythmias remains to be clarified. We imply the following: as the intraventricular echo beats occurred in nearly 60% of the cases studied, they can be considered a model arrhythmia. We expand the hypothesis of an essential local conduction delay within the peripheral Purkinje network near the site of stimulation after premature ventricular stimulation leading to a local re-entry phenomenon to the genesis of some forms of clinically observed ventricular extrasystoles and tachycardias[25]. We infer from our results that intraventricular echo phenomena based on a macro-re-entry circuit including the main bundle branches occur rarely.

References

1. Antoni, H. (1975). Elektrophysiologische Äquivalente bei Herzrhythmusströrungen. *Verh. Dtsch. Ges. Inn. Med.*, **81**, 69
2. Moe, G. K. (1975). Evidence for re-entry as a mechanism of cardiac arrhythmias. *Rev. Physiol. Biochem. Pharmacol.*, **72**, 56
3. Akhtar, M., Damato, A. N., Batsford, W. P., Ruskin, J. N., Ogunkelu, J. B. and Vargas, G. (1974). Demonstration of re-entry within the His–Purkinje system in man. *Circulation*, **50**, 1150
4. Durrer, D. and Wellens, H. J. (1974). The Wolff–Parkinson–White syndrome. Anno 1973. *Eur. J. Cardiol.*, **1**, 347
5. Zipes, D. P., De Joseph, R. L. and Rothbaum, D. A. (1974). Unusual properties of accessory pathways. *Circulation*, **49**, 1200
6. Fleischmann, D., Pop, T. and De Bakker, J. M. T. (1975). Zur Frage der Entstehung ventrikulärer Extrasystolen. Kreiserregung im intraventrikulären Leitungssystem. *Herz. Kreisl.*, **7**, 82
7. Fleischmann, D., Pop, T. and De Bakker, J. M. T. (1976). Re-entry mechanism within the *His–Purkinje system in man during extrasystolic stimulation of the right ventricle. In:* Lüderitz (ed.). *Cardiac Pacing*, (Berlin: Springer) p. 194
8. Schuilenburg, R. M. (1976). Patterns of V–A conduction in the human heart in the presence of normal and abnormal A–V conduction. In: *The Conduction System of the Heart* (Leiden: Stenfert Kroese) p. 485
9. Wellens, H. J. J., Wesdorp, J. C., Duren, D. R. and Lie, K. I. (1976). Second degree block during reciprocal atrioventricular nodal tachycardia. *Circulation*, **53**, 595
10. Han, J. and Moe, G. (1964). Non-uniform recovery of excitability in ventricular muscle. *Circ. Res.*, **14**, 44
11. Janse, M. J. (1971). The effect of changes in heart rate on the refractory period of the heart. Thesis. Amsterdam. Mondeel-Offsetdruckerij
12. Moore, E. N. and Spear, J. F. (1973). Local block and re-entry. In: Dreifus and Likoff (eds.). *Cardiac Arrhythmias.* (New York: Grune and Stratton) p. 71
13. Sasynuik, B. J. and Mendez, C. (1971). A mechanism for re-entry in canine ventricular tissue. *Circ. Res., **28**, 3
14. De Bakker, J. M. T., Fleischmann, D., Pop, T. and Effert, S. (1977). Programmierbarer Elektrostimulator zur Abklärung von Herzrhythmusstörungen. *Z. Kardiol.* (In preparation.)
15. Van Dam, R. T. V., Hoffman, B. F. and Stuckey, J. H. (1964). Recovery of excitability and of impulse propagation in the *in situ* canine conduction system. *Am. J. Cardiol.*, **14**, 184
16. Hoffman, B. F., Kao, C. Y. and Suckling, E. E. (1957). Refractoriness in cardiac muscle. *Am. J. Physiol.*, **190**, 473
17. Kao, C. Y. and Hoffman, B. F. (1958). Graded and decremental response in heart muscle fibers. *Am. J. Physiol.*, **194**, 187
18. Hoffmann, B. F. and Cranefield, P. F. (1960). *Electrophysiology of the Heart.* New York: McGraw-Hill)
19. Moore, E. N., Preston, J. B. and Moe, G. K. (1965). Duration of transmembrane action potentials and functional refractory periods of canine false tendon and ventricular myocardium. *Circ. Res.*, **17**, 259
20. Mendez, C., Müller, W. F., Merideth, J. and Moe, G. K. (1969). Interaction of transmembrane potentials in canine Purkinje fibers and at Purkinje fiber–muscle junctions. *Circ. Res.*, **24**, 361

21. Myerburg, R. J., Stewart, J. W. and Hoffman, B. F. (1970). Electrophysiological properties of the canine peripheral A–V conducting system. *Circ. Res.*, **26,** 36

22. Wit, A. C., Cranefield, P. F. and Hoffman, B. F. (1972). Slow conduction and re-entry in the ventricular conduction system. II. Single and sustained circus movement in networks of canine and bovine fibers. *Circ. Res.*, **30,** 11

23. Wit, A. C., Hoffman, B. F. and Cranefield, P. F. (1972). Slow conduction and re-entry in the ventricular conducting system. I. Return extrasystole in canine Purkinje fibers. *Circ. Res.*, **30,** 1

24. Abildskov, J. A. (1976). Effects of activation sequence on the local recovery of ventricular excitability in the dog. *Circ. Res.*, **38,** 240

25. Wellens, H. J. J., Lie, K. J. and Durrer, D. (1974). Further observations on ventricular tachycardia studied by electrical stimulation of the heart. Chronic recurrent ventricular tachycardia and ventricular tachycardia during acute myocardial infarction. *Circulation,* **49,** 647

19
Reciprocation between Pacemaker Sites: Re-entrant Parasystole?*

G. K. MOE, J. JALIFE and W. J. MUELLER†

Masonic Medical Research Laboratory, Utica, New York

Premature contractions that fit the classical criteria for parasystolic rhythms must be the result of pacemaker activity in an impulse-generating focus 'protected' by entrance block against invasion from the surrounding tissue. Such a focus can initiate a manifest premature activation when it discharges during electrical diastole, and must fail to do so when the surrounding tissue is refractory; i.e. the pattern of ectopic activity should exhibit a simple interference dissociation from the dominant pacemaker rhythm.

Some intellectual reservations develop when attempts are made to explain departures from the expected behaviour. For example, an expected ectopic response may fail to appear on schedule. One may postulate, not too convincingly: (1) the ectopic focus is not *precisely* rhythmic; or (2) the degree of block that confers protection (entrance block) is severe enough to result in occasional exit block as well. These are, of course, valid and incontestable explanations, but a further complication arises when ventricular premature beats that appear to be coupled at a fixed interval to the normal QRS complex in one sample of the electrocardiogram, become frankly parasystolic, or almost so, in another sample, although the site of origin appears to be the same[1]

In a carefully reasoned study of the shift between 'extrasystolic' (bigeminal) and parasystolic rhythms in a number of clinical cases, Schamroth and Marriott[1] proposed a model in which a period of enhanced excitability

* Supported in part by a grant from the National Heart and Lung Institute, HL–15759.
† Associate professor of physiology and director, Bioelectronics and Computer Sciences Laboratory, SUNY Upstate Medical Center, Syracuse, N.Y.

following closely upon the T wave of a normal activation could, in effect, lock an ectopic pacemaker to the normal complex for more or less extended periods of bigeminy and 'concealed' bigeminy.

We propose to show that the interactions between pacemakers can explain many of the characteristics of parasystolic activity, and that certain patterns of dysrhythmic activity are obligatory results of electrotonic influences transmitted across the region of impaired conductivity that separates an ectopic focus from the surrounding myocardium.

The excitability of a tissue, as measured by the inverse of the current strength necessary to initiate a propagated response, depends upon the difference between the resting membrane potential and the so-called threshold potential, and upon the membrane conductance. During pacemaker activity (slow diastolic or 'phase 4' depolarization) in Purkinje fibres, the membrane potential slowly approaches the threshold potential. At the same time, membrane conductance diminishes. Both of these factors will enhance the electrical excitability of the pacemaker as phase 4 depolarization progresses.

In an ectopic pacemaker within the ventricles, protected by one-way block in a region of impaired conductivity, there must nevertheless be an intracellular electrical communication across the blocked area, or else the ectopic event could not escape. It follows that the normal depolarization of the myocardium can exert an influence across the zone of impaired conduction, and that the resulting electrotonic depolarization in the pacemaker cells could influence the course of phase 4 depolarization within them.

A subthreshold depolarizing current pulse applied early in the course of phase 4 depolarization will delay the next spontaneous discharge of a pacemaker in Purkinje fibres[2]. The depolarisation will become progressively greater as membrane conductance decreases later in phase 4. An electrotonic depolarization occurring late in phase 4 may reach threshold and evoke a premature regenerative response; i.e. it should 'capture' the pacemaker[3].

BIOLOGICAL MODEL

To study this general hypothesis in a model relevant to the behaviour of a parasystolic focus, false tendons excised from dog ventricles were mounted in a three-chamber perfusion apparatus, in which the central chamber, perfused with sucrose, provided the zone of impaired conduction.

In initial experiments, pacemaker activity in chamber 1 was enhanced by perfusion with a modified Tyrode's solution ($K^+ = 2$ mM) containing norepinephrine (10^{-7} g/ml). Pacemaker activity at a much lower frequency persisted in the tissue beyond the gap (chamber 3), perfused with Tyrode's solution containing 4 mM K^+. Each spontaneous discharge of the faster pacemaker was accompanied by a low amplitude depolarization in the segment of fibre in chamber 3. The amplitude of these electronic depolarization increased as they occurred progressively later in the cycle (Figure 19.1). When spontaneous

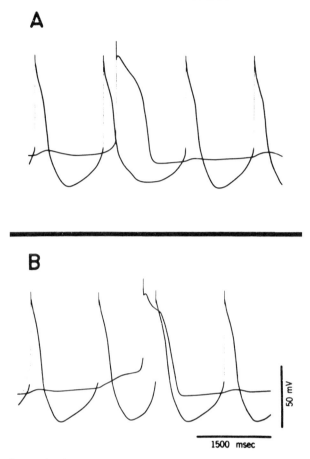

Figure 19.1 Interaction between spontaneous pacemakers. Dog false tendon, sucrose-gap preparation. Transmembrane action potentials recorded from fibre in chamber 3 (upper trace) and chamber 1 (lower trace). Intrinsic cycle length of the faster pacemaker, 1400 msec. Average cycle length of the slower pacemaker in chamber 3, 3800 msec. Note that electrotonic depolarizations recorded in chamber 3 increase in amplitude as slow diastolic depolarization progresses

depolarization of the slow pacemaker had progressed sufficiently, the electrotonic depolarization reached threshold and 'captured' the slower pacemaker, but only after a significant latency. In panel A of Figure 19.1 the latency was *ca.* 250 msec. The electrotonic evidence of the chamber 3 discharge is reflected by a failure of complete repolarization in chamber 1, and is followed by a delay of more than 22% in the next spontaneous discharge. In panel B, the latency between the chambers increased to almost 900 msec; the captured response in chamber 3 occurred later in the cycle of the faster pacemaker, and accelerated the subsequent response by 16%.

Reciprocal interactions between two spontaneously active pacemakers do not permit a systematic study of the magnitude of the electrotonic influence as a function of its temporal position in the cycle. Additional experiments were conducted in which the complete pacemaker cycle of the fibre segment in chamber 1 could be scanned by evoked action potentials in chamber 3, or by depolarizing current pulses. During the first half of the pacemaker cycle, depolarizations prolong the cycle by progressively increasing amounts. Beyond the midpoint, the influence is abruptly reversed, resulting in acceleration of similar degree (Figure 19.2).

The following conclusions may be drawn from these experiments: (1) An electrotonically mediated depolarization, subthreshold during the early stages

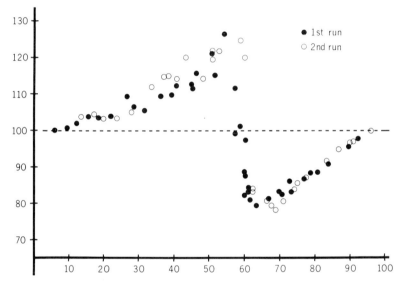

Figure 19.2 Delay and acceleration of the spontaneous cycle length of a chamber 1 pacemaker in response to evoked action potentials in chamber 3. Stimuli were applied to fibre in chamber 3 every 10–15 spontaneous beats. Ordinate: percentage increase or decrease of pacemaker cycle as a function of test stimulus interval (expressed as percentage of the intrinsic cycle length of the pacemaker). (From Jalife and Moe[3] reproduced with permission of The American Heart Association)

of a pacemaker cycle, will reach threshold as the membrane potential and membrane conductance decrease later in the cycle. (2) The resulting triggered response of the pacemaker would not occur unless phase 4 depolarization were progressing; i.e. the electrotonic influence would remain subthreshold. (3) The 'trigger' is, therefore, analogous to a slowly developing stimulus, and not the result of slow propagation of a wave front through the area of depressed conduction. (4) The pacemaker 'protected' by the sucrose gap is nevertheless influenced by events beyond the gap. (5) The influence may be negative (delay of a subsequent discharge), or positive (acceleration of the next 'spontaneous' depolarization).

It follows from these conclusions that so long as an intracellular ionic pathway exists between a pacemaker and its environment, an ectopic focus will fire at a cycle length that is variable and dependent on the timing of events in the surrounding tissue. In other words, the protection of an ectopic pacemaker is not complete; rhythms that are not rigidly 'parasystolic' may nonetheless be due to the modulated activity of an ectopic pacemaker.

MATHEMATICAL MODEL

With these principles in mind, a mathematical model was devised to illustrate the behaviour of an ectopic focus subjected to various degrees of electrotonic modulation[4]. The programmed rules were: (1) 'normal' action potentials of supraventricular origin can accelerate or decelerate a 'protected' ectopic pacemaker by varying degrees, depending on their position in the pacemaker cycle; (2) a discharge of the pacemaker, whether delayed, triggered, or spontaneous, can be propagated to the 'ventricle' as a premature beat, or as a fusion beat, except during the ventricular refractory period; (3) a manifest premature beat must be followed by a fully compensatory pause.

The model was programmed on a digital computer, using the form of the curve of influence experimentally recorded in the Purkinje fibre model, but with the positive and negative influences limited to a maximum of 15%. To mimic the effect of changes in heart rate, the intrinsic cycle length of the 'ectopic pacemaker' was varied by small increments from 1.5 times the 'SA nodal' cycle to 3.75. At each EP/SN ratio the program was allowed to continue until a repetitive pattern of responses was established.

A number of mathematically obligatory patterns emerge as the EP/SA ratio is varied. We shall consider primarily ratios above and below those at which a manifest bigeminal rhythm occurs. Qualitatively similar conclusions apply also to ratios that lead to trigeminal and quadrigeminal patterns.

(1) Because the ectopic pacemaker can be either accelerated or decelerated by activity in the surrounding tissue, the ectopic focus can be entrained by the dominant pacemaker. The dimensions of the entrainment phase depend, of course, on the programmed amplitude of the electrotonic influence and the point in the cycle at which maximal delay gives way to maximal abbreviation. The relationships plotted in Figure 19.3 illustrate the patterns that appear as the ratio of cycle lengths is altered.

Entrainment at a ratio of 2:1 in the illustrated example begins at a ratio (*intrinsic* ectopic cycle length to SA cycle length) of 1.75 and extends to 2.35. During the earliest part of the phase of entrainment, the intermediate responses of SA nodal origin fall within the zone of maximal delay, and the ectopic cycle length is prolonged. The pacemaker fires simultaneously with every other SA response, as a fusion beat. As the ratio of cycle lengths is increased (equivalent

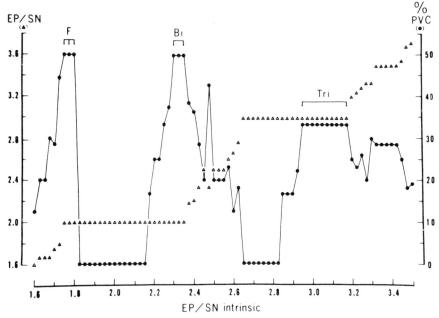

Figure 19.3 Response patterns of mathematical model as a function of intrinsic EP/SN ratio. Triangles, *operative* ratio, scale at left; solid circles, percent of manifest premature beats ('PVC'), scale at right. (F) fusion beats; (Bi) manifest bigeminy; (Tri) manifest trigeminy. Computer program with maximal electrotonic influence limited to ±15%; crossover point at 60% of the intrinsic ectopic cycle

to an acceleration of the basic heart rate), the discharge of the ectopic focus occurs progressively later within the RP of the ventricle; no manifest ectopic activity is apparent although the entrainment is still fixed at 2:1. Eventually, overt ectopic activity appears as a hexageminal rhythm, giving way to quadrigeminy, then alternating quadrigeminy and bigeminy, and eventually bigeminy. The stable bigeminal rhythms occurred only during a narrow range (ratios in the range 2.3–2.35), and only at the right hand edge of the entrainment zone. At higher ratios, the ectopic pacemaker breaks away from its bondage; intermittent bigeminal couplets now alternate with pentageminal patterns; a narrow zone of stable pentageminal rhythm appears at ratios of 2.5–2.55. This pattern gives way in turn to octageminy (ratio 2.6), and eventually, as each ectopic discharge falls within the ventricular refractory period, to complete silence. During the silent period (ratio 2.65–2.825), the ectopic focus is entrained at the 3:1 ratio, an entrainment that lasts up to the ratio of 3.175. The last portion of this zone appears as a stable trigeminal rhythm.

The implications of this model in the interpretation of clinical records are obvious. During an episode of apparently stable bigeminal rhythm, a slight deceleration of the SA nodal frequency will lead to periods of 'concealed bigeminy', during which only odd numbers of sinus beats are interposed between the manifest ectopic beats[1]. This will be true, in fact it *must* be true, so long as the ectopic focus is entrained in a 2:1 pattern. An example based on the model is simulated in Figure 19.4. Conversely, acceleration of the SA nodal frequency will lead to parasystolic patterns in which couplets and higher ratios are interspersed, and even numbers of sinus beats are often interposed. Further acceleration results in a 'silent' period.

At the next higher level of entrainment, 3:1, the relevant rules again apply. The frank trigeminal rhythm is much less sensitive to slight changes in frequency, but ratios below the zone of stability yield periods of the 2–5–8–11 pattern characteristic of concealed trigeminy; ratios above the stable zone yield patterns which depart from the rule (e.g. 2, 3 and 6 intervening sinus beats in each complete period).

The experimental conditions necessary for the production of a stable bigeminal pattern in the sucrose-gap model are not easy to maintain; this is, in fact, predictable from the mathematical model. We were able to demonstrate, however, that acceleration of the dominant (driven) impulse generator caused interectopic periods containing 1, 2 or 4 intervening 'normal' beats, progressing to disappearance of manifest extrasystoles, while slight deceleration resulted in 'concealed' bigeminy with only odd numbers of intervening responses, and, again a silent period.

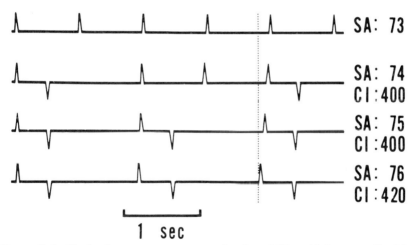

Figure 19.4 Simulated response pattern as a function of SA nodal frequency, listed in beats/min at right. CI = Coupling interval. Normal ventricular responses, upright pips; manifest extrasystoles, downward pips. Based on a computer program designed to match case 2 of Schamroth and Marriott[1] (see Figure 19.5)

CLINICAL APPLICATION

These results permit a semiquantitative re-examination of a number of published records of parasystolic rhythms. We have chosen case 2 in the report by Schamroth and Marriott[1] because it is illustrated by quite long continuous records, obtained on several occasions. These records are particularly amenable to analysis because slight changes in the heart rate caused well-defined alterations in the ectopic pattern.

When the basic pattern was bigeminal (three or four couplets in a row) a slight increase in heart rate led to progressive prolongation of the coupling interval, followed by interectopic intervals containing even numbers of sinus beats. When the heart rate decreased slightly, the characteristic pattern of concealed bigeminy appeared. The range of heart rates within which the bigeminal pattern was manifest was narrow (ca. 88–94 beats/min). Within this range, however, we can assume that a *stable* bigeminal rhythm would be further constrained; we make then a starting assumption that the range is ca. $\pm 2\%$ of the mean rate. This range would imply that the electrotonic influence can be no more than $\pm 15\%$, and it permits an estimate of the ratio, EP/SN, of ca. $2.3 - 2.35$. The intrinsic ectopic cycle must then be ca. 1570 msec. From this value one can estimate (probably within an error range of $\pm 10\%$) the time of appearance of successive discharges of the ectopic pacemaker during a 'silent' period; and, in fact, construct a curve that gives reasonable quantitative values to the amplitude of the electrotonic influence as a function of its position in the ectopic cycle.

This estimate appears in Figure 19.5. This is not presented as a unique solution of the interactions in this case, but it is compatible with those episodes of parasystole both 'above' and 'below' the EP/SN ratio at which manifest bigeminy (the 'extrasystolic rhythm') appeared in the published description.

In a similar analysis of many published and unpublished examples of 'slightly irregular' parasystole, the predictive success rate has been high enough to lend firm support to the original hypothesis. We can therefore say with some assurance:

(1) Variations in the apparent ectopic cycle length of a parasystolic pacemaker are obligatory and predictable results of electrotonic influences exerted across the area of impaired conduction.

(2) Drifting of the ectopic pattern from bigeminy to concealed bigeminy to silence is to be expected when the heart rate decreases; a shift from bigeminy to other patterns not characteristic of bigeminal rhythm must accompany *acceleration* of the heart rate, in a zone in which 2:1 entrainment of the pacemaker is lost.

(3) Similar events are demonstrable on both sides of a zone of trigeminal rhythm.

(4) Analysis of rhythms not diagnosed as parasystolic may nevertheless reveal a fundamentally rhythmic ectopic basis.

(5) Because the width of the range of heart rates in which a stable bigeminal rhythm may occur is relatively narrow, it follows that the coupling interval of the ectopic beats will be relatively fixed. It follows further that fixed coupling cannot be taken as evidence for re-entrant excitation, a conclusion previously

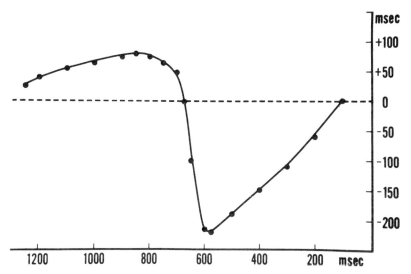

Figure 19.5 Electrotonic influence of normal ventricular beats on pacemaker cycle, derived from analysis of case 2 of Schamroth and Marriott[1]. Ordinates, estimated shift of intrinsic pacemaker cycle induced by normal beats occurring within that cycle. Temporal position expressed on abscissa as milliseconds prior to expected ectopic discharge. The curve was constructed from three of the figures in the published description, and it 'fits' the episodes of bigeminy, concealed bigeminy (deceleration of the SA frequency) and loss of 2:1 entrainment (acceleration of the SA frequency), assuming an intrinsic ectopic cycle of 1570 msec. Circles do not represent numerical observations, but are plotted as an 'eyeball' reconstruction of the estimated influence

reached by Langendorf and Pick[5].

In the title we questioned whether parasystole could in fact be re-entrant. We do not mean to suggest re-entry in the concept of a closed circus loop, although we should not exclude that as a special case; but rather to consider the reciprocal electrotonic influences across a zone of impaired conduction as a kind of re-entry. For example, a depolarization of the ventricle occurring beyond the midpoint of the ectopic cycle will accelerate the ensuing discharge; the ventricular response is not propagated across the blocked area in the sense of a grossly decelerated wave front; there is more likely a true latency between the two segments of tissue. When, after a latent period of considerable duration, the pacemaker eventually fires, a closely coupled premature beat may be reciprocally generated in the ventricle.

Faced with a bigeminal or trigeminal rhythm with fixed coupling, how then can one determine whether the ectopic activity is re-entrant or parasystolic? This question was considered by Langendorf and Pick in 1967[5] and is also implicit in the analysis by Schamroth and Marriott[1]. If the rhythm is parasystolic, a very gradual acceleration of the heart rate, readily induced by intra-atrial pacing electrodes, must lead to progressive prolongation of the coupling interval, followed by a break to pentageminal periods; a gradual deceleration (induced by carotid sinus pressure) should cause abbreviation of the coupling interval, followed by patterns indicative of concealed bigeminy. Further alteration of the heart rate, in either direction, should lead to disappearance of manifest ectopic activity. We can see no reason why a re-entrant focus should behave in the same way.

How can one establish whether an apparently random ectopic focus is in fact the expression of an intrinsically rhythmic 'parasystolic' pacemaker? Wide deviations from a fixed cycle length will occur if the amplitude of the electrotonic influence is great, but entrainment of the pacemaker must still occur. Very gradual acceleration or deceleration should then reveal a zone during which bigeminal or trigeminal coupling occurs. The behaviour of the ectopic focus in response to variations in heart rate can then reveal, not only the intrinsic cycle length of the pacemaker, but also an approximation of the degree of interaction with the surrounding tissue.

Acknowledgement

This work was supported in part by a grant from the National Heart and Lung Institute, HL–15759.

References

1. Schamroth, L. and Marriott, H. J. L. (1961). Intermittent ventricular parasystole with observations on its relationship to extrasystolic bigeminy. *Am. J. Cardiol.*, **7**, 799
2. Weidmann, S. (1951). Effect of current flow on the membrane potential of cardiac muscle. *J. Physiol. (London)*, **115**, 227
3. Jalife, J. and Moe, C. K. (1976). Effect of electrotonic potentials on pacemaker activity of canine Purkinje fibers in relation to parasystole. *Cir. Res.*, **39**, 801
4. Jalife, J., Mueller, W. J., Moe, B. and Moe, G. K. (1977). A mathematical model of parasystole and its application to clinical examples. (Submitted to Circulation)
5. Langendorf, R. and Pick, A. (1967). Parasystole with fixed coupling. *Circulation*, **35**, 304

Section V
Treatment of Re-entrant Arrhythmias

20
Effects of Pharmacological Agents on Mechanisms Responsible for Re-entry

M. R. ROSEN

Departments of Pharmacology and Paediatrics,
Columbia University College of Physicians and Surgeons, New York

Theoretically, there are several means for pharmacological suppression of re-entrant arrhythmias. These means all have at their core an attempt to alter the apparently fine balance between abnormal conduction and refractoriness that is present in a re-entrant circuit. The theoretical means for abolishing re-entry due to unidirectional block and retrograde conduction[1] can be considered by referring to Figure 20.1. For successful pharmacotherapy here it is necessary either to improve antegrade conduction through a depressed segment of the conducting system until such time as it participates effectively in antegrade activation B, or further depress conduction until there is bidirectional block and a failure of both antegrade and retrograde propagation C. For the situation in B to develop a drug would have to hyperpolarize cardiac fibres D or decrease the slope of phase 4 depolarization of fibres in a depressed segment thereby enhancing the propagation of impulses arriving through this segment E. A decrease in the action potential duration of fibres having abnormally long action potential durations also could enhance antegrade propagation F. For bidirectional block to occur, as shown in C, fibres would have to be depolarized until propagation failed resulting in bidirectional block G, or the action potential duration (and effective refractory period) would have to be further prolonged, leading to total failure of propagation as in H. Hence, within the framework of unidirectional block and re-entry, the slowing or speeding of conduction within a depressed segment and/or the increase or decrease of action potential duration and refractoriness all contribute to the termination of re-entry.

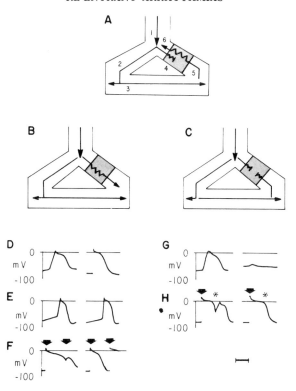

Figure 20.1 A: Model for unidirectional block and re-entry. Activation arriving at a distal portion of the Purkinje system[1] proceeds through two terminal Purkinje fibres. One of these fibres[2] is normal and activation proceeds through it to the myocardium[3]. The other terminal fibre is depressed (shaded area) and antegrade activation is blocked[4]. Activation proceeding through the myocardium enters the depressed segment in a retrograde direction[5], propagates through it and re-enters the proximal conducting system[6].

B: Suppression of unidirectional block and re-entry by enhancement of antegrade conduction. If antegrade activation proceeds through the depressed segment (shaded area) before a retrogradely propagated wave form arrives, then re-entry will not occur.

C: Suppression of unidirectional block and re-entry by induction of bidirectional block. In this case both antegrade and retrograde propagation through the depressed segment (shaded area) are blocked and, as a result, re-entry cannot occur.

D: The left panel shows an action potential from a depressed segment of Purkinje fibre. The resting membrane potential (RMP) is low as are action potential amplitude and upstroke velocity. The right panel shows the effects of epinephrine, 1×10^{-7} M. The fibre has been hyperpolarized, its amplitude and upstroke velocity have been increased. These changes are associated with enhancement of conduction and might result in the conversion of the diagram in A to that in B. Hyperpolarization of depressed cardiac fibres has also been described with lidocaine, diphenylhydantoin, acetylcholine and digitalis.

E: Left panel: Marked phase 4 depolarization results in initiation of the action potential at a low level of membrane potential. Amplitude and upstroke velocity are low. On the right, lidocaine ($4 \mu g/ml$) has been added to the perfusate. The slope of phase 4 is decreased, the action potential is initiated at a higher level of membrane potential than previously and its amplitude and upstroke velocity are increased. Conduction in this situation, too, would be expected to improve

Other mechanisms such as reflection and summation have been described as contributing to the initiation and propagation of re-entrant arrhythmias[1]. For both of these mechanisms—as for unidirectional block and re-entry the level of membrane potential, the conduction velocity and the duration of the action potential and effective refractory period are crucial to the occurrence of re-entry. As in the case of unidirectional block and re-entry, any intervention which alters conduction and/or refractoriness should contribute to the termination of this arrhythmia.

On interacting with cardiac tissues a drug must alter the balance that exists between conduction and refractoriness, and thereby alter propagation through the re-entrant pathway. To do this the drug may act: (1) at the site of origin of the arrhythmia (i.e. on the depressed segment); (2) on the variably depressed tissues that may be present between the totally abnormal zone and normal tissues; and/or (3) on normal tissues that are present elsewhere in the re-entrant pathway. Any one of the actions shown in Figure 20.1 should be antiarrhythmic, as should combinations thereof, and hence we expect that drugs which are effective against re-entrant rhythms will have some of the following effects:

(1) Depress conduction of the action potential within the re-entrant loop. If the drug is sufficient to decrease resting membrane potential and/or the excitability of cardiac fibres in the re-entrant pathway it may render the action

---

resulting in improvement of the situation in A to that in B. Similar effects have been attributed to quinidine, procaine amide, diphenylhydantoin, acetylcholine, and β-receptor blocking agents.

F: Left panel: The action potential duration is abnormally long such that a 2:1 block of activation is occurring. (Normal stimuli are indicated by arrows; the second stimulus in the series occurs before the effective refractory period of the segment has terminated.) Lidocaine (4 μg/ml) induces marked shortening of action potential duration (and the effective refractory period). As a result, antegrade propagation now proceeds normally. This situation too results in the conduction pattern shown in B. In addition to lidocaine, diphenylhydantoin, and propranolol decrease action potential duration.

G: Left panel: As in D. On the right superfusion of the preparation with procaine amide, 30μg/ml has further depolarized the fibre and, in addition, has depressed conduction. In this case an action potential no longer is initiated in response to the stimulus. Such a situation—which has also been described for quinidine and, under certain circumstances lidocaine, would result in bidirectional conduction block as in C. In fibres which are markedly depressed and slow responses are occurring procaine amide has no effect on the action potential. In this situation, however, verapamil, in low concentrations, will depress action potential amplitude, upstroke velocity and conduction.

H: Left panel: The arrow indicates a normally initiated and propagated action potential. The asterisk indicates a prematurely initiated action potential which occurs after the end of the effective refractory period and is propagated.

The right panel shows the effect of procaine amide (30 μg/ml). The durations of the action potential and effective refractory period have increased. As a result, the premature depolarization arises before termination of refractoriness and cannot be propagated. This, too, could induce a situation like that in C. The same effect is seen with quinidine.

All records in this Figure were traced from experimental recordings and retouched. For references to drug actions, see text

potential a poorer stimulus for further propagation, thereby completely depressing conduction in the re-entrant loop. If the drug does not alter resting potential or excitability but, nonetheless, decreases the inward current responsible for the action potential, then, again the action potential will lose efficacy as a stimulus and propagation will fail. Such an effect may be exerted on the rapid inward (sodium) current or the slow inward current carried primarily by calcium.

(2) Prolong refractoriness of fibres in the re-entrant loop. Such an effect, if of sufficient magnitude, would render the fibre refractory to propagation of impulses through the re-entrant loop.

(3) Enhance conduction. This may occur as a result of hyperpolarization of cardiac fibres as has been described for agents such as catecholamines[2]. The increase in membrane potential is associated with enhancement of action potential amplitude and upstroke velocity, and an increase in conduction velocity. Alternatively, this effect may occur in situations in which a drug decreases action potential duration. By shortening an abnormally long action potential, a drug may increase the level of membrane potential at which an action potential is initiated and normalize its conduction.

The pharmacological agents used in the treatment of cardiac arrhythmias all can modify certain of the factors described as important in the genesis of the re-entrant arrhythmias. These factors (conduction through the re-entrant loop, refractoriness of the fibres involved) are altered in a different fashion by each of the drugs involved. The drugs to be discussed here include quinidine, procaine amide, lidocaine, verapamil and propranolol.

LIDOCAINE

Although the interactions between healthy and diseased fibres, in all likelihood are responsible for the occurrence of re-entrant arrhythmias, to date studies of the cellular electrophysiologic actions of lidocaine have been performed mainly on normal cardiac tissues. Bigger and Mandel[3,4] and Davis and Temte[5] reported that lidocaine had little or no effect on phase 0 depolarization or conduction in normal canine Purkinje fibres until high concentrations ($11-50\,\mu g/ml$) were used. Bigger and Mandel[4] also found that lidocaine improved conduction across the Purkinje fibre–papillary muscle junction when the drug acted on partly depolarized fibres. They proposed that this action might abolish re-entrant arrhythmias, through the restoration of normal conduction in areas of unidirectional conduction block. Singh and Vaughan Williams[6] in studies of rabbit atrial and ventricular tissues, indicated that lidocaine in concentrations $<10\,\mu g/ml$ has only a depressant effect on myocardial action potentials, decreasing their amplitude and phase 0 upstroke velocity ($\dot{V}_{max}$), and therefore presumably slowing conduction. This depressant effect was enhanced as the extracellular potassium concentration was increased to >3 mM.

These differences described for the effects of lidocaine emphasize that, depending on the species of animal and type of tissue studied as well as on the experimental protocol, rather different observations of drug effects may be made. For example, in stretched cardiac fibres, lidocaine has been shown to increase potassium conductance, resulting in significant hyperpolarization and improved conduction[7]. Alternatively, studies of lidocaine effects on Purkinje fibres surviving in regions of extensive experimental myocardial infarction[8] have shown that the low maximum diastolic potential, amplitude and $\dot{V}_{max}$ of such fibres are further depressed by therapeutic lidocaine concentrations. Lidocaine-induced improvement in these transmembrane potentials has not been observed, indicating that lidocaine probably does not hyperpolarize cardiac cells which have a low resting membrane potential due to ischaemia or infarction.

Lidocaine markedly shortens the action potential duration and the effective refractory period of Purkinje fibres[3]. The magnitude of this effect varies with the location of the Purkinje fibre within the specialized conducting system[9] and is greatest at the area of maximum action potential duration in the Purkinje system. Although the decrease of action potential duration induced by lidocaine is accompanied by shortening of the effective refractory period, several studies indicate that the refractory period does not decrease as much as the action potential. This may be due to a drug-induced delay in the reactivation of the sodium carrier responsible for phase 0[10]. As a result, after lidocaine administration, the earliest premature response that can be propagated arises at a more negative level of membrane potential and conducts at a more rapid velocity than the earliest premature impulse elicited before the drug was present.

By decreasing the duration of the action potential and of refractoriness at sites of longer duration to a greater extent than at sites of shorter duration lidocaine could eliminate the unidirectional conduction block of early premature impulses which initiate re-entry. Although premature depolarizations still might occur, they would be less likely to induce re-entry and sustained re-entrant tachycardia. It should be noted that this description still is hypothetical and requires experimental verification.

QUINIDINE AND PROCAINE AMIDE

Quinidine and procaine amide have similar effects on the transmembrane potentials and electrical activity of cardiac fibres. Most of these effects are exerted directly by the drugs but some are due to drug-induced modifications of autonomic responses.

As with lidocaine, most of the effects of quinidine and procaine amide have been described for normal cardiac cells and only recently has systematic investigation of their actions on depressed or diseased fibres been initiated. In concentrations approximating the therapeutic range quinidine and procaine amide induce a dose-dependent decrease in the $\dot{V}_{max}$ and the action potential amplitude of atrial and ventricular muscle and Purkinje fibres[11]. These concentrations do not decrease the resting potential or maximum diastolic potential. The effects on the action potential upstroke appear to result from a direct action on the mechanism controlling the voltage and time-dependent increase in sodium conductance[12,13]. Most investigators have found that, for a given concentration of drug, the decrease in responsiveness is increased by elevating extracellular potassium concentration $[K^+]_0$ and diminished by lowering $[K^+]_0$[14].

Quinidine and procaine amide both appear to shift the threshold potential for initiation of the action potential to less negative values[12]. As a result, more stimulus current is needed to initiate an action potential from the normal level of resting potential. Because of the effects on both the action potential upstroke and threshold potential, conduction velocity usually is decreased progressively as drug concentration rises. There is one exception to this statement. If conduction is measured in specialized conducting fibres which demonstrate marked phase 4 depolarization, low concentrations of either quinidine or procaine amide may increase the speed of impulse propagation[15] (Figure 20.1(e)). This occurs for the following reason: in the presence of marked phase 4 depolarization, the action potential upstroke is initiated at a low membrane potential. Hence, the $\dot{V}_{max}$ and action potential amplitude are low and the impulse propagates slowly. Low drug concentrations will markedly decrease the slope of phase 4 depolarisation and permit the action potential to be initiated at a more negative level of membrane potential. The increase in membrane potential at the moment of excitation outweighs the direct effect of a low concentration of drug on inward sodium current and as a result the action potential improves and conduction velocity increases.

In studies of isolated preparations of diseased human atrium, procaine amide exerts a variable effect on the action potential of specialized conducting fibres[16]. In fibres with normal action potential amplitudes and upstroke velocities, there is a dose-dependent decrease in these parameters. In partially depolarized fibres, having somewhat lower action potential amplitudes and upstroke velocities, there is a slightly greater depressant effect. However, in markedly depressed fibres generating slow response action potentials even high concentrations of procaine amide ($100 \mu g/ml$) have little or no effect[16].

Both quinidine and procaine amide prolong the action potential duration and the duration of refractoriness in atrial and ventricular muscle and Purkinje fibres[11,12,17]. These direct effects are modified to some extent both by their ability to attenuate the effects of catecholamines and acetylcholine on the myocardium and by any drug-induced changes in rate.

The effects of these drugs on action potential duration also are influenced by $[K^+]_0$ in that prolongation is more marked at lower values of $[K^+]_0$. In addition, the magnitude of the drug effect on action potential duration varies with the anatomical location of fibres in the His–Purkinje system. The change is more marked for fibres initially demonstrating the shortest action potentials[17]. The overall effect is thus to make the action potential duration more uniform over the entire length of the His–Purkinje system.

VERAPAMIL

Verapamil has a markedly different mechanism of action than the drugs thus far described. It blocks the slow inward current carried primarily by Ca^{2+} and a slow current carried by Na^+[18]. Hence, its primary action appears to be on the slow channel that has been implicated in the genesis of re-entrant rhythms in cardiac fibres with low levels of membrane potential.

As mentioned, procaine amide, quinidine and lidocaine have local anaesthetic effects during phase 0 depolarization and interfere with sodium entry in cells with sodium-dependent action potentials[19]. This action depresses conduction, and this may be a major factor underlying the efficacy of these drugs in the therapy of atrial and ventricular arrhythmias. Verapamil, on the other hand, has little or no effect on action potential amplitude or $\dot{V}_{max}$ in cells with normal sodium dependent action potentials in the ventricular specialised conducting system and the atria.

In normal Purkinje fibres, low concentrations of verapamil (*ca.* 1 mg/1) shift the plateau phase of repolarization to more negative potential levels but do not significantly alter the overall duration of the action potential[20]. Further the effective refractory period of normal Purkinje fibres is not significantly changed[21]. Only in high concentrations (5–10 mg/l) does verapamil prolong the repolarization time and effective refractory period of normal Purkinje fibres and depress action potential amplitude and $\dot{V}_{max}$[21]. Therefore it is unlikely that verapamil exerts its antiarrhythmic effects by virtue of its action on the electrophysiologic properties of normal cells.

The most pronounced electrophysiologic effects of verapamil are exerted on cardiac fibres with slow response action potentials. Microelectrode studies of isolated, superfused cardiac tissue obtained at surgery from diseased human atria have demonstrated such slow responses[16]. Whereas verapamil does not significantly alter the normal atrial action potential, it markedly depresses amplitude, $\dot{V}_{max}$ and conduction in the depressed atrial fibres. These effects probably are due to inhibition of the slow inward current. The depression of action potential amplitude, $\dot{V}_{max}$ and conduction may abolish re-entry in these diseased atria.

Verapamil also exerts potent depressant effects on sinus and atrioventricular nodal function and in low concentrations it prolongs the effective refractory period of the atrioventricular node[22]. A study on the isolated, superfused rabbit right atrium has suggested a mechanism by which verapamil may abolish certain supraventricular tachycardias[23]. Whereas premature impulses conduct slowly through the node and re-enter the atrium prior to exposure to verapamil, after verapamil conduction of these premature impulses is blocked in the node and re-entry is prevented. This effect of verapamil occurs in concentrations (*ca.*

0.1 mg/l) which do not significantly modify conduction of the normal atrial impulse, and may be due to a prolongation in the time dependence for recovery of excitability of AV nodal cells. A similar effect may occur in the sinus node, although it has not been demonstrated.

Verapamil depresses the amplitude of action potentials in the upper and mid-AV node without altering resting potential[23]. This effect is more pronounced at rapid atrial rates. Such an electrophysiologic effect is probably the cause for the depression and block of conduction through the AV node (particularly at rapid atrial rates) which occurs after verapamil administration[24].

PROPRANOLOL

In this discussion we shall consider one β-adrenergic blocking agent, propranolol, as a prototype for this group of compounds. This is because propranolol is the most widely used of the β-blockers at the present time. It also has been shown to have more of a direct membrane effect on cardiac fibres than many of the other β-blockers available.

Most clinical and experimental evidence suggests that it is the β-blocking and not the direct membrane effects of β-blockers in general and propranolol in particular that is responsible for their antiarrhythmic action[25]. The direct membrane effects of propranolol occur at concentrations 10–100 times greater than those necessary for β-blockade. At concentrations of 3 $\mu g/ml$ and greater propranolol depresses action potential amplitude, $\dot{V}_{max}$ and conduction in normal atrial, ventricular and Purkinje fibres and accelerates repolarization[26–29]. These effects probably are due to a drug-induced decrease in Na conductance[30]. In low (β-receptor blocking) concentrations propranolol does not affect action potential amplitude, $\dot{V}_{max}$ and repolarization when these tissues are not being superfused with catecholamines.

In the presence of catecholamines the effect of β-receptor blockade is more complex. β-Antagonists will reverse the acceleratory effects on repolarization of the β-agonist, isoproterenol[31]. The effects of norepinephrine, a mixed α- and β-agonist, and β-receptor blockade on ventricular muscle fibres have not been well-defined. Evidence from studies on the intact heart suggests that β-adrenergic stimulation accelerates repolarization and shortens the refractory period. β-Receptor blockade thus should prolong action potential duration and refractoriness in the presence of catecholamines[31]. This may be a mechanism of antiarrhythmic action, particularly against re-entrant ventricular arrhythmias resulting from dispersion of ventricular refractoriness due to sympathetic activation.

The spectrum of clinical efficacy of β-blockers without direct membrane effects seems to be the same as that of the blockers having a direct membrane effect[25,31]. The actions of these drugs on conduction depend on several factors including: (1) whether catecholamines are present and, if so, the effects the catecholamines are exerting on the action potential; (2) the type of tissue and its condition, i.e. are action potentials normal or are they depressed; and (3) the presence or absence of direct effects of the drug.

In summary, the effective clinical concentrations of the β-blockers, including propranolol, as well as the similarity of clinical efficacy of drugs having variable degrees of direct membrane effect suggest that it is, in fact, β-blockade that is important for the antiarrhythmic action of these drugs. While it is possible that direct membrane effects of certain of these drugs are exerted on markedly depressed or slow response fibres at low β-blocking concentrations, this still is open to conjecture.

EFFECTS OF ANTIARRHYTHMIC DRUGS ON AUTOMATICITY

Re-entrant rhythms may be initiated by premature beats initiated by automatic foci. Hence, it is possible that in some situations drugs may modify the occurrence of re-entrant arrhythmias by depressing automatic foci. All the drugs described can depress automaticity, although by different mechanisms. In the case of lidocaine, procaine amide and quinidine, the slope of phase 4 depolarization of fibres having the fast response is depressed[19]. Studies have shown that lidocaine decreases the slope of phase 4 by increasing the outward potassium current that occurs during electrical diastole[32] while procaine amide may decrease the inward current carried by sodium[33]. Studies of the effects of these drugs on automaticity of slow response fibres are still in progress. Although it has been shown for human atria that procaine amide has no effect on slow response automaticity[16], information concerning lidocaine and quinidine is still not available.

Verapamil in low concentrations suppresses automaticity of fibres having the slow response[34]. In addition, it appears to modify fast response automaticity[26], especially in situations in which fibres with the fast response have been treated with toxic concentrations of digitalis[34]. Low (β-blocking) concentrations of the β-adrenergic antagonists do not alter automaticity of fast response fibres. However, they do counteract the positive chronotropic effects of catecholamines on fast response fibres[31]. Similarly, β-blockers will counteract the effects of catecholamines on slow response automaticity. Although high (direct membrane depressant) concentrations of β-blockers will depress automaticity of fibres having the fast response it is unlikely that such effects are of clinical importance[37].

CONCLUSIONS

In summary, we have seen that re-entrant rhythms resulting from abnormal conduction can be suppressed by drugs which alter conduction and/or refractoriness. In addition, drugs may prevent the occurrence of those re-entrant rhythms which are initiated by automatic foci by suppressing the automaticity of these fibres. As we have discussed, the mechanisms of action of the drugs do differ, explaining in part the difference in efficacy of the various drugs. However, many questions still remain concerning the extent to which various mechanisms (such as the slow response and the depressed fast response) are responsible for arrhythmias and also concerning the effects of various drugs on these mechanisms. Until further information is obtained concerning these questions we will be unable to state firmly the relative importance of the various drug effects described above in the prevention and treatment of re-entrant rhythms.

Acknowledgement

Part of this work was supported by USPHS–NHLBI grant HL–12738 and a grant from the New York Heart Association.

References

1. Cranefield, P. F., Wit, A. L. and Hoffman, B. F. (1973). Genesis of cardiac arrhythmias. *Circulation*, **47**, 190
2. Hoffman, B. F. and Singer, D. H. (1967). Appraisal of the effects of catecholamines on cardiac electrical activity. In: N. Moran (ed.). *New Adrenergic Blocking Drugs: Their Pharmacological Biochemical and Clinical Actions. Ann. N.Y. Acad, Sci.*, **139**, 914.
3. Bigger, J. T., Jr. and Mandel, W. J. (1970). Effect of lidocaine on transmembrane potentials of ventricular muscle and Purkinje fibers. *J. Clin. Invest.*, **49**, 63
4. Bigger, J. T., Jr. and Mandel, W. J. (1970). Effect of lidocaine on canine Purkinje fibers and at the ventricular muscle–Purkinje fiber junction. *J. Pharmacol. Exp. Ther.*, **172**, 239
5. Davis, L. D. and Temte, J. F. (1969). Electrophysiological actions of lidocaine on canine ventricular muscle and Purkinje fibres. *Circ. Res.*, **24**, 639
6. Singh, B. N. and Vaughan Williams, E. M. (1971). Effects of altering potassium concentration on the action of lidocaine and diphenylhydantoin on rabbit atrial and ventricular muscle. *Circ. Res.*, **29**, 286
8. Sasyniuk, B. I. and Kus, T. (1974). Comparison of the effects of lidocaine on electrophysiological properties of normal Purkinje fibers and those surviving acute myocardial infarction (abstr.) *Fed. Proc.*, **33**, 476
9. Wittig, J., Harrison, L. A. and Wallace, A. G. (1973). Electrophysiological effects of lidocaine on distal Purkinje fibers of canine heart. *Am. Heart J.*, **86**, 69
10. Vaughan Williams, E. M. Classification of antiarrhythmic drugs. In: Sandoe, E., Flensted-Jensen, E. and Olesen, K. H. (eds.). *Symposium on Cardiac Arrhythmias,* Sweden, 1970, Astra, pp. 449–472
11. Hoffman, B. F. (1958). Action of quinidine and procaine amide on single fibers of dog ventricle and specialized conducting system. *Anais Acad. Brasil, Cienc.*, **29**, 365
12. Weidmann, S. (1955). Effects of calcium ions and local anesthetics on electrical properties of Purkinje fibers. *J. Physiol.*, **129**, 568
13. Singh, B. N. and Hauswirth, O. (1974). Comparative mechanisms of action of antiarrhythmic drugs. *Am. Heart J.*, **87**, 367
14. Watanabe, Y., Dreifus, L. and Likoff, W. (1963). Electrophysiological antagonism and synergism of potassium and antiarrhythmic agents. *Am. J. Cardiol.*, **12**, 702
15. Singer, D. H. and Ten Eick, R. E. (1969). Pharmacology of cardiac arrhythmias. *Progr. Cardiovasc. Dis.*, **11**, 488
16. Hordof, A., Edie, R., Malm, J. and Rosen, M. (1975). Effects of procaine amide and verapamil on electrophysiologic properties of human atrial tissues. *Pediatr. Res.*, **9**, 267
17. Rosen, M., Gelband, H., Merker, C. and Hoffman, B. (1973). Effects of procaine amide on the electrophysiologic properties of the canine ventricular conducting system. *J. Pharmacol. Exp. Ther.*, **185**, 438

18. Shigenobu, K., Schneider, J. A. and Sperelakis, N. (1974). Verapamil blockade of slow Na$^+$ and Ca^{2+} responses in myocardial cells. *J. Pharmacol. Exp. Ther.*, **190**, 280

19. Rosen, M. R. and Hoffman, B. F. (1973). Mechanisms of action of antiarrhythmic drugs. *Circ. Res.*, **32**, 1

20. Cranefield, P. F., Aronson, R. S. and Wit, A. L. (1974). Effect of verapamil on the normal action potential and on a calcium-dependent slow response of canine cardiac Purkinje fibers. *Circ. Res.*, **34**, 204

21. Rosen, M. R., Ilvento, J. P., Gelband, H. and Merker, C. (1974). Effects of verapamil on electrophysiologic properties of canine cardiac Purkinje fibers. *J. Pharmacol. Exp. Ther.*, **189**, 414

22. Zipes, D. P. and Fischer, J. C. (1974). Effects of agents which inhibit the slow channel on sinus node automaticity and atrioventricular conduction in the dog. *Circ. Res.*, **34**, 184

23. Wit, A. L. and Cranefield, P. F. (1974). The effects of verapamil on the sinoatrial and atrioventricular nodes of the rabbit and the mechanism by which it arrests re-entrant AV nodal tachycardia. *Circ. Res.*, **35**, 413

24. Wit, A. L. and Cranefield, P. F. (1974). Verapamil inhibition of the slow response: a mechanism for its effectiveness against re-entrant AV nodal tachycardia. *Circulation* (Suppl. III) 49 and 50: III-146

25. Wit, A. L., Hoffman, B. F. and Rosen, M. R. (1975). Electrophysiology and pharmacology of cardiac arrhythmias. IX. Cardiac electrophysiologic effects of beta-adrenergic receptor stimulation and blockade, Part B. *Am. Heart J.*, **90**, 665

26. Davis, L. D. and Temte, J. V. (1968). Effects of propranolol on the transmembrane potentials of ventricular muscle and Purkinje fibers in the dog. *Circ. Res.*, **23**, 661

27. Vaughan Williams, E. M. (1966). Mode of action of beta-receptor antagonists on cardiac muscle. *Am. J. Cardiol.*, **18**, 399

28. Wit, A. L. and Bassett, A. L. (1971). Electrical and mechanical effects of alprenolol on isolated heart muscle. *Fed. Proc.*, **30**, 393

29. Pitt, W. A. and Cox, A. R. (1968). The effect of the β-adrenergic antagonist propranolol on rabbit atrial cells with the use of the ultramicroelectrode technique. *Am. Heart J.*, **76**, 242

30. Tarr, M., Luckstead, E. F., Turewicz, P. A. and Haas, H. G. (1973). Effect of propranolol on the fast inward sodium current in frog atrial muscle. *J. Pharmacol. Exp. Ther.*, **184**, 599

31. Wit, A. L., Hoffman, B. F. and Rosen, M. R. (1975). Electrophysiology and pharmacology of cardiac arrhythmias. IX. Cardiac electrophysiologic effects of beta-adrenergic receptor stimulation and blockade. Part C. *Am. Heart J.*, **90**, 795

32. Arnsdorf, M. F. and Bigger, J. T., Jr. (1972). Effect of lidocaine hydrochloride on membrane conductance in mammalian cardiac Purkinje fibers. *J. Clin. Invest.*, **51**, 2252

33. Weld, F. M. and Bigger, J. T., Jr. (1972). Effect of procaine amide on membrane conductance of cardiac Purkinje fibers. *Circulation* (Abstr.), **46**, II-39

34. Rosen, M. R., Wit, A. L. and Hoffman, B. F. (1975). Electrophysiology and pharmacology of cardiac arrhythmias. VI. Cardiac effects of verapamil. *Am. Heart J.*, **89**, 665

21
Chronic Electrophysiological Study in Patients with Recurrent Paroxysmal Tachycardia: a New Method for Developing Successful Oral Antiarrhythmic Therapy

D. WU, C. R. WYNDHAM, P. DENES, F. AMAT-Y-LEON, R. H. MILLER, R. C. DHINGRA and K. M. ROSEN

Section of Cardiology, Department of Medicine, Abraham Lincoln School of Medicine, University of Illinois College of Medicine, West Side Veterans' Administration Hospital, Chicago, Illinois

INTRODUCTION

In most patients with paroxysmal supraventricular tachycardia (PSVT) and some with paroxysmal ventricular tachycardia (PVT), the arrhythmia can be reproduced in the catheterization laboratory utilizing electrical stimulation of the heart[1-4]. The ability to reproduce this arrhythmia has allowed the acute pharmacological study of antiarrhythmic drugs in patients with paroxysmal tachycardia. Thus, agents such as propranolol, digitalis, procaine amide and quinidine have been administered during electrophysiological studies in patients having arrhythmias in order to determine the presence or absence of antiarrhythmic actions, and in an attempt to define the mechanism of action of these agents in specific arrhythmias[2,5-9].

Since these are acute studies with intravenous administration of drugs, the clinical relevance of findings to chronic oral antiarrhythmic action is not known. Wellens and his co-workers demonstrated that patients with PSVT manifesting beneficial effects of intravenous ouabain maintained these effects when studied two weeks later on oral digoxin[9]. However, his study did not provide information concerning the relevance of initial and subsequent study to future incidence of spontaneous paroxysmal tachycardia on digoxin therapy.

In the present study, we report a method by which patients with incapacitating paroxysmal arrhythmias can be studied with multiple antiarrhythmic agents, singly or in combination, intravenously and orally. We have attempted to delineate optimal oral drug therapy, and relate this to subsequent clinical course over a short-term follow-up period. Our data suggest that rational antiarrhythmic therapy determined with chronic electrophysiological studies will be successful in therapy of recurrent paroxysmal tachycardia.

METHODS

Three patients, two with paroxysmal supraventricular tachycardia and one with paroxysmal ventricular tachycardia, underwent a chronic electrophysiological study in order to evaluate the effects of sequential antiarrhythmic drug administration on the induction of paroxysmal tachycardia. All three patients fulfilled the following criteria: (1) documented recurrent paroxysmal tachycardia necessitating multiple hospital visits or admissions; (2) severe symptoms associated with recurrent tachycardias; (3) histories of failure of oral antiarrhythmic therapy; and (4) signing of informed consent for chronic electrophysiological study.

An initial electrophysiological study was performed with the patients in the post-absorptive, non-sedated state and with all cardiac drugs discontinued at least 72 hours prior to study. A tripolar electrode catheter was passed percutaneously via a femoral vein and placed at the tricuspid valve for His bundle recording[10]. A hexapolar electrode catheter was introduced via an antecubital vein and advanced to the right ventricular apex. The distal two electrodes were utilized for ventricular stimulation, the middle two electrodes for atrial stimulation, and the proximal two electrodes for recording of atrial electrograms. Multiple electrocardiographic leads as well as additional intracardiac electrograms were simultaneously recorded on a multichannel oscilloscopic recorder (Electronics for Medicine DR-16, White Plains, New York) at paper speeds of 100 and 200 mm/sec. Recordings were also stored on an eight-channel tape system for further analysis. Extra-stimuli were delivered via a digital programmable stimulator (manufactured by M. Bloom, Philadelphia).

The initial study included complete electrophysiological evaluation with rapid atrial and ventricular pacing, atrial and ventricular extra-stimulus testing, and recording of multiple atrial sites during induced tachycardia. During the initial study, one pharmacological agent was also studied. At the conclusion of the initial study, the hexapolar catheter was left in place for subsequent daily arrhythmia induction, with testing of sequential parenteral and then oral antiarrhythmic drugs. The sequence of drugs studied was determined by previous drug history (significant side effects eliminated a drug from the protocol), the mechanism of tachycardia noted at initial study, and the drug response at initial study. If striking beneficial effects were observed with a particular antiarrhythmic agent or combination of agents, the patient was placed on that drug orally with daily incremental increase in doses in order to define optimal dose. Blood samples were taken for the measurements of drug levels. The patient was then placed on the proposed effective antiarrhythmic regimen, as defined by the above studies, and was then discharged and followed.

All patients tolerated the study well without significant morbidity or discomfort.

RESULTS

Case 1

This was a 58-year-old female referred to the University of Illinois Hospital because of frequent recurrent PSVT of many years duration. In the 18 months prior to admission, episodes of PSVT occurred with a frequency of approximately once per week, and were associated with diaphoresis, chest discomfort and dyspnea. PSVT episodes necessitated multiple emergency room visits and frequent admission for arrhythmia conversion. Numerous single and multiple antiarrhythmic drug regimens had failed to prevent PSVT recurrence. Cardiac examination revealed moderate hypertension. Electrocardiograms during sinus rhythm showed left ventricular hypertrophy.

Electrophysiological studies are summarized in Table 21.1. Initial study revealed dual pathway AV nodal re-entrant PSVT[2,8]. Sustained PSVT (PSVT lasting longer than 2 min) induction could be obtained with cessation of atrial pacing at 170/min, and with atrial extrastimulus testing (driven cycle length of 400 msec) at A_1-A_2 coupling intervals between 280 and 210 msec (Figure 21.1, top panel). Ouabain (0.75 mg) (0.01 mg/kg) was given intravenously and the study was repeated 30 min later. Post-ouabain study revealed that PSVT could still be induced with cessation of atrial pacing at 160/min, and with atrial extrastimulus technique at A_1-A_2 coupling intervals of 370 and 290 msec (driven cycle length of 400msec). However, the ability to sustain PSVT was totally abolished with ouabain, episodes of PSVT lasting no longer than six beats (Figure 21.1, second panel).

On days 2 and 3, the patient was given oral digoxin 0.5 mg/day. Electrophysiological study (with inducing catheter) was repeated 3 hours after the last dose of oral digoxin on day three and a blood sample was taken for measurement of serum digoxin level. This study revealed that sustained PSVT could still be induced with either atrial pacing or atrial extrastimulus technique. Serum digoxin level was 0.8 ng/ml.

Oral digoxin doses were increased to 0.75 mg/day and the study was

Table 21.1 Electrophysiological findings in Case 1

Day		Blood level (ng/ml)	Echoes + PSVT with AP (beats/min)	AEST (msec)		CL of PSVT (msec)	Ability to sustain PSVT
				CL	EZ (A_1-A_2) − (A_1-A_2)		
1	Control	(—)	yes (170)	400	280–210	335	yes
	Ouabain (0.75 mg i.v.)	(—)	yes (160)	400	370–290	342	no
3	Digoxin (0.5 mg/day)	0.8	yes (150)	400	375–230	362	yes
7	Digoxin (0.75 mg/day)	0.24	yes (150)	600	none	375	no

Abbreviations: PSVT = Paroxysmal supraventricular tachycardia; AP = Atrial pacing; AEST = Atrial extra-stimulus technique; CL = Driving cycle length; EZ = Echo zone.

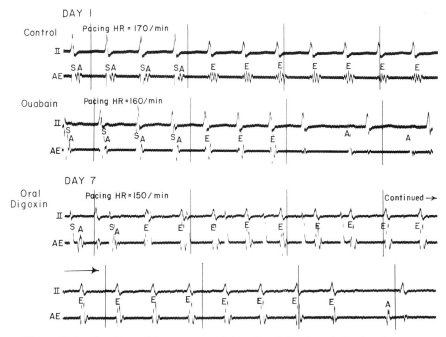

Figure 21.1 The effects of intravenous ouabain and oral digoxin on induction of paroxysmal supraventricular tachycardia (PSVT) in case one. In each panel, electrocardiographic lead II and atrial electrogram (AE) are shown. S, A and E are respectively stimulus artifact, atrial response and atrial echo. Time lines are at one second and paper speed is 100 mm/sec in this and subsequent illustrations.

The top panel shows induction of sustained PSVT with rapid atrial pacing at a paced heart rate (HR) of 170/min on day one before ouabain administration. The second panel shows induction of non-sustained self-terminating PSVT at atrial paced rate of 160/min after 0.75 mg intravenous ouabain. The third and fourth panels are continuous tracings showing induction of non-sustained self-terminating PSVT at an atrial paced rate of 150/min on day seven or oral digoxin 0.75 mg/day

repeated four hours after the last dose of digoxin on day 7. On day 7, only non-sustaining self-terminating PSVT could be induced with rapid atrial pacing at a rate of 150/min and echo zones could no longer be defined with extrastimulus technique (Figure 21.1, third and fourth panels). Serum digoxin level was 2.4 ng/ml.

In summary, ouabain totally abolished the ability to sustain paroxysmal supraventricular tachycardia. Oral digoxin 0.5 mg/day with a blood level of 0.8 ng/ml had no effect. Oral digoxin 0.75 mg/day with blood level of 2.4 ng/ml abolished the ability to sustain tachycardia. Because of this, the patient was discharged on oral digoxin 0.75 mg/day. She has tolerated this dose without side effects and has had only one short episode of PSVT for a follow-up period of 7 months since discharge. Serum digoxin levels during the follow-up period have ranged from 1 to 2.4 ng/ml.

Case 2

This was a 70-year-old female referred to the University of Illinois Hospital because of recurrent PSVT for many years. Episodes lasted for 2–15 hours and were associated with severe dizziness requiring hospital admission approximately once every 2 months. Therapy with digoxin 0.25 mg/day, quinidine up to 800 mg/day, and propranolol up to 120 mg/day was unsuccessin controlling her PSVT. Cardiac examination was within normal limits. Electrocardiograms during sinus rhythm revealed non-specific ST–T changes.

Electrophysiological studies are summarized in Table 21.2. Initial study on day one revealed inability to induce PSVT (Figure 21.2, top panel). However, induction of sustained dual pathway AV nodal re-entrant PSVT was successful after 0.5 mg intravenous atropine. PSVT could be induced following cessation of rapid atrial pacing (160/min) and with atrial extrastimulus technique (echo zone at A_1–A_2 coupling intervals of 330–230 msec) (Figure 21.2, 2nd panel). On day 2, control study demonstrated induction of sustained PSVT with atrial pacing (200/min) and with atrial extrastimulus technique (echo zone at coupling intervals of 290–210 msec). Ouabain 0.7 mg (0.01 mg/kg) was administered intravenously and the study was repeated 30 min later. Post-ouabain study revealed inability to induce PSVT, but persistence of an echo zone (A_1–A_2 of 320–315 msec). On day 3, control study showed no PSVT induction. However, an echo zone was defined at A_1–A_2 of 310–290 msec. Propranolol (5 mg) was administered intravenously. Post-propranolol study revealed total abolition of the echo zone. The patient was then placed on oral digoxin 0.5 mg/day and the study was repeated on day 9. Study on day 9 while on oral digoxin (0.5 mg/day) revealed no PSVT induction or echo zone. Atropine (0.5 mg) was given intravenously and the study was repeated. Post-atropine study (on oral digoxin) revealed induction of nonsustained, self-terminating PSVT with rapid atrial pacing (150/min) and with atrial extrastimulus technique (echo zone at A_1–A_2 of 370–300 msec). After this, propranolol (5 mg) was given intravenously and the study was repeated. Post-propranolol study (on oral digoxin and post atropine) revealed no echo zone or PSVT induction. Oral digoxin (0.5 mg/day) was continued and oral propranolol (20 mg every 6 hours) was added. The study was repeated on day 10. This revealed no echo zone (or PSVT) both before and after 0.5 mg intravenous atropine (Figure 21.2, 3rd and 4th panels).

In summary, the combination of oral digoxin and propranolol totally suppressed the echo phenomenon and paroxysmal tachycardia after atropinization. The patient was then discharged on oral digoxin (0.5 mg) and propranolol (80 mg/day). She has had no PSVT for six months since discharge.

Case 3

This was a 22-year-old male referred to the University of Illinois Hospital because of recurrent paroxysmal ventricular tachycardia for 3 years. Episodes of PVT were associated with severe dizziness and occasional syncope. PVT

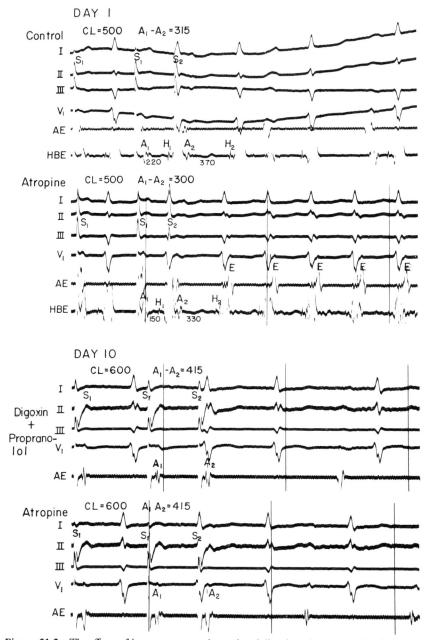

Figure 21.2 The effects of intravenous atropine and oral digoxin and propranolol on induction of PSVT in case two. In each panel, multiple electrocardiograms and atrial electrogram (AE) are shown. In the upper two panels, His bundle electrograms (HBE) are also shown. S_1, A_1 and H_1 are, respectively, the stimulus artifact, atrial and His bundle responses of the driven beats; S_2, A_2 and H_2 are, respectively, the stimulus artifact, atrial and His bundle responses of the test beat.

occurred approximately once a month and had always required therapeutic intervention with either lidocaine administration or cardioversion. Antiarrhythmic therapy with propranolol (up to 160 mg/day) and quinidine (up to 1.2 g/day) failed to prevent PVT. Complete cardiac work-up including echocardiogram, cardiac catheterization and coronary arteriography was normal. Electrocardiograms during sinus rhythm were within normal limits.

Electrophysiological studies are summarized in Table 21.3. Initial studies revealed induction of sustained PVT (PVT lasting longer than 2 minutes) following cessation of rapid atrial pacing at a rate of 150/min. The cycle length of PVT was 370 msec. Attempted conversion with closely coupled single or double ventricular extra-stimulus was unsuccessful. A 100 mg intravenous bolus of lidocaine followed by continuous infusion of 2 mg/min was administered. Spontaneous conversion to sinus rhythm was not noted for the subsequent 20 min. However, the PVT could then be converted easily with timed single ventricular stimulation. Post-lidocaine studies revealed that sustained PVT could still be induced with both rapid atrial or ventricular pacing at a rate of 150/min, and with ventricular extrastimulus technique. The cycle length of the ventricular tachycardia remained 370 msec. Induced PVT could always be converted with timed ventricular stimulation. On day 2, sustained ventricular tachycardia with a cycle length of 360 msec was induced with rapid ventricular pacing at a rate of 160/min and with ventricular extra-stimulus technique (Figure 21.3, 1st and 2nd panels). On this day, PVT could be converted to sinus rhythm with timed ventricular stimulation. After control study, PVT was induced and procaine amide (750 mg) was administered intravenously over 15 min. PVT cycle length lengthened to 480 msec. Spontaneous conversion to sinus rhythm after a prolonged period of PVT was noted. However, this was followed by spontaneous recurrence of sustained ventricular tachycardia following two sinus beats (Figure 21.3, 3rd and 4th panels). The same phenomenon also occurred following conversion with timed ventricular stimulation. Lidocaine (100 mg i.v. bolus) was given and sustained sinus rhythm was restored with timed ventricular stimulation.

On day 3, sustained PVT was induced with ventricular pacing at a rate of 160/min, and was converted to sinus rhythm with timed ventricular stimulation. After control study, sustained PVT was induced and disopyramide phosphate (norpace) 200 mg. i.v. bolus followed by 0.33 mg/min (20 mg/hour)

The driven cycle length (CL) and A_1–A_2 coupling intervals are listed on the top of each panel; A_1–H_1 and A_2–H_2 intervals are listed on the bottom of the upper two panels.

The first panel shows no induction of PSVT at A_1–A_2 of 315 msec (the shortest A_1–A_2 at which A_2 was conducted to the His bundle) on day one before atropine administration. The second panel shows induction of sustained PSVT at A_1–A_2 of 300 msec after 0.5 mg intravenous atropine.

The third and fourth panels show inability to induce PSVT before (third panel) and after (fourth panel) 0.5 mg intravenous atropine on day 10 while the patient was on oral digoxin (0.5 mg/day) and propranolol (80 mg/day)

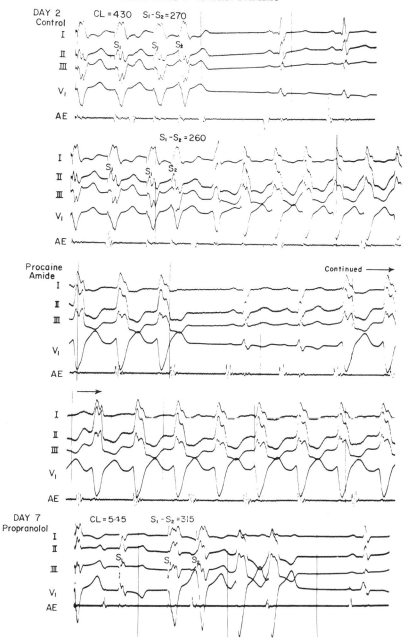

Figure 21.3 The effects of intravenous procaine amide and oral propranolol on induction of paroxysmal ventricular tachycardia (PVT) in case three. Shown are multiple electrocardiographic leads and atrial electrogram (AE). The driven cycle length (CL) and coupling intervals (S_1–S_2) are listed.

The first to fourth panels are studies before (first and second panels) and after (third and fourth

infusion was administered. Thirty minutes after disopyramide, the cycle length of ventricular tachycardia lengthened to 410 msec. Electrical conversion to sinus rhythm with timed ventricular stimulation was again followed by spontaneous recurrence of ventricular tachycardia after two to three sinus beats. Sinus rhythm was restored with timed ventricular stimulation after lidocaine (100 mg i.v. bolus).

On day 4, sustained PVT with a cycle length of 380 msec occurred spontaneously while the patient was being transferred to the electrophysiological laboratory. Attempted electrical conversion with timed ventricular stimulation was unsuccessful. Diphenylhydantoin (350 mg i.v.) was administered over a 5-minute period without change in the cycle length of PVT. However, spontaneous conversion to sinus rhythm was obtained 6 minutes following diphenylhydantoin administration. Post-diphenylhydantoin study revealed induction of sustained PVT with both atrial and ventricular pacing at a rate of 130/min. PVT episodes could always be converted to sinus rhythm with timed ventricular stimulation.

On day 5, sustained PVT with a cycle length of 355 msec was induced with atrial and ventricular pacing at a rate of 150/min, and with ventricular extrastimulus technique. PVT could be terminated with timed ventricular stimulation. After control study, PVT was induced and propranolol (12 mg; 0.1 mg/kg) was administered intravenously over 12 min. The cycle length of ventricular tachycardia lengthened slightly to 380 msec and spontaneous conversion to sinus rhythm was obtained 17 min after propranolol. Post-propranolol study revealed that only non-sustained PVT (20–30 beats of PVT) could be induced with atrial or ventricular pacing at a rate of 130/min and with ventricular extrastimulus technique. Following this the patient was placed on oral propranolol 60 mg every six hours and the study was repeated. On day 7 (240 mg/day of oral propranolol), only non-sustained self-terminating PVT could be induced with rapid ventricular pacing at a rate of 140/min, and with ventricular extrastimulus technique (Figure 21.3, 5th panel). Sustained ventricular tachycardia did not occur. Oral propranolol was then increased to 100 mg every 6 hours and the study was repeated on day 8, with identical results. After this, oral propranolol 400 mg/day was continued, diphenylhydantoin 100 mg every 6 hours was added following a loading dose of 300 mg, and the study repeated on day 9. Self-terminating PVT with a cycle length of 375 msec could still be induced with ventricular pacing at a rate of 140/min,

---

panels) procaine amide on day 2. Note induction of sustained PVT with ventricular extrastimulus at S_1–S_2 coupling interval of 260 msec (CL–430 msec) before procaine amide administration (second panel), and transient spontaneous termination to sinus rhythm with self induction of sustained PVT after two sinus beats following intravenous procaine amide (750 mg) administration (third and fourth panels). The fifth panel shows induction of non-sustained self-terminating PVT with ventricular extrastimulus technique on day 7, while the patient was placed on 240 mg oral propranolol.

Table 21.2 Electrophysiological findings in Case 2

Day	Echoes + PSVT with AP (beats/min)	AEST (msec)		CL of PSVT (msec)	Ability to sustain PSVT
		CL	EZ $(A_1-A_2) - (A_1-A_2)$		
1	Control	no	500	none	(—)	(—)
	Atropine (0.5 mg i.v.)	yes (160)	500	330–230	340	yes
2	Control	yes (200)	600	290–210	340	yes
	Ouabain (0.7 mg i.v.)	yes (160)	600	320–315	(—)	echoes only
3	Control	yes (160)	600	310–290	(—)	echoes only
	Propranolol (5 mg i.v.)	no	600	none	(—)	(—)
9	Digoxin (0.5 mg/day)	no	600	none	(—)	(—)
	Atropine (0.5 mg i.v.)	yes (150)	600	370–300	392	no
	Propranolol (5 mg i.v.)	no	600	none	(—)	(—)
10	Digoxin (0.5 mg/day) + Propranolol (80 mg/day)	no	500	none	(—)	(—)
	Atropine (0.5 mg i.v.)	no	500	none	(—)	(—)

Abbreviations: PSVT = Paroxysmal supraventricular tachycardia; AP = Atrial pacing; AEST = Atrial extra-stimulus technique; CL = Driving cycle length; EZ = Echo zone.

and with ventricular extrastimulus technique. Ability to sustain ventricular tachycardia was not noted.

In summary, lidocaine always potentiated conversion of PVT with timed ventricular stimulation. Procaine amide and disopyramide potentiated PVT induction and made conversion difficult. Intravenous propranolol converted PVT, and prevented sustained PVT induction. Similar results were obtained with oral propranolol 240 and 400 mg/day. Intravenous diphenylhydantoin facilitated electrical conversion with ventricular stimulation. However, oral diphenylhydantoin did not potentiate the effects of oral propranolol. Since oral propranolol in a dose of 240 mg/day prevented induction of sustained PVT, the patient was discharged on this drug regimen. The patient has tolerated the drug well and has been totally free of PVT for 13 months since discharge.

DISCUSSION

Recent electrophysiological studies have suggested that most patients with PSVT and some patients with PVT have re-entrant tachycardia[1-4]. Current concepts of re-entrance suggest that re-entry depends upon unidirectional block of one pathway, with slow conduction in a second pathway, allowing the recovery of the previously blocked pathway for re-excitation[11-17]. When sustained re-entrance occur, paroxysmal tachycardia results. In the cardiac catheterization laboratory, re-entrant paroxysmal tachycardia can frequently be reproduced with: (1) critically timed atrial or ventricular extrastimuli with definition of an echo zone; (2) following sudden cessation of rapid atrial or ventricular pacing at critical pacing rates[1-4,18-19]. Termination of paroxysmal tachycardia can frequently be obtained with critically timed single or double atrial or ventricular extrastimuli. Ability to reproduce and terminate paroxysmal tachycardia in the catheterization laboratory has provided a means of studying mechanisms of tachycardia, as well as the effects of antiarrhythmic drugs.

Paroxysmal supraventricular tachycardia

Re-entrant paroxysmal supraventricular tachycardia can occur in the sinus node[20-21], atria[21], AV node[1,2,8,18], and between the AV node–His bundle pathway and a manifest or concealed accessory pathway (Kent bundle)[5-7,22]. Recent electrophysiological studies have demonstrated that antiarrhythmic agents effective in one type of arrhythmia may enhance or potentiate other types of arrhythmias[2,8]. In addition, with the same type of arrhythmia, a given antiarrhythmic agent might be effective in one patient, and ineffective or even deleterious in another patient[2,8]. If electrophysiological studies in the catheterization laboratory could reflect the effects of chronic drug administration, these studies would facilitate management of patients with troublesome paroxysmal tachycardia.

In case one of the present study, a patient with AV nodal re-entrant PSVT, a

Table 21.3 Electrophysiological findings in Case 3

Day	Blood level	VT induction with VP (beats/min)	VEST CL	VEST ZI (V₁−V₂)−(V₁−V₂)	CL of VT (msec)	Termination of VT with VEST	Spontaneous termination of VT after drug	Ability to sustain VT
1 Control Lidocaine (100 mg bolus + 2 mg/min)	(—)	yes (150)	(—)	(—)	370	no	(—)	yes
2 Control	(—)	yes (150)	600	250–220	370	yes	no	yes
Procaine amide (750 mg i.v.)	0	yes (160)	430	260–195	360	yes	(—)	yes
2.6 μg/ml (5 min) 4.5 μg/ml (10 min) 9.75 μg/ml (15 min)		(—)	(—)	(—)	480	no	yes	yes
3 Lidocaine (100 mg i.v.)	(—)	(—)	(—)	(—)	415	yes	no	yes
Control	0	yes (160)	430	0	370	yes	(—)	yes
Disopyramide phosphate (240 mg bolus + 0.33 mg/min) 2.75 μg/ml (30 ml)		(—)	(—)	(—)	410	no	no	yes
Lidocaine (100 mg bolus)	(—)	(—)	(—)	(—)	385	yes	no	yes

#	Drug (dose)	0	spontaneous induction						
4	Control		yes (130)	(—)	(—)	380	no	(—)	yes
	Diphenyl-hydantoin (350 mg i.v.)	6.2 µg/ml (5 min) 4 µg/ml (7 ml)				375	yes	yes	yes
5	Control		yes (150)	600	270–230	355	yes	(—)	yes
	Prcpranolol (12 mg i.v.)	(—)	yes (130)	600	510–380	380		yes	no
7	Prcpranolol (240 mg/day)	173 ng/ml	yes (140)	545	420–300	370		(—)	no
8	Propranolol (400 mg/day)	338 ng/m	yes (140)	545	410–260	360		(—)	no
9	Propranolol (400 mg/day) + Diphenyl-hydantoin (400 mg/day)	173 ng/m 2.2 µg/ml	yes (140)	545	350–290	375		(—)	no

Abbreviations: VT = Ventricular tachycardia; VP = Ventricular pacing; VEST = Ventricular extrastimulus technique; CL = Cycle length; ZI = Zone of VT induction.

discrepancy of acute ouabain effects and chronic digoxin administration at a dose of 0.25 mg/day existed. However, with subsequent studies at higher doses of oral digoxin, it became apparent that the discrepancy was due to an inadequate blood level at a digoxin dose of 0.5 mg/day or less. At a digoxin dose of 0.75 mg/day, digoxin effectively abolished the echo zone and the ability to sustain PSVT. Follow-up study in this patient demonstrated that electrophysiological study in the catheterization laboratory reflected the response to chronic drug administration. In this patient, it could be argued that the final dose of digoxin utilized could have been achieved by measuring serum levels alone. However, chronic electrophysiological demonstration of effectiveness of 0.75 mg/day of oral digoxin eliminated a prolonged period of trial and error in determining the optimum therapeutic dose.

In case two of the present study, a patient also with AV nodal re-entrant PSVT, the ability to induce and sustain PSVT varied from day to day, suggesting that autonomic tone influenced the functional properties of the re-entrant pathways. However, PSVT could always be induced after atropine, suggesting that vagolysis facilitated PSVT induction[23]. In this patient, who responded to intravenous and oral combined therapy with digoxin and propranolol, prospective follow-up study demonstrated that electrophysiological studies in the catheterization laboratory could reflect the response to chronic drug administration.

Both cases one and two are consistent with our recent studies regarding effects of propranolol and ouabain on the induction of AV nodal re-entrant PSVT, and with the study of Wellens et al. on the effect of digitalis in patients with PSVT[2,8,9].

Ventricular tachycardia

Re-entrant ventricular tachycardia can presumably occur in the bundle branches or fascicles (macro-re-entrance), distal His–Purkinje tissues, or ventricular muscle (micro-re-entrance), and perhaps around a ventricular aneurysm[3,4,24]. Antiarrhythmic agents which change the critical relationships of refractory periods and conduction times in the re-entrant circuit may affect the ability to initiate or sustain ventricular tachycardia. It is likely that antiarrhythmic agents which suppress tachycardia in some patients may enhance or potentiate the tachycardia in other patients, and that in the same patient, some agents may be beneficial, while other agents, deleterious. Case 3 of the present study represents such a case. It should be noted that in this patient, both procaine amide and disopyramide potentiated tachycardia induction and made conversion difficult. Both drugs predisposed to spontaneous induction of tachycardia during sinus rhythm. These effects are best explained by postulating that both procaine amide and disopyramide phosphate increase the refractory period of an area of unidirectional block, and delayed conduction times allowing development of sustained ventricular tachycardia during sinus rhythm[25,26]. In this patient, lidocaine, diphenylhydantoin and propranolol facilitated conversion of tachycardia and/or suppressed the ability to sustain tachycardia. Lidocaine and diphenylhydantoin could shorten refractory periods of an area of unidirectional block, and enhance conduction times in the re-entrant circuit, resulting in changes in the critical relationships making sustained re-entrance impossible[27,28]. Propranolol could change the critical relationships of the re-entrant circuit via β-blocking action and/or quinidine-like effect, making sustained re-entrance impossible[29]. Follow-up study in this patient demonstrated that electrophysiological study in the catheterization laboratory correlated well with subsequent drug response.

Clinical implications

This study is not a systematic study of mechanisms of either PSVT or PVT, since it is concerned with only two PSVT patients and one PVT patient. No generalizations should be drawn regarding the effectiveness of specific antiarrhythmic agents in regard to management of other patients with similar arrhythmias. The study does suggest that paradoxical responses to antiarrhythmic agents can be expected.

The present study presents a new method for studying the effects of antiarrhythmic agents in patients with recurrent paroxysmal tachycardia. We have demonstrated that electrophysiological studies in the catheterization laboratory can predict the development of rational therapeutic programs and should be useful in patients with troublesome arrhythmias that are reproducible in the catheterization laboratory. The use of daily arrhythmia induction, with single and combined drug administration, can obviate the necessity for prolonged periods of trial and error in attempting to achieve satisfactory control of refractory recurrent sporadic paroxysmal tachycardias. The method should also allow delineation of a group of patients refractory to all drug management, who are thus candidates for sophisticated electrical modalities of therapy or surgical intervention[30,31].

References

1. Bigger, J. T. and Goldreyer, B. N. (1970). The mechanism of supraventricular tachycardia. *Circulation*, **42**, 673
2. Wu, D., Denes, P., Dhingra, R. C., Khan, A. and Rosen, K. M. (1974). The effects of propranolol on induction of AV nodal re-entrant paroxysmal tachycardia. *Circulation*, **50**, 665
3. Wellens, J. H., Schuilenburg, R. M. and Durrer, D. (1972). Electrical stimulation of the heart in patients with ventricular tachycardia. *Circulation*, **46**, 216
4. Spurrell, R. A. J., Sowton, E. and Deuchar, D. C. (1973). Ventricular tachycardia in four patients evaluated by programmed electrical stimulation of the heart and treated in two patients by surgical division of the anterior radiation of the left bundle branch. *Br. Heart J.*, **35**, 1014

5. Rosen, K. M., Barwolf, C., Ehsani, A. and Rahimtoola, S. H. (1972). Effect of lidocaine and propranolol on the normal and anomalous pathways in patients with pre-excitation. *Am. J. Cardiol*, **30**, 801

6. Wellens, H. J. and Durrer, D. (1974). The effect of procaine amide, quinidine gluconate and ajmaline in the Wolff–Parkinson–White syndrome. *Circulation*, **50**, 114

7. Wellens, H. J. and Durrer, D. (1973). Effect of digitalis on atrioventricular conduction and circus movement tachycardias in patients with the Wolff–Parkinson–White syndrome. *Circulation*, **47**, 1229

8. Wu, D., Wyndham, C., Amat-y-Leon, F., Denes, P., Dhingra, R. C. and Rosen, K. M. (1975). The effects of ouabain on induction of atrioventricular nodal re-entrant paroxysmal supraventricular tachycardia. *Circulation*, **52**, 201

9. Wellens, J. H., Duren, D. R., Liem, K. L. and Lie, K. I. (1975). Effect of digitalis in patients with paroxysmal atrioventricular nodal tachycardia. *Circulation*, **52**, 779

10. Scherlag, B. J., Lau, S. H., Helfant, R. H., Stein, E., Berkowitz, W. S. and Damato, A. N. (1969). Catheter technique for recording His bundle activity in man. *Circulation*, **39**, 13

11. Moe, G. K., Preston, J. B. and Burlington, H. (1956). Physiologic evidence for a dual AV transmission system. *Circ. Res.*, **4**, 357

12. Mendez, C. and Moe, G. K. (1966). Demonstration of a dual AV nodal conduction system in the isolated rabbit heart. *Circ. Res.*, **19**, 378

13. Denes, P., Wu, D., Dhingra, R., Chuquimia, R. and Rosen, K. M. (1973). Demonstration of dual AV nodal pathways in patients with paroxysmal supraventricular tachycardia. *Circulation*, **48**, 549

14. Wu, D., Denes, P., Dhingra, R. C., Wyndham, C. and Rosen, K. M. (1975). Determinants of fast and slow pathway conduction in patients with dual AV nodal pathways. *Circ. Res.*, **36**, 782

15. Wu, D., Denes, P., Wyndham, C., Amat-y-Leon, F., Dhingra, R. C. and Rosen, K. M. (1975). Demonstration of dual atrioventricular nodal pathways utilizing a ventricular extrastimulus in patients with atrioventricular nodal re-entrant paroxysmal supraventricular tachycardia. *Circulation*, **52**, 789

16. Cranefield, P. F., Wit, A. L. and Hoffman, B. F. (1973). Genesis of cardiac arrhythmias. *Circulation*, **47**, 190

17. Wit, A. L., Hoffman, B. F. and Cranefield, P. F. (1972). Slow conduction and re-entry in the ventricular conduction system. I. Return extra-systole in canine Purkinje fibres. *Circ. Res.*, **30**, 1

18. Goldreyer, B. N. and Bigger, J. T. (1971). Site of reentry in paroxysmal supraventricular tachycardia in man. *Circulation*, **43**, 15

19. Goldreyer, B. N. and Damato, A. N. (1971). The essential role of atrioventricular conduction delay in the initiation of paroxysmal supraventricular tachycardia. *Circulation*, **43**, 679

20. Narula, O. S. (1974). Sinus node reentry: a mechanism for supraventricular tachycardia in man. *Circulation*, **50**, 1114

21. Wu, D., Amat-y-Leon, F., Denes, P., Dhingra, R. C., Pietras, R. J. and Rosen, K. M. (1975). Demonstration of sustained sinus and atrial re-entry as a mechanism of paroxysmal supraventricular tachycardia. *Circulation*, **51**, 234

22. Zipes, D. P., De Joseph, R. L. and Rothbaum, D. A. (1974). Unusual properties of accessory pathways. *Circulation*, **49**, 1200

23. Akhtar, M., Damato, A. N., Batsford, W. P., Caracta, A. R., Ruskin, J. N., Weisfogel, G. M. and Lau, S. H. (1975). Induction of atrioventricular reentrant tachycardia after atropine. *Am. J. Cardiol.*, **36**, 286

24. Akhtar, M., Damato, A. N., Batsford, W. P., Ruskin, J. N., Ogunkeln, B. and Vargas, G. (1974). Demonstration of re-entry within the His–Purkinje system in man. *Circulation*, **50**, 1150

25. Rosen, M. R., Gelband, H. and Hoffman, B. F. (1972). Canine electrocardiographic and cardiac electrophysiologic changes induced by procaine amide. *Circulation*, **46**, 528

26. Yeh, K. B., Sung, P. K. and Scherlag, B. J. (1973). Effects of disopyramide on electrophysiological and mechanical properties of the heart. *J. Pharm. Sci.*, **62**, 1924

27. Davis, L. D. and Temte, J. V. (1969). Electrophysiological actions of lidocaine on canine ventricular muscle and Purkinje fibres. *Circ. Res.*, **24**, 639

28. Bigger, J., Jr., Bassett, A. and Hoffman, B. (1968). Electrophysiological effects of diphenylhydantoin on canine Purkinje fibres. *Circ. Res.*, **22**, 221

29. Wit, A. L., Hoffman, B. F. and Rosen, M. R. (1975). Electrophysiology and pharmacology of cardiac arrhythmias. IX. Cardiac electrophysiologic effects of β-adrenergic receptor stimulation and blockade. Part B. *Am. Heart J.*, **90**, 665

30. Goyal, S. L., Lichstein, E., Gupta, P. K. and Chadda, K. D. (1975). Refractory reentrant atrial tachycardia: Successful treatment with a permanent radio frequency triggered atrial pacemaker. *Am. J. Med.*, **58**, 586

31. Fontaine, G., Guiraudon, G., Frank, R., Gerbaux, A., Costeau, J., Barillon, A., Gay, J., Cabrol, C. and Facquet, J. (1975). La cartographie épicardique et le traitement chirurgical par simple ventriculotomie de certaines tachycardies ventriculaires rebelles par réentrée. *Arch. Mal. Coeur Vaiss.*, **2**, 113

22
Effects of Various Drugs on Ventricular Conduction Delay and Ventricular Arrhythmias during Myocardial Ischaemia in the Dog

D. P. ZIPES, V. ELHARRAR, R. J. NOBLE, W. E. GAUM,
P. J. TROUP and A. FASOLA

*Krannert Institute of Cardiology, Department of Medicine,
Department of Pharmacology, Indiana University School of Medicine,
and the Veterans' Administration Hospital, Indianapolis, Indiana*

Delayed activation of the ischaemic myocardium has been noted by many investigators[1,2] and, in recent studies[3-6], attempts have been made to quantify the extent of conduction delay and correlate it with the incidence of ventricular tachyarrhythmias which occurred at the time of coronary artery occlusion. It was found that drugs which increased the extent of conduction delay produced by myocardial ischaemia either had no effect on the incidence or time to onset of ventricular arrhythmias[7], or could actually be associated with a reduction in the number of ventricular extrasystoles[6]. Since conduction delay has an important influence on the genesis of arrhythmias[8,9], we felt that the results of these studies might reflect the effect of drugs which only minimally altered the extent of conduction delay and that other possible antiarrhythmic effects of these drugs could counterbalance the slight increase in conduction delay which they produced. Therefore, we performed similar studies, using drugs which we found to alter dramatically the extent of ischaemia-induced conduction delay. Drugs tested included quinidine and aprindine, a new antiarrhythmic agent, and, because the electrophysiologic changes resulting from myocardial ischaemia appear conducive to generation of the 'slow response'[9-11] we evaluated the effects of verapamil and isoproterenol on myocardial conduction during ischaemia.

To eliminate the effects of anaesthesia and open-chest conditions, we also performed additional studies in closed-chest dogs receiving oral doses of aprindine, and in another group of closed-chest dogs given i.v. aprindine immediately after and 24 hours after LAD occlusion.

Methods

Open-chest studies

Mongrel dogs weighing 10–25 kg were anaesthetized with sodium secobarbital (30 mg/kg i.v.). Following intubation and ventilation with a Harvard respirator, a left lateral thoracotomy was performed and the heart was cradled in the pericardium. A heating blanket was used to maintain normothermia. Fluid losses incurred during the experiment were replaced by infusing lactate Ringer's solution (200 ml/h) into an external jugular vein. The blood pressure was monitored with a catheter inserted into the carotid artery and connected to a Statham 23BD strain gauge transducer.

Acute myocardial ischaemia was produced by one-stage, complete occlusion of the left anterior descending coronary artery (LAD), 2–3 cm distal to its origin, using a non-traumatic arterial clamp or an umbilical tape. Dogs were subjected to three ischaemic episodes of 6 min duration each and allowed to recover for 30 min in between ligations.

Multipolar plaque electrodes were sutured on the epicardium of a normal zone (NZ) not affected by myocardial ischaemia and on the epicardium of the potentially ischaemic zone (IZ). NZ was located at the base of the right ventricle and IZ was located at the bifurcation of the LAD and its first diagonal branch. Plunge electrodes were used to record endocardial activity of the ischaemic zone, at a site directly beneath the IZ epicardial recording electrode. Bipolar electrograms from IZ and NZ were amplified (Electronics for Medicine DR 8), filtered (40–500 Hz) and displayed on a memory oscilloscope (Tektronix D11) along with a lead II electrocardiogram at a sweep speed of 20 msec/div. Data were also recorded on a 4-channel FM tape recorder (Hewlett Packard) for later replay and analysis. The time interval from the onset of the major deflection of the bipolar electrogram (Q–Eg interval) recorded from IZ and NZ was measured.

The sinus node was crushed and the atrium was paced at a cycle length (CL) of 500 msec. To study the effect of heart rate on the Q–Eg intervals during myocardial ischaemia, the atrium was paced at a CL of 500 msec for 5 min, and then the CL was decreased from 500 to 400 msec for 30 sec and then to 300 msec for an additional 30 sec. At this point, the coronary occlusion was released and atrial pacing again resumed at a CL of 500 msec. If ventricular fibrillation occurred, the heart was defibrillated within 10–15 sec with a 5–10 watt-second DC shock (American Optical Company).

The effect of the following drugs on ischaemia-induced conduction delay was determined: aprindine* (2.85 mg/kg, $n = 11$ dogs); quinidine (8 mg/kg $n = 8$ dogs); verapamil† (0.2 mg/kg, $n = 8$ dogs) and isoproterenol (0.2 μg/kg/min, $n = 7$ dogs). Aprindine, quinidine and verapamil were each administered in eight equally divided doses over a period of 15 min. Drug administration was completed 6 min before the second period of LAD occlusion was begun.

The following two exceptions to the above protocol were made to accommodate the specific effects of verapamil and isoproterenol. Because the negative dromotropic effect of verapamil on atrio–ventricular (A–V) conduction might have prevented 1:1 A–V transmission to the ventricles while driving the atrium at rapid rates[12], dogs included in the verapamil group were paced from the base of the right ventricle through the multipolar plaque electrode sewn in the NZ. The second exception dealt with the isoproterenol group. Infusion (i.v.) of isoproterenol was begun 5 min before the second period of LAD occlusion and maintained until the occlusion was released. Moreover, in this group, the atrium was paced at a CL of 300 msec throughout the entire 6 min of LAD occlusion.

Closed chest studies—oral aprindine

Through a lateral thoracotomy, a balloon occluder was placed around the LAD and an atrial pacing electrode was sewn on the right atrial epicardium in ten dogs. One week after they recovered from surgery, the dogs were sedated with morphine (1.5 mg/kg) and valium (1.0 mg/kg). The balloon was inflated and the atrium was paced at a CL of 500 msec for 5 min, and then the CL was decreased from 500 to 400 msec for 30 sec and then to 300 msec for an additional 30 sec. At this point, atrial pacing was stopped, the balloon deflated and the animal allowed to recover. ST segment elevation in a V_5 lead confirmed the presence of acute ischaemia during balloon inflation. These studies were done in the same dogs before aprindine administration, after administering aprindine 5.6, 4.2, 2.8, 1.4 and 1.4 mg/kg on consecutive days, and again after administering 7.5 mg/kg daily for five days. If ventricular fibrillation developed, the balloon was deflated, atrial pacing stopped, and the animal rapidly defibrillated (Malkin Instrument Co.).

Closed chest studies—i.v. aprindine

A separate group of seven dogs was subjected to a 15 min balloon occlusion of the LAD while pacing the right atrium at a CL of 500 msec for the first 14 min then at a CL of 400 msec for 30 sec, and then at a CL of 300 msec for 30 sec. A control occlusion was performed without aprindine administration. The

* Generously supplied by Eli Lilly Company
† Generously supplied by Knoll Pharmaceutical Company

balloon was then deflated and the animal allowed to recover. Twenty-four hours later, the 15 min LAD occlusion was repeated and aprindine (2.85 mg/kg) was administered intravenously over a 5 min period beginning just *after* occluding the LAD. The balloon was deflated and the animal allowed to recover. Finally, 1 week later in this same group of dogs, the LAD was occluded for 24 hours and aprindine (2.85 mg/kg) was administered intravenously at that time. The spontaneous cardiac rhythm was recorded for 1 hour before and 1 hour after administering the drug and the number of ventricular extrasystoles in each 15 min interval was counted.

RESULTS

Open chest studies—control values

The typical changes in electrogram amplitude, duration and activation time following coronary occlusion are illustrated in Figure 22.1 which was obtained from one dog. No changes occurred in the electrogram recorded from the normal zone. However, loss of amplitude, increased duration and delayed activation in relation to the onset of the QRS complex were usual findings in the electrogram recorded from the epicardial ischaemic zone. The delay in activation of the ischaemic zone (ΔQ–IZ) was usually manifest after 2–3 min of LAD occlusion and progressed with time. Under these specific conditions, i.e., 5 min after LAD occlusion while pacing the atrium at a cycle length of 500 msec, the mean ΔQ–IZ in 27 dogs (excluding the isoproterenol treated group) was 19 msec. Conduction delays observed at the endocardial IZ were generally much less marked than those observed at the epicardium, and averaged only 5 msec.

Decreasing the cycle length to 400 and 300 msec resulted in more marked delay in activation of the ischaemic zone (Figure 22.1). Moreover, loss of any discernible deflection, despite high amplification, occurred commonly at these shorter cycle lengths and prevented measurement of Q–IZ time interval. Faster heart rates were also associated with the development of various degrees of block at the recording site and ventricular arrhythmias, which included premature ventricular extrasystoles, ventricular tachycardia and ventricular fibrillation. Seven of 27 dogs exhibited these ventricular arrhythmias during the control ligation, but only two did so during the first 5 min while pacing at a CL of 500 msec.

Open-chest studies—effects of drug pretreatment on ΔQ–IZ and incidence of arrhythmias

Figure 22.2 shows the effect of aprindine on conduction delay observed after 6 min of LAD ligation after pacing at a CL of 500 msec for 5 min, at a CL of 400 msec for 30 sec and then at a CL of 300 msec for 30 sec. Figure 22.2 also illustrates the difficulties in measuring conduction delay at this CL. In the left

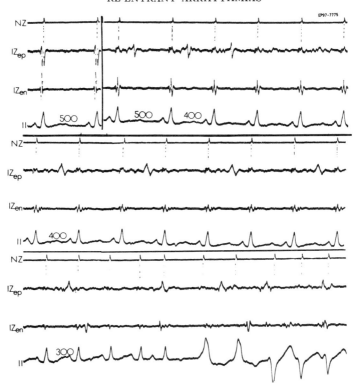

Figure 22.1 Precipitation of ventricular tachycardia in a dog following a 5 min occlusion of the left anterior descending coronary artery. Right atrial pacing at progressively shorter cycle lengths results in increasing conduction delay and block in the ischaemic zone, as recorded with epicardial (IZ_{ep}) and plunge endocardial (IZ_{en}) electrodes. Top left panel, control; top right panel, shortening cycle length from 500 to 400 msec following occlusion; middle panel, after pacing for 30 sec at a cycle length of 400 msec; bottom panel, after just starting to pace at a cycle length of 300 msec. A premature atrial depolarization is followed by the emergence of ventricular tachycardia which progressed to ventricular fibrillation. Electrogram recorded in the normal zone (NZ) shows no change. Time lines, 1 sec; paper speed, 100 mm/sec; numbers in msec; right atrial electrogram not shown. (From D. P. Zipes (1975). *Circulation*, **51–52**, 120, reproduced by permission of the American Heart Association)

panel are shown the control recordings (prior to LAD ligation), before (upper panel) and after (middle and lower panels) aprindine administration. The same recordings following 6 min of LAD occlusion are shown on the right. Prior to aprindine administration, ischaemia flattened the epicardial electrogram recorded at IZ_{ep} and delayed its activation; the endocardial IZ was also delayed, but less so; no change was seen in the NZ (top right panel). Repeat ligation of the LAD, begun 6 min after aprindine was administered (middle right panel), delayed further the activation at IZ_{ep} and IZ_{en}; both electrograms flattened, particularly IZ_{en} and accurate measurement of the extent of the conduction delay became impossible. Thus, aprindine increased ischaemia-induced

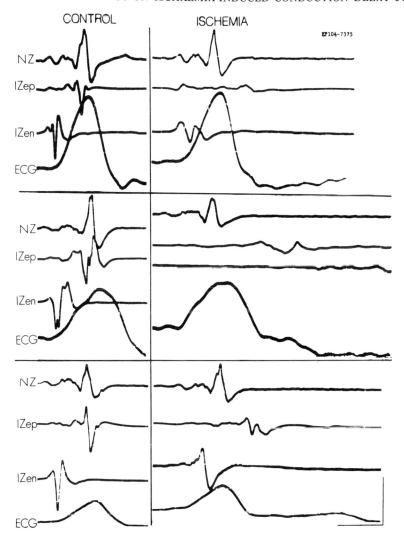

Figure 22.2 Effect of aprindine on conduction delay produced by a 6 min occlusion of the LAD after pacing at a cycle length of 500 msec for 5 min, 400 msec for 30 sec and 300 msec for 30 sec. NZ, IZ_{ep} and IZ_{en} are, respectively, bipolar electrograms recorded from the epicardium of a normal zone and the ischaemic zone and from the endocardium of the ischaemic zone. Left and right panels were obtained prior to and after 6 min of coronary occlusion, before (top panels), 12 min after (middle panels) and 48 min after (lower panels) aprindine administration (2.85 mg/kg). Note that the 6 min LAD occlusion, 12 min after aprindine administration, produced an increased degree of conduction delay when compared to before or 48 min after aprindine administration. Calibrations: Horizontal bar: 40 msec; vertical bar: 0.5 V for NZ; 1.0 V for IZ_{ep} in middle right panel, 5.0 V in lower left panel and 2.0 V in remainder; 1.0 V for IZ_{en} in left panels, 0.5 V in right panels; 0.2 V for ECG in top and middle panels, 0.5 V in bottom panels

conduction delay in this example more markedly at IZ_{en} than at IZ_{en} 12 min after drug administration. Forty-eight minutes after aprindine was administered, a third LAD ligation produced conduction delay comparable to that obtained before aprindine administration (bottom right panel). In this dog, ventricular arrhythmias did not occur when the atrial CL was decreased to 400 and 300 msec during the control occlusion or at 48 min after aprindine administration, whereas ventricular fibrillation occurred during the second LAD occlusion immediately after recording the middle right panel, while pacing at a CL of 300 msec.

Aprindine-induced ventricular fibrillation occurred in a fashion similar to that produced by ischaemia alone, and probably represents an intensification of the ischaemia-produced conduction delay. The onset of ventricular tachycardia and fibrillation began without premature ventricular extrasystoles occurring during the vulnerable period. As seen in Figure 22.3, displayed in a fashion similar to Figure 22.1, LAD occlusion following aprindine administration resulted in progressive fractionation of the electrogram recorded in the ischaemic zone, culminating in the onset of ventricular tachycardia which progressed to ventricular fibrillation.

The effects of cycle length on aprindine-induced conduction delay following LAD occlusion can be seen more dramatically by analysis of single cycles at

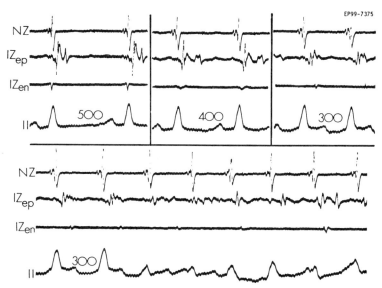

Figure 22.3 Progressive delayed activation of the ischaemic zone epicardium and endocardium produced by occlusion of the LAD after administration of aprindine. Right atrial pacing at a cycle length of 500 msec for 5 min (top left panel), then 400 msec for 30 sec (top middle panel), then 300 msec for 30 sec (top right and lower panels). Note progressive delay and fractionation of conduction as the cycle length is shortened, with the subsequent development of ventricular tachycardia that progressed to ventricular fibrillation. Conventions as in Figure 22.1

rapid sweep speeds (Figure 22.4). After 5 min of LAD occlusion (top panel), the epicardial electrogram (IZ$_{ep}$) recorded from ischaemic zone exhibited conduction delay and fragmentation with little change in the electrogram recorded from the endocardium (IZ$_{en}$) directly beneath it. Shortening the atrial pacing cycle length to 400 msec and 300 msec intensified the conduction delay and fractionation at both IZ$_{ep}$ and IZ$_{en}$. In dogs which developed ventricular tachycardia prior to developing ventricular fibrillation, stopping atrial pacing prevented the subsequent development of ventricular fibrillation (Figure 22.5).

Verapamil pretreatment reduced the extent of conduction delay following LAD occlusion and prevented ischaemia-induced fractionation of the electrogram. Quinidine and isoproterenol had very little effect on the degree of conduction delay produced by ischaemia alone, and in the dogs that developed ventricular tachycardia or ventricular fibrillation, progressive conduction delay in the ischaemic zone was no different from the conduction delay which occurred before drug administration.

Aprindine prolonged ΔQ–IZ from a mean value of 11.5 msec to a mean value of 30.5 msec ($p < 0.05$, paired analysis) whereas verapamil decreased ΔQ–IZ from a mean value of 21 to 10 msec ($p < 0.05$). Pretreatment with isoproterenol or quinidine did not significantly alter the conduction delay produced by myocardial ischaemia. Values returned toward control at 47–48 min after drug administration. Aprindine increased the incidence of ventricular tachycardia or ventricular fibrillation (VT–VF) from 1/11 to 8/11. In the quinidine group, two out of eight dogs developed ventricular fibrillation prior to quinidine administration, and these same dogs fibrillated after quinidine administration. Verapamil pretreatment reduced the incidence of VT–VF from 3/8 to 0/8. In the isoproterenol group, 2/7 dogs had VT–VF during the control ischaemic period, and these same dogs plus a third developed VT–VF during the second LAD occlusion while infusing isoproterenol.

The same dog(s) which developed VT–VF before drug administration did so 47–48 min after drug administration for all four drugs with the following exceptions: one verapamil treated dog which had VT–VF before drug administration did not develop VT–VF at 47–48 min after drug administration and one isoproterenol treated dog which developed VT–VF during treatment also developed VT–VF 47–48 min after treatment.

Closed chest studies—oral aprindine

None of the 10 dogs developed ventricular tachycardia or ventricular fibrillation during balloon occlusion of the LAD prior to aprindine administration. However, following the decremental dosing schedule of aprindine orally on consecutive days, 1/10 dogs developed ventricular fibrillation after LAD occlusion and was defibrillated. When aprindine was given orally at a dose of 7.5 mg/kg daily for 5 days, 4/10 dogs developed ventricular fibrillation after balloon occlusion of the LAD on the fifth day.

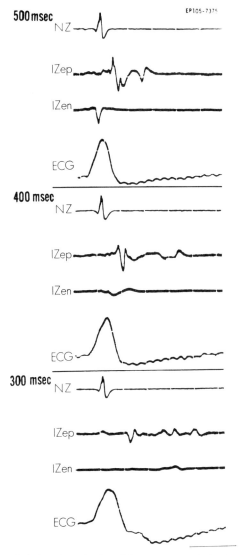

Figure 22.4 Ischaemia-induced conduction delay at progressively shorter right atrial cycle lengths after aprindine administration. Conventions as in Figure 22.1. Calibration: Horizontal bar: 100 msec

Closed chest studies—IV aprindine

During the initial control occlusion, 1/7 dogs developed ventricular fibrillation, and could not be resuscitated; one dog developed ventricular tachycardia that terminated spontaneously. When aprindine was given *after* the LAD occlusion to this group of dogs, 1/6 dogs developed ventricular fibrillation. This was the

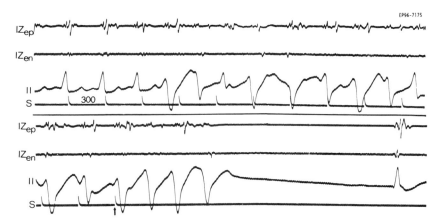

Figure 22.5 Precipitation and termination of ventricular tachycardia, following a 6 min LAD occlusion, after aprindine administration. Five seconds after beginning right atrial pacing at a cycle length of 300 msec the epicardial (IZ_{ep}) and endocardial (IZ_{en}) electrograms recorded from left ventricular ischaemic zone became markedly fragmented, indicating conduction delay and block at this site. Following cessation of right atrial pacing (arrow, lower panel) ventricular tachycardia persisted briefly and then spontaneously terminated. Note decreased fragmentation and increased amplitude in the electrograms of the AV junctional escape beat. Continuous recording; paper speed 100 mm/sec; numbers in msec

same dog which had developed ventricular tachycardia during the control occlusion and the dog could not be resuscitated. Two dogs developed ventricular fibrillation during the 24-hour occlusion and could not be resuscitated. In the remaining three survivors given aprindine 24 hours after LAD occlusion, all dogs exhibited a marked reduction in the number of ventricular extrasystoles (Figure 22.6), particularly in the first 30 min after aprindine administration.

Thus, the preliminary data from the closed chest studies suggest that a sufficiently high oral dose of aprindine administered *prior* to LAD occlusion increased the incidence of ventricular fibrillation following coronary occlusion, that aprindine given immediately *after* LAD occlusion did not increase the in-

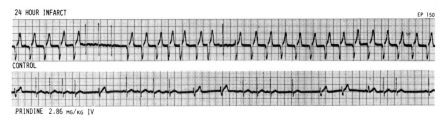

Figure 22.6 Effect of aprindine on ventricular arrhythmias 24 hours following LAD occlusion. (top) representative tracing prior to aprindine administration; (bottom) representative tracing following aprindine administration

cidence of ventricular fibrillation resulting from coronary occlusion and that aprindine given 24 hours after LAD occlusion exerted marked antiarrhythmic effects.

DISCUSSION

Although various changes in the ventricular electrogram during myocardial ischaemia have long been studied[1,2], it is only recently that several investigators[3-6] have attempted to relate the extent of conduction delay recorded in the subepicardial electrogram with the development of early ventricular arrhythmias that follow coronary occlusion. The marked delay in activation time recorded in the subepicardium of the IZ and/or the persistence of electrical activity beyond the T wave of the electrocardiogram provides suggestive evidence implicating a re-entrant mechanism as the basis of these early arrhythmias[5,8-10]. This is reinforced by the finding that ventricular automaticity does not appear to be enhanced early after coronary occlusion[13].

If a relationship actually exists between the extent of conduction delay and the incidence of ventricular arrhythmias, one might expect that drugs which increase the degree of conduction delay should also increase the incidence of VT–VF while drugs which decrease the degree of conduction delay should decrease the incidence of VT–VF. However, Hope et al.[7], in documenting the effects of lidocaine, procaine amide and propranolol on ischaemia-induced conduction delay and ventricular arrhythmias, found that lidocaine hastened the time course of conduction delay in the IZ and reduced, although not significantly, the time to onset of ventricular arrhythmias. Procaine amide and propranolol minimally increased the extent of conduction delay but did not affect the incidence of ventricular arrhythmias. Kupersmith et al. examined the effects of lidocaine[14] propranolol[6] and verapamil[15] during acute myocardial ischaemia and reported that all three drugs slowed intraventricular conduction only in the ischaemic myocardium. However, while lidocaine and propranolol reduced the incidence of arrhythmias, verapamil had no such antiarrhythmic effect.

Our present study has demonstrated that both aprindine and verapamil markedly alter the extent of ischaemia-induced conduction delay. Moreover, it was shown that prolongation of the ΔQ—IZ interval was associated with an increased incidence of ventricular arrhythmias, whereas a decrease in the ΔQ–IZ interval was associated with decreased incidence of ventricular arrhythmias. Quinidine and isoproterenol, which did not significantly alter the ΔQ–IZ interval, had no effect on the incidence of ventricular arrhythmias.

Thus, our data differ from the previously reported studies in that we found a direct relationship between a drug intervention which markedly increased (aprindine) or decreased (verapamil) the extent of ischaemia-induced conduction delay and the incidence of VT–VF. Drugs which only minimally increased the degree of conduction delay (isoproterenol, quinidine) did not alter the incidence of ventricular arrhythmias.

The discrepancy between our data and the other reports may be explained by the magnitude of the conduction delay changes produced by aprindine and verapamil. It is probable that antiarrhythmic agents exert diverse actions on the ischaemic myocardium and that some of these actions may be 'arrhythmogenic', e.g. increasing the amount of conduction delay and other effects may be 'antiarrhythmic', e.g. equalizing action potential and refractory period durations between ischaemic and non-ischaemic tissue. The effect on the incidence of ventricular arrhythmias will depend on whether antiarrhythmic or arrhythmogenic factors predominate. Therefore, drugs which *markedly* lengthen or shorten the degree of conduction delay may have this factor predominate and thus affect the development of VT–VF.

Conduction delay in the ischaemic or infarcted myocardium may influence the development of arrhythmias by creasing an island of asynchronous activation in which all elements cannot conduct uniformly. In this study, we precipitated ventricular arrhythmias by rapid pacing which results in an increased degree of ischaemia, more conduction delay, and very likely prevents each of the elements in the ischaemic or infarcted area from being able to conduct in a 1 : 1 response to each stimulus. This factor probably creates areas of block and thus sets the stage for the development of re-entrant arrhythmias. It is of interest that less conduction delay occurred at the endocardial surface of the myocardium than at the epicardial surface. Such heterogeneity may contribute further to the genesis of ventricular arrhythmias and may be explained by the presence of viable Purkinje fibres and a viable inner shell of endocardium, nourished by the effects of cavity blood[16,17], which help preserve near normal endocardial conduction acutely.

In considering the effects of an antiarrhythmic agent on re-entrant arrhythmias, it has been suggested that a drug which creates unidirectional block may initiate arrhythmias while a drug which converts the unidirectional block to a bidirectional block suppresses re-entrant arrhythmias. Such concepts, when applied to the conduction delay which occurs during myocardial ischaemia, in all probability represent an oversimplification since conduction through the three-dimensional matrix of the ischaemiac or infarcted ventricular myocardium, particularly when influenced by drugs, is considerably more complex[5]. Indeed, measurement of conduction delay with a single electrogram in the ischaemic zone can be considered only as a guide to the slow, tortuous, complex conduction occurring in that area.

Slow response

The effects of verapamil and isoproterenol on the ischaemia-induced conduction delay were contrary to our initial predictions, in view of the conjecture that the slow response, thought to be mediated by a slow inward calcium (or sodium) current, was responsible for impulse propagation in the ischaemic zone[9–11]. If this concept were true, then slow channel blockers like verapamil[18] would be expected to slow further conduction through the ischaemic myocardium whereas isoproterenol, a slow channel agonist[19], might be expected to improve conduction.

However, since the specific electrophysiologic action of a drug may not be the sole factor which governs its effect on the extent of ischaemia-induced conduction delay, or the incidence of VT–VF, a consideration of other effects, such as haemodynamic or metabolic changes, is essential. If the degree of ischaemia influences the extent of conduction delay and development of VT–VF, then the effects of verapamil may be explained by a reduction in the size of the ischaemic injury, mediated either by haemodynamic or metabolic factors. Experimental data exist to support this possibility[20,21]. Any direct effect of verapamil to block the slow response[18] and prolong the conduction delay could be offset by a reduction in the extent of ischaemia, which would serve to improve conduction.

The deleterious effect of positive inotropic agents, including isoproterenol administration, during myocardial ischaemia has been demonstrated by ST segment mapping[22]. However, in the present study, isoproterenol was not found to alter significantly ischaemia-induced conduction delay and the incidence of ventricular arrhythmias. It is possible that improved conduction in the ischaemic myocardium caused by isoproterenol was counterbalanced by extension of the infarct size, so that no net change in the degree of ischaemia-induced conduction delay was observed.

Experimental model

The validity of the open or closed chest dog as an experimental model in which to evaluate the electrophysiological effect of drugs on conduction in the ischaemic myocardium is thus affected by the possible metabolic or haemodynamic action of these drugs, which may influence infarct size. In addition, since it is likely that the concentration of the drug perfusing the ischaemic area will influence the results in a dose–response relationship, the method of drug administration becomes critical. Problems related to the drug distribution into the ischaemic myocardium were avoided in the acute occlusion model by administering drugs before occlusion of the LAD. However, it is possible that this methodology may result in excessively high concentration of the drug trapped in the ischaemic area. Drugs given after coronary artery occlusion may result in concentrations which are too low. It appears quite clear from the difference between our results and those of Kupersmith *et al.*[15], regarding the effects of verapamil, that whether the drug is administered before or after coronary artery ligation has an important influence not only on the magnitude, but also on the direction of the effects. Which method of testing provides data more relevant to the clinical situation is unknown. Patients already taking a drug at the time of myocardial infarction may be more comparable to the experimental model in which the drug is given prior coronary artery occlusion, while those patients receiving the drug intravenously after an infarction may be more comparable to the experimental model in which the drug is given after the coronary artery is occluded. It is probable, however, that both forms of drug administration need to be investigated in the experimental model before valid conclusions can be drawn.

Finally, data from this study support the observation that the pathogenesis of arrhythmias development acutely after LAD occlusion differs from the mechanism(s) giving rise to ventricular arrhythmias 24 hours after occlusion. Thus, antiarrhythmic agents such as aprindine may exert arrhythmogenic or antiarrhythmic effects, depending on when the drug is administered in relation to the time of coronary occlusion. In this study, aprindine appeared to exert arrhythmogenic effects when given i.v. or orally (the latter in sufficiently high, toxic doses) *prior* to LAD occlusion, was neutral when given i.v. *after* LAD occlusion, and exerted antiarrhythmic effects when given i.v. *24 hours after* LAD occlusion.

Acknowledgement
Supported in part by the Herman C. Krannert Fund; and by Grants HL–06308, HL–05363, HL–07182 and HL–18795 from the National Heart, Lung and Blood Institute of the National Institutes of Health and the Eli Lilly & Company.

References

1. Wilson, F. N., Johnston, F. D., Hill, I. G. W. (1935). The form of the electrocardiogram in experimental myocardial infarction. IV. Additional observations on the later effects produced by ligation of the anterior descending branch of the left coronary artery. *Am. Heart J.*, **10,** 1025

2. Durrer, D., Van Lier, A. A. W. and Buller, J. (1964). Epicardial and intramural excitation in chronic myocardial infarction. *Am. Heart J.*, **68,** 765

3. Williams, D. O., Scherlag, B. J., Hope, R. R., El-Sherif, N. and Lazzara, R. (1974). The pathophysiology of malignant ventricular arrhythmias during acute myocardial ischemia. *Circulation,* **50,** 1163

4. Waldo, A. L. and Kaiser, G. A. (1973). Study of ventricular arrhythmias associated with acute myocardial infarction in the canine heart. *Circulation,* **47,** 1122

5. Boineau, J. P. and Cox, J. L. (1973). Slow ventricular activation in acute myocardial infarction: A source of reentrant premature ventricular contraction. *Circulation,* **48,** 702

6. Kupersmith, J., Shiang, H., Litvak, R. S. and Herman, M. V. (1976). Electrophysiological and antiarrhythmic effects of propranolol in canine acute myocardial ischemia. *Circ. Res.,* **38,** 302

7. Hope, R. R., Williams, D. O., El-Sherif, N., Lazzara, R. and Scherlag, B. J. (1974). The efficacy of antiarrhythmic agents during acute myocardial ischemia and role of the heart rate. *Circulation,* **50,** 507

8. Scherlag, B. J., Helfant, R. H., Haft, J. I. and Damato, A. N. (1970). Electrophysiology underlying ventricular arrhythmias due to coronary ligation. *Am. J. Physiol.,* **219,** 1665

9. Cranefield, P. F. (1975). *The Conduction of The Cardiac Impulse.* (Mt. Kisco, N.Y.: Futura Publishing Co)

10. Wit, A. L. and Friedman, P. L. (1975). Basis for ventricular arrhythmias accompanying myocardial infarction. *Arc. Intern. Med.,* **135,** 459

11. Zipes, D. P., Besch, H. R. and Watanabe, A. M. (1975). Role of the slow current in cardiac electrophysiology. *Circulation,* **51,** 761

12. Zipes, D. P. and Fischer, J. C. (1974). Effects of agents which inhibit the slow channel on the sinus node automaticity and atrioventricular conduction in the dog. *Circ. Res.,* **34,** 184

13. Scherlag, B. J., El-Sherif, N., Hope, R. and Lazzara, R. (1974). Characterization and localization of ventricular arrhythmias resulting from myocardial ischemia and infarction. *Circ. Res.,* **35,** 372

14. Kupersmith, J., Antman, E. M. and Hoffman, B. F. (1975). *In vivo* electrophysiological effects of lidocaine in canine acute myocardial infarction. *Circ. Res., 36,* 84

15. Kupersmith, J., Shiang, H., Litwak, R. S. and Herman, M. V. (1976). Electrophysiologic effects of verapamil in canine myocardial ischemia. *Am. J. Cardiol.* (abstract) *37,* 149

16. Lazzara, R., El-Sherif, N. and Scherlag, B. J. (1974). Early and late effects of coronary artery occlusion on canine Purkinje fibers. *Circ. Res., 35,* 391

17. Friedman, P. L., Stewart, J. R., Fenoglio, J. J. and Wit, A. L. (1973). Survival of subendocardial Purkinje fibers after extensive myocardial infarction in dogs. *Circ. Res., 33,* 597

18. Kohlhardt, M., Bauer, B., Krause, H. and Fleckenstein, A. (1972). New selective inhibitors of the transmembrane Ca conductivity in mammalian myocardial fibers. Studies with the voltage clamp technique. *Experientia (Basel), 28,* 288

19. Pappano, A. J. (1970). Calcium-dependent action potentials produced by catecholamines in guinea pig atrial muscle fibers depolarized by potassium. *Circ. Res., 27,* 379

20. Smith, H. J., Singh, B. N., Nisbet, H. D. and Norris, R. M. (1975). Effect of verapamil on infarct size following experimental coronary occlusion. *Cardiovasc. Res., 9,* 569

21. Smith, H. J., Goldstein, R. A., Griffith, J. M., Kent, K. M. and Epstein, S. E. (1976). Selective depression of ischemic myocardium by verapamil. *Am. J. Cardiol.* (abstract), *37,* 174

22. Maroko, P. R., Kjekshus, J. K., Sobel, B. E., Watanabe, T., Covell, J. W., Ross, J., Jr. and Braunwald, E. (1971). Factors influencing infarct size following experimental coronary artery occlusions. *Circulation, 43,* 67

23
The Use of Programmed Pacing Techniques in the Management of Re-entrant Tachycardias

R. A. J. SPURRELL,

St. Bartholomew's Hospital, London

Over the last few years the use of intracardiac recordings associated with programmed electrical stimulation of the heart has demonstrated that a re-entrant mechanism is the basis for many cases of tachycardia in man[1-3]. In such situations it has been found that suitably timed single or double premature beats can consistently terminate tachycardias of this type.

Using programmed pacing techniques the approach to therapy can be divided into the prevention of paroxysms of tachycardia and the termination of such tachycardias once initiated.

PREVENTION OF RE-ENTRANT SUPRAVENTRICULAR TACHYCARDIAS USING PROGRAMMED PACING

Coumel[4] has shown that simultaneous atrial and ventricular pacing has led to suppression of paroxysms of re-entrant tachycardia. A refinement of this principle is to use an atrial synchronous pacing system with a short atrioventricular (AV) delay. The principles of such a system are illustrated in Figure 23.1. Panel A represents activation of the heart with the pacemaker switched off and Panel B with it switched on. It will be seen that the first two beats in Panel A are sinus beats but the third beat is an atrial premature beat which is conducted to the ventricles with a long AV delay such that re-entry can occur and a re-entry

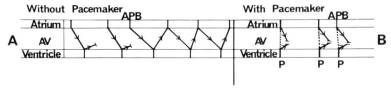

Figure 23.1 Diagram demonstrating the theoretical function of an atrial synchronous pacemaker with a short AV delay. APB = atrial premature beat; P = pacing stimulus

supraventricular tachycardia is initiated. In Panel B, with the pacemaker functioning, the first two beats are sinus beats but because the atrial synchronous pacemaker has a short AV delay each sinus is rapidly followed by a triggered ventricular beat. The third beat is an atrial premature beat which would normally have initiated a tachycardia but because a triggered ventricular premature beat is initiated by the atrial premature beat, this ventricular premature beat is conducted retrogradely into the re-entrant circuit and prevents initiation of the tachycardia.

Such a system was implanted in a patient with recurrent bouts of paroxysmal supraventricular tachycardia. The pacemaker, a Devices 4271*, was an implantable atrial synchronous pacemaker with an AV delay of 30 msec. It was designed such that it could not trigger ventricular premature beats at atrial premature beat coupling times of <300 msec and in this way the patient was protected from a rapid ventricular rate should an atrial arrhythmia with a rate in excess of 200/min occur. In this patient an epicardial electrode was sutured to the back of the left atrium, where an adequate atrial signal was obtained and a second electrode was sutured to the front of the right ventricle. Both electrodes were connected to the pacemaker which was implanted subcutaneously.

Figure 23.2 is a recording obtained from the above patient showing the system functioning. The first two beats are sinus beats and the resultant atrial potential can be seen on the RAE. Each sinus beat is followed by a triggered ventricular premature beat response. The third beat is an induced atrial premature beat with a coupling time of 365 msec. This atrial premature beat is followed by a ventricular premature beat response and no tachycardia is initiated. The fourth beat is again a sinus beat with its ventricular premature beat reponse. At a pre-implant study it was demonstrated that atrial premature beats with coupling times in the range 320–390 msec could initiate tachycardias and therefore a premature beat at 365 msec should have initiated a tachycardia. Pre-operatively this patient suffered from 10–15 attacks of tachycardia per week, but following implantation of this system, apart from one early documented attack of tachycardia, the patient remained free of tachycardias for a period of 2.5 years at which time he died from a myocardial infarction. Further details of this system are reported by Spurrell *et al.*[5].

---

*Devices Instruments Ltd., Welwyn Garden City, Herts., England

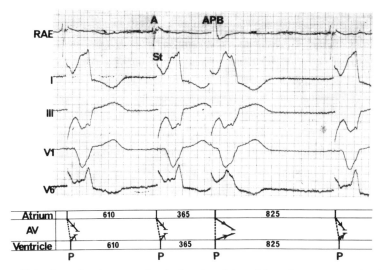

Figure 23.2   Recording demonstrating the function of the atrial synchronous pacemaker during sinus rhythm and following an induced premature beat with a coupling time of 365 msec. RAE = right atrial electrogram

THE USE OF PROGRAMMED PACING FOR THE TERMINATION OF ESTABLISHED RE-ENTRANT TACHYCARDIAS

An ideal pacing system for tachycardia termination would be one in which the pacemaker senses when tachycardia has occurred and then fires in a single or double, appropriately timed, ventricular premature beat, terminates the tachycardia, at which time the pacemaker would switch itself off.

Figure 23.3 is a recording obtained from a patient with a paroxysmal supraventricular tachycardia. The first four QRS complexes are occurring during tachycardia. The fourth potential on the atrial electrogram is an atrial premature beat with a coupling time of 210 msec; this terminates the tachycardia and the last three beats are sinus beats. Unfortunately it has been found that the position in which the premature beat can terminate the tachycardia varies over *ca.* 30 msec in any one patient during different attacks and therefore an automatic pacing system firing in a single premature beat at a preset coupling time could not be expected to consistently terminate the attack. For this reason Spurrell *et al.*[6] used bursts of high frequency stimuli in order to cover a wider area of the cardiac cycle and in this way increase the likelihood of producing an atrial premature beat at a suitable time. Figure 23.4 is a recording obtained from a patient with a paroxysmal re-entrant supraventricular tachycardia. The first four beats are the last four of the tachycardia. Following the third retrograde atrial potential, as seen on the two atrial electrograms, there occurs a burst of high frequency stimuli (HFS) at 100 stimuli/sec over a period of 100 msec and occurring with a delay from the preceding atrial poten-

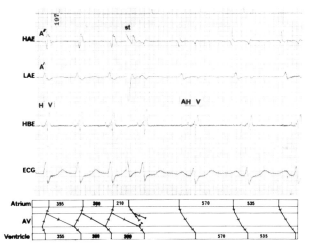

Figure 23.3 Recording showing the termination of a re-entry supraventricular tachycardia by a single atrial premature beat. HAE = high right atrial electrogram; LAE = low right atrial electrogram; HBE = His bundle electrogram; ECG = surface electrocardiogram; AV = atrioventricular region; A = retrograde atrial potential; H = His potential; V = ventricular potential as seen on the HBE; St = pacing stimulus artefact; A = antegrade atrial potential as seen on the HBE

tial of 165 msec. This burst of HFS produces an atrial premature beat which terminates the tachycardia and the last two beats are the first two beats of sinus rhythm.

In many patients two atrial premature beats are required to terminate their tachycardia and under these circumstances bursts of HFS of longer duration (up to 250 msec) may be required to terminate the attack.

This system has been shown to terminate tachycardia with a high degree of consistency. Atrial fibrillation has been induced rarely but when it occurs it usually terminates the re-entrant tachycardia and is itself short-lived.

This system has only been used as an external pacemaker and not developed into an implantable form because of certain limitations in its mode of action. Many patients can only have their tachycardias terminated by appropriately timed ventricular premature beats and the HFS would obviously be potentially dangerous in this situation. Therefore a system was developed which could be used for producing appropriately timed single or double atrial or ventricular premature beats.

The Devices 4272 and 4273 fulfilled the above requirements. A pacing electrode is positioned in the appropriate chamber to be stimulated. Spontaneous cardiac activity is continually sensed and when tachycardia occurs, i.e. the cycle length shortens below a certain preset value, the output circuit of the pacemaker is activated which proceeds to fire a premature stimulus triggered from the intracardiac potential with a present coupling time such that the

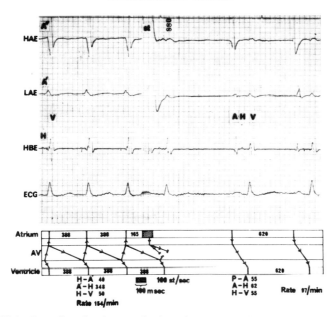

Figure 23.4 Recording showing termination of a supraventricular tachycardia using high frequency stimuli (HFS) of 100 msec duration

stimulus falls just inside the refractory period of the atria or ventricles, whichever is being stimulated. Following this first stimulus a further stimulus is induced about every second but each time the coupling time is increased by 5 msec. This continues until 100 msec of the cardiac cycle is scanned and the pacemaker then recycles and scans again. However, at some stage in the scan, after the stimulus begins to fall outside the refractory period of the stimulated chamber, an appropriate premature beat will usually occur which terminates the tachycardia and the output circuit of the pacemaker is then switched off. If a patient requires two premature beats to terminate the tachycardia then the scan can occur with two premature stimuli, a constant coupling time being maintained between the two stimuli.

Figure 23.5 is a recording demonstrating the termination of a tachycardia using the scanning pacemaker with one premature stimuli. The first part of the recording shows the tachycardia. There are four pacing stimuli seen, the first occurring within the refractory period of the ventricle and occurs 185 msec after the preceding spontaneous ventricular beat. The second and third stimuli also occur within the refractory period, the second delayed to 190 msec and the third to 195 msec. The fourth pacing stimulus is delayed to 200 msec which is outside the refractory period of the ventricle and so a ventricular premature beat is produced which terminates the attack of tachycardia, the last two beats are sinus beats and the pacemaker stops scanning.

Figure 23.6 demonstrates the same principle occurring but in a patient who

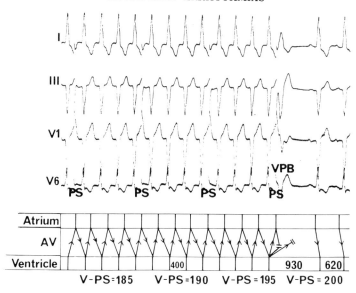

Figure 23.5 Recording demonstrating the termination of a supraventricular tachycardia in a patient with L-transposition of the great arteries using the scanning pacing system to induce single ventricular premature beats. VPB = ventricular premature beat; PS = pacing stimulus artefact; V–PS = time in msec from the onset of ventricular activation to the pacing stimulus

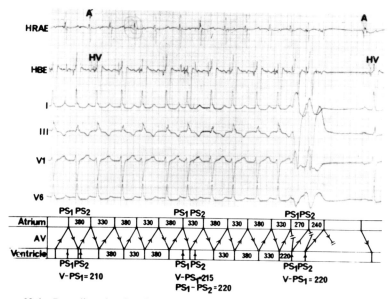

Figure 23.6 Recording showing the termination of a supraventricular tachycardia using the scanning pacemaker to produce double ventricular premature beats. HRAE = high right atrial electrogram; PS₁–PS₂ = time in milliseconds between the two induced pacing stimuli

required two ventricular premature beats to terminate the tachycardia. In this situation a pair of stimuli PS_1 and PS_2 with a fixed coupling time of 220 msec scan the cardiac cycle during tachycardia until the third pair delayed out to 220 msec produces two correctly timed ventricular premature beats which terminate the tachycardia. The last beat is the first beat of sinus rhythm and the scan has stopped.

This system has the benefit that it can be used for both atrial and ventricular stimulation. It has been used successfully many times in the laboratory but two patients suffering from drug resistant recurrent attacks of paroxysmal re-entrant supraventricular tachycardia have had permanent endocardial pacing electrodes positioned in their ventricles and these electrodes have been exteriorized following a long subcutaneous course in the abdomen and attached to a Devices 4273 miniscan. Both patients had the systems in excess of two years, and in both patients spontaneous attacks of tachycardia are rapidly terminated by the pacemaker. One patient required single ventricular premature beats and the other paired ventricular premature beats. Both patients were able to return to a normal life. In one patient, however, the system finally had to be removed because of repeated electrode fractures in the electrode extensions. In the other patient the system continues to work satisfactorily.

Development is in progress for this system to be totally implantable.

References

1. Durrer, D., Schuilenburg, R. M. and Wellens, H. J. J. (1969). The role of the atrioventricular junction in the genesis of arrhythmias in the human heart. *Proceedings of the Koninklijke Nederlandse Akademie van Wetenschappen te Amsterdam,* **72,** 515
2. Bigger, J. T. and Goldreyer, B. N. (1970). The mechanism of supraventricular tachycardia. *Circulation,* **42,** 673
3. Wellens, H. J. J. (1971). *Electrical Stimulation of the Heart in the Study and Treatment of Tachycardias.* (Leiden: Stenfert Kroese), p. 40
4. Coumel, P. (1970). Management of paroxysmal tachycardia. Symposium on Cardiac Arrhythmias. E. Sandoe, E. Flensted-Jensen and K. H. Olesen (eds.). (Ab. Astra, Södertalje, Sweden) p. 783
5. Spurrell, R. A. J. and Sowton, E. (1976). An implanted atrial synchronous pacemaker with a short atrioventricular delay for the prevention of paroxysmal supraventricular tachycardia. *J. Electrocardiol.,* **9,** 89
6. Spurrell, R. A. J. and Sowton, E. (1975). The use of high frequency stimulation (HFS) in the management of paroxysmal supraventricular tachycardia. *J. Electrocardiol.,* **8,** 287

24
Stimulation Studies and Epicardial Mapping in Ventricular Tachycardia: Study of Mechanisms and Selection for Surgery

G. FONTAINE, G. GUIRAUDON, R. FRANK, J. VEDEL, Y. GROSGOGEAT, C. CABROL and J. FACQUET

Services de Cardiologie Centre et de Chirurgie Cardiovasculaire, Hôpital de la Pitié Salpêtrière Paris XIII

Treatment of severe ventricular tachycardia (VT) may be attempted by the use of antiarrhythmic agents[1-3], cardiac pacing[4-7], or surgery. If surgery is advocated, it may consist of excision of abnormal tissue (aneurysmectomy)[8,9], myocardial revascularization[10], or ventriculotomy[11,12]. In our institution, the latter technique, guided by data obtained from epicardial mapping, has been used as a last resort in cases of life-threatening arrhythmias, refractory to other forms of therapy.

Since May 1973, 57 consecutive cases were investigated at the Department of Electrocardiology of the Hôpital de la Salpêtrière. 39 of them had been referred by other hospitals for evaluation and possible surgical treatment of recurrent VT. This accounts for the fact that, in this selected series, the various aetiologies are not represented in the same proportions as in other clinical series[13-15].

For reasons previously discussed[12], our cases were classified into two categories characterized by the main clinical features mentioned in Table 24.1.

In 29 instances, the rhythm disturbance appeared as a complication of

Table 24.1

		VT started or interrupted by electrical stimulation	Operated upon	Presence of late potentials	Ventriculotomy		Uninterpretable data
					success	failure	
VT following myocardial infarction: 29 cases		26/27	13	1	1	1	11
VT unrelated to ischaemic heart disease 28 cases	Permanent VT: 17 cases	17	7	7	7	0	0
	Bouts of VT: 9 cases	0	2	0	0	2	0
	Accelerated idioventricular rhythm: 3 cases	0	1	0	0	1	0

chronic ischaemic heart disease or myocardial infarction (from 15 days to 10 years old). Thirteen of these patients were operated upon.

In 28 instances, the VT was not associated with coronary artery disease; ten of these subjects were submitted to surgery.

The present report is not intended to describe the surgical results which have been summarized in the Table 24.1 and discussed, at length, in a previous report[12]. The aim of our paper is to present some findings obtained by stimulation studies and epicardial mapping[11,12], both in sinus rhythm and during VT. They yield new information regarding the mechanisms of this rhythm disturbance, the pathways of abnormal activation, and the genesis of delayed potentials. They permit a better selection of those patients who are suitable for surgery, furthermore they allow the description of a new syndrome which we have denominated 'arrhythmogenic right ventricular dysplasia', and which is a subdivision of the more general so-called 'post-excitation syndrome'.

Studies on the mechanism of VT have started from deductive analysis of electrocardiograms. Ischaemia-induced arrhythmias were later used as an experimental model to approach this problem[16-23]. More recently, sophisticated clinical electrophysiological methods of investigation[6,24,25], observations made on patients treated by permanent pacemakers[4,7], as well as electrophysiological studies carried out in the operating theatre[26], have considerably furthered our understanding of this rhythm disturbance.

Basically, two different mechanisms have been proposed to explain the genesis of VT. Focal increased automaticity used to be considered the most frequent phenomenon. Nowadays, re-entry, due to slow conduction, gains more and more popularity every day[24].

The Wolff–Parkinson–White syndrome represents a remarkable model to study re-entry. Careful observation of the delta wave as well as the results of intracavitary recordings, generally make it possible to localize rather easily the pathway of re-entrant excitation[27]. The situation is totally different in VT where the usual techniques of investigation remain unsatisfactory and epicardial mapping is needed. The latter method not only provides an overall picture of total cardiac excitation, but also yields data of considerable importance by the analysis of the signal recorded at each epicardial site[29]. The data obtained by epicardial mapping put together with the results of the conventional electrocardiogram and of the programmed electrical stimulation studies have renewed our outlook upon VT.

MECHANISMS OF VT

Analysis of data obtained by programmed electrical stimulation

In 1972, Wellens, Schuilenburg and Durrer[24], were able, by using appropriately timed ventricular stimuli, to initiate or to interrupt episodes of VT in five cases of whom four suffered from chronic ischaemic heart disease. This observation suggested that VT reflected re-entrant phenomena. In 1974[25], the same group reported on results gathered from 20 patients who were subdivided into two groups. The first group consisted of eleven cases of chronic myocardial infarction and of three cases of idiopathic VT. In those patients, it was generally possible to initiate and to stop the arrhythmia by electrical stimulation. The second group contained six patients studied within the first 24 hours of an acute myocardial infarction. All responded as if they had an ectopic focus.

In 1976, Denes et al.[28] studied 17 consecutive cases of recurrent VT. In two of them, VT could be repetitively induced by electrical stimulation. In another four, only a single episode of VT could be induced. It was thus possible to initiate VT episodes in 35% of the studied cases. In a recent publication, Derrida[30] showed that VT could be induced in 47% of 32 cases. Wellens et al.[6] obtained the same result in 58% of their 50 patients. In our series, the rate of success was still higher since, among the 29 subjects with VT related to chronic ischaemic heart disease, we were able to initiate episodes of tachycardia in 26 of the 27 cases, in whom electrical stimulation was carried out. In the second group, with normal coronary vessels, initiation of VT was possible in only 61% of cases.

In addition to differences in the selection of patients, the unusually high percentage of cases in whom VT episodes could be induced in our series might be accounted for by the technique which we used. Initially, the electrocardiological investigations were carried out in the operating room[26]. Very often, tachycardia could only be started after several minutes of stimulation at a rate close to that of the spontaneous VT. This feature was initially thought to be related to anaesthesia, but later was also encountered in the catheter laboratory. At the present time, for the preoperative investigations, we start by trying the extrastimulus technique at a basic pacing rate of 80–100/min. In case of failure, the ventricles are then overdriven at the highest rate acceptable by the patient, i.e. usually ca. 150/min. Every fifth minute, the extrastimulus technique is again tried out. If we fail to induce the tachycardia within 30 min, ventricular stimuli are fired at 200–300/min by bursts of 2 or 3 sec separated by intervals of 1–3 sec. All manoeuvres are abandoned if VT cannot be started within 45 min. This attitude is admittedly purely empirical and it has its shortcomings. Some episodes of VT have such a high ventricular rate that they can only be stopped after having been slowed by an antiarrhythmic agent. One subject of our second group underwent the whole protocol without developing VT under electrical stimulation. However, on reinvestigation a few weeks later, at a time when he had spontaneous episodes of tachycardia, it was possible to start and to stop the arrhythmia at will. In another instance, VT could not be started by apical stimulation but whenever it appeared spontaneously, it could be easily interrupted by bursts of ventricular stimuli. One has therefore to be most careful in the interpretation of the electrophysiological data and to refrain from hasty conclusions as regards their specificity for the identification of the mechanisms of VT.

The situation is still less clear if one remembers the recent experimental work by Cranefield and Wit[31]who showed that an automatic activity can be triggered by one single stimulus.

There are indeed in the data obtained during electrophysiological investigations, many features which point to the existence of re-entrant mechanisms. The site of stimulation is, for example, of critical importance. Stimulation can stop the arrhythmia only when the site of pacing is sufficiently close to the pathway of the circus movement[32]. Furthermore, in a patient showing a large "tachycardia zone", an inverse relation was found between the prematurity of the tachycardia initiating premature beat and the delay between the premature beat and the first beat of tachycardia[6,33]. Finally, the basic cycle length also plays a significant role. According to Wellens et al.[6], VT is easier to start at relatively slow or rapid heart rates which confirms experimental data by Chadda et al.[34]. All these features, considered as evidence in favour of re-entry are found with a high incidence in VT occurring in the chronic phase of myocardial infarction in man, i.e. at least five weeks after the acute episode.

Considering only the practical viewpoint, the data obtained by programmed electrical stimulation techniques allow two conclusions to be drawn: (1) In chronic ischaemic heart disease, for example five weeks after a myocardial infarction, it is almost always possible to interrupt VT by electrical stimulation. This technique could therefore be of interest in the coronary care unit where it might replace d.c. shock[27]. One should, however, be aware that incidents may occur. Electrical stimulation may, in some cases, lead to ventricular fibrillation which can only be corrected by electrical shock. In the operating theatre, programmed electrical stimulation is also useful to trigger the arrhythmia before epicardial mapping. (2) Data obtained by programmed electrical stimulation studies may also help in the selection for surgery. In this respect, it appears that among patients with VT unrelated to ischaemic heart disease, two subgroups may be identified. In the first subgroup, VT can be started and stopped by stimulation techniques. In our experience, seven such patients were operated upon with excellent results. In the second subgroup, electrical stimulation can neither start nor stop the arrhythmia. An operation was attempted in three of these cases and the results were unsatisfactory. In one of these subjects, VT was almost continuous. Pre-operative investigations had shown that a single stimulus, at the apex of the right ventricle could interrupt the VT during 2 or 3 sec, but the tachycardia would then resume and show identical rate and morphology of ventricular complexes. These features had erroneously been interpreted as indicative of a re-entrant mechanism[12]. In the remaining two cases, there were bouts of ventricular tachycardia, the origin of which was found along the anterior interventricular groove[35].

Analysis of epicardial recordings
Epicardial activation maps failed to provide a definite answer regarding the

mechanisms of the tachycardia in the majority of our cases. The epicardial activation sequence was explored during VT in the dog by Kastor et al.[36]. They observed the activation fronts to spread in a concentric manner over the epicardium from an epicardial location. We obtained similar results in 1973, by stimulating the heart at one or two different sites[37]. Concentric spread of activation was also seen by Horowitz, Spear and Moore in 1976, in their investigation of ischaemia-induced arrhythmias in the dog heart[38]. These authors were unable to draw conclusions regarding the precise mechanisms of the rhythm disturbance, but noticed that the site of origin was located along the margin between the normal and ischaemic zones. Intramural and endocardial recordings demonstrated that the actual point of origin was within the distal ramifications of the His–Purkinje system. A similar picture was obtained by Gallagher et al. in their study of an episode of VT originating from the margin of a large ventricular aneurysm[39]. In the first case of Spurrell's series, it is again on the border of an infarcted zone that the earliest epicardial activation site was found[11]. Most of our observations go along the same line[35]. These features might, in fact, seem to favour the hypothesis of an ectopic focus of hyperexcitability.

In a remarkable experimental work, Allessie, Bonke and their co-workers[39,40] were recently able to map the initiation of a re-entrant loop in a preparation of atrial myocardium. Their results are comparable to those reported in the second observation by Spurrell et al.[11], in which the activation fronts seemed to reverse in direction over the pulmonary infundibulum: there were thus two zones, lying side by side, that were activated with a time difference of 120 msec during a tachycardic cycle of 280 msec. No intermediate values in activation times could be demonstrated in between those two regions with an interelectrode distance of 2 mm.

In our series, one case also suggests the possibility of a circus movement. The patient was a lady with a paper thin right ventricle (Uhl's syndrome) and her clinical data have been previously described (Reference 41, case no. 6). Due to the size of the heart and her poor haemodynamic condition, it was only possible to obtain an epicardial mapping of the anterior aspect of the right ventricle. On the infundibular region, fragmented potentials were found throughout the interval separating the fast components related to the QRS complexes which indicated marked slowing of conduction during tachycardia. Furthermore, on certain points, potentials made up of two consecutive components were recorded, a pattern similar to that described by Spurrell et al.[11] (Figure 24.1). Re-entry is likely in this case but cannot however be asserted since data on the first cycles of the VT are missing. There is indeed no clearcut evidence that the later activity gives rise to the earlier one. A zone of focal block cannot be ruled out especially if one considers that the time delay between the two components of the epicardial potential is shorter than the duration of the ventricular refractory period, thus pointing to the idea that two very closely located zones might have been activated independently.

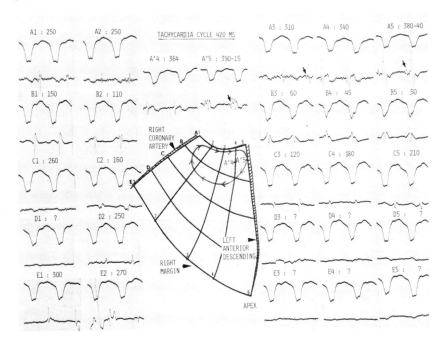

Figure 24.1   Epicardial potentials during an episode of ventricular tachycardia in a case of paper thin right ventricle (Uhl's syndrome). The grid covers the anterior aspect of the right ventricle from the root of the great vessels to the right border. Epicardial recordings are made by means of bipolar electrodes (1 mm apart). The activation time (indicated in msec) is measured from the onset of QRS in the inverted lead I. Points where potentials were too small to allow precise measurements are indicated by a question mark. Potentials made up of two separate components can be seen during tachycardia in those leads indicated by an arrow (A_3, A_5 and A_5'). From the measured activation times, the hypothetical loop followed by the circus movement has been drawn

RE-ENTRY AND SPECIFIC CONDUCTION SYSTEM

In their initial report, the Amsterdam group[24] put forward the hypothesis that the re-entrant pathway could use the bundle branches, the Purkinje system, fibrotic ventricular muscle, or a combination of these. Starting from the bifascicular representation of the intraventricular conduction system, Spurrell et al.[33], as well as Blanchot and Warin[42] imagined various intraventricular circuits and explained the marked morphological QRS alterations which may occur during tachycardia by changes in the activation pathways along the conduction fascicles. Guerot et al.[43] proposed the diagnosis of a re-entry phenomenon from one bundle branch to the other in a case where the initiation of VT by a single atrial premature beat was dependent on the occurrence of a functional right bundle branch block of the conducted atrial beat. He stressed, however, the unusual character of this type of observation. Wellens *et al.*[25] also used the same hypothesis to explain that, in one of their cases, an episode of VT could be interrupted by an atrial premature beat which was not transmitted to the ventricles. They also underlined the unusual character of their observation and mentioned that the tachycardia could have been interrupted by a sudden stretch of the various structures incorporated in the tachycardia circuit, due to the mechanical effects of the atrial premature contraction.

Recently, Akhtar *et al.*[44] reported re-entry in the His–Purkinje system as a possible mechanism for the genesis of ventricular ectopic beats following timed ventricular stimuli. On the contrary, Touboul *et al.*[45] described a patient in whom VT could be induced by a premature atrial beat transmitted to the ventricles without aberration of intraventricular conduction, which suggested that the site of origin of the VT was located away from the conduction system. Wellens *et al.*[6] recently discussed the results obtained by Akhtar and his co-workers[44]. They stressed that in patients with a wide tachycardia zone, late premature beats initiating tachycardia were not followed by a His bundle electrogram (His bundle activity being probably hidden in the QRS complex), in contrast to early premature beats which initiated tachycardia. They concluded that activation of the His bundle may be a concomitant phenomenon and not helpful in delineating the re-entry circuit during ventricular tachycardia. Likewise, when the His bundle potentials can be observed during tachycardia their actual location is of little help to identify the site of origin of the rhythm disturbance[6,46].

Epicardial mapping makes it possible to localize: (1) the site of origin of the abnormal rhythm in VT; (2) the sites of origin of initial activation during normal sinus rhythm. In the latter condition, the zones of epicardial breakthrough are located at the endpoints of the right bundle branch and ramifications of the left bundle; the epicardial picture is closely correlated with the image obtained on the endocardial surface[47]. It is therefore of interest to compare the two different patterns of excitation during VT and sinus rhythm. To date, no coincidence was observed between the areas of earliest epicardial activity during sinus rhythm and the areas of initial activation during VT. This feature indicates that participation of the specific conduction system is unlikely. One should realize however that, due to their properties of fast conductivity, the distal Purkinje fibres, if they are invaded, could induce, at a distance, a secondary zone of epicardial breakthrough, as was found in one of our cases[41].

From a study of the orientation of the initial QRS vectors in premature beats, Burchell *et al.*[48] concluded that the site of origin was most frequently located away from the specific conducting system, which accounts for the multiform configuration of most ectopic beats. One may thus conclude that, at the present stage of our knowledge, the specific conduction system seems to play a minor role, if any, in most instances of sustained VT, whatever the aetiology. This, of course, does not rule out the possibility of the specific system playing a significant role in the first or last cycles of a tachycardic episode[43,45].

THE POST-EXCITATION PHENOMENON

Post-excitation is said to occur when late epicardial potentials (ε-wave) are observed after the end of ventricular depolarization as judged from the standard electrocardiographic leads (Figures 24.2–24.5). Post-excitation is the manifestation of delayed activation in a group of fibres and the consequence of a severe, although very localized, conduction disturbance (Figure 24.2). Late potentials were first recorded by Durrer et al.[49] in the ischaemic dog myocardium and later, also, found in the human[50-52].

A late potential, recorded at the margin of a healed myocardial infarction, which had not attracted attention at that time could be seen in one of our first investigated cases (Figure 24.2)[37]. In 1973, Boineau and Cox[53] demonstrated within a zone of ischaemic myocardium in the dog, late potentials occurring ca. 250 msec after the onset of depolarization recorded on the surface leads. Late potentials were also observed at the epicardial surface of a patient with VT un-

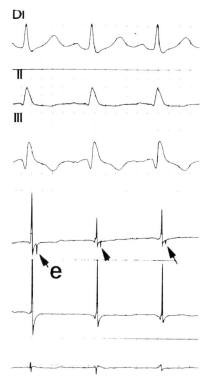

Figure 24.2 Late potential recorded on the epicardial surface in a patient with a previous history of posterior myocardial infarction. This picture is reproduced from Fontaine et al.[20]. On the first epicardial lead, the potential is made up to two components; the late potential (ε-wave) is indicated by an arrow; it is limited to a very small area since electrodes situated 2 mm away (lower two traces) fail to record it

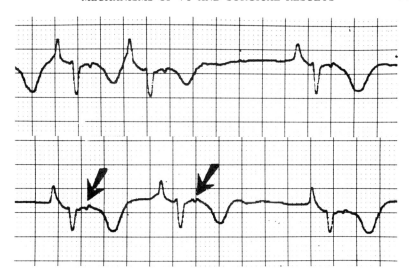

Figure 24.3 ε-Wave recorded from the body surface by two precordial electrodes positioned on both sides of the xyphoid extremity. The ε-wave is indicated by an arrow

related to ischaemic heart disease. They occurred 80 msec after the end of the QRS complex[27]. In the same subject, late potentials were further delayed after a ventricular ectopic beat (190 msec after ventricular ectopic beat as opposed to 70 msec during sinus rhythm)[26]. In our patient with the paper thin right ventricle, the ε-wave appeared with a delay of 300 msec[12].

In one of our cases, in whom VT was due to ischaemic heart disease, late potentials recorded along the border of a fibrous scar located at the postero-

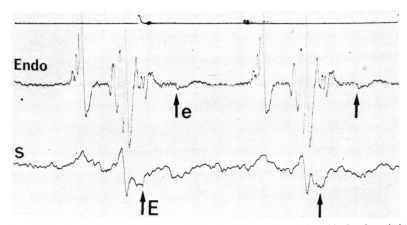

Figure 24.4 Arrhythmogenic right ventricular dysplasia syndrome. On a bipolar thoracic lead (S), late potentials (indicated by an arrow) are seen in spite of considerable muscular activity. An intracavitary bipolar lead (electrodes located 6 cm apart) shows post-excitation waves which occur much later than on the surface lead

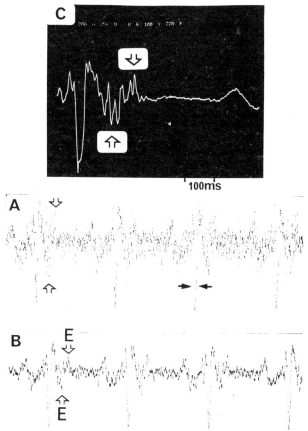

Figure 24.5 Surface lead in one case of arrhythmogenic right ventricular dysplasia. (a) Bipolar thoracic lead greatly amplified. The QRS complexes (horizontal arrows) are lost in the noise produced by muscular activity. (b) Same trace after analogic filtering. (c) Trace obtained after averaging using a digital technique

inferior aspect of the left ventricle were found to induce responses propagated to the whole ventricular mass[35], thus confirming experimental data by Boineau and Cox[54] and Scherlag et al.[23,55,56]. Self-sustained VT was also observed in the same individual. It was thus demonstrated that late potentials can reactivate the surrounding myocardium after the end of the refractory period and initiate sustained VT. The major conduction delay, which is responsible for the rhythm disturbance is maintained throughout the tachycardic episode and may explain the presence of potentials made up of two separate components which we have observed on several occasions during tachycardia (Figure 24.1). Variations in the pattern of the spread of activation may inversely interrupt the tachycardic episode or produce various changes in its characteristics.

In our series, out of the 13 cases with VT complicating a myocardial infarction, late epicardial potential were found in only one instance[35]. On the contrary, they were observed in seven out of ten cases with VT unrelated to ischaemic heart disease. In the remaining three patients, the criteria for a re-entrant arrhythmia were not fulfilled during the pre-operative electrophysiological investigations and none of these subjects benefited from the operation.

It is our feeling that the presence of late potentials in VT unrelated to ischaemic heart disease and, even to a certain extent, in VT complicating a myocardial infarction, in itself, favours the existence of a re-entrant mechanism[57,58]. The main characteristics of these late potentials are as follows: (1) The epicardial potential consists of, at least, two successive components, one being synchronous with the reference QRS complex and the other or others occurring late after the end of ventricular depolarization as judged from the surface tracing. (2) If the electrode position remains unchanged, the consistency in morphology from beat to beat of these two components indicates that the activation circuit is remarkably stable. (3) Most frequently, the second, delayed, potential is fairly close to the potential synchronous with the QRS complex. One cannot exclude, however, that even later potentials might exist and be missed either because they are not present on any point of the grid, or else because they are situated within the depth of the myocardial muscle. The latest potential we ever saw occurred after the top of the T wave, the delay being approximately equal to the duration of the refractory period of the normal myocardium. (4) Late potentials may, if they are sufficiently late, re-excite the neighbouring cells and induce an ectopic beat. (5) Late potentials can be observed during episodes of VT.

The initiation of a re-entrant tachycardia may be explained by the existence of late potentials according to three hypothetical mechanisms. (1) The delay of appearance of late potentials may increase, either spontaneously or under some extrinsic influence, and become longer than the refractory period of adjacent tissues, thus giving rise to a propagated response (ectopic beat). (2) The same phenomenon would result, should the refractory period of adjacent tissues be suddenly shortened. Both mechanisms (1) and (2), might, of course, occur simultaneously. (3) A focal block in tissues with abnormal conduction could also induce a similar series of events. Development of block in a given region may allow activation conducted normally to the adjacent zones to re-enter later through the previously blocked segment[59,60].

By an analysis of the data obtained from the operated and non-operated cases, we think it possible to postulate a syndrome which we would like to denominate 'arrhythmogenic right ventricular dysplasia'. This syndrome which was suspected by Sebastien et al.[15] may be defined as follows by its main characteristics:

(1) Presence of the post-excitation phenomenon, i.e. demonstration of late potentials which can be depicted in different ways: (a) on the right chest leads of the standard electrocardiogram as can be seen in the paper-thin right ventricle; (b) by averaging techniques using digital methods; (c) by intracavitary

recordings if the catheter-electrode is close enough to the abnormal region; (d) by epicardial mapping, on the thin right ventricular wall.

The post-excitation phenomenon may account for some unspecific alterations of the electrocardiogram during sinus rhythm.

(2) Recognition of episodes of VT whose particular features are worth being noted: (a) The QRS complexes during VT show a left ventricular delay; (b) the episodes of VT can be started or interrupted by electrical stimulation provided the technique is properly used; (c) the site of origin of the VT is consistent with abnormalities found at angiocardiography.

(3) Presence of abnormalities at angiography. They consist of localized bulges seen in the right infundibular region or of irregularities along the ventricular wall, generally observed in the infundibulum of the right ventricle or else in the apical or diaphragmatic portions.

(4) Recognition, during the operative procedure, of areas of wall thinning in the right ventricle. This thinning may involve the whole right ventricular wall

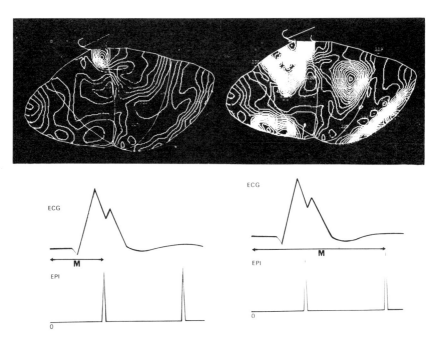

Figure 24.6 Post-excitation syndrome. Epicardial mapping. To the left, mapping was performed in sinus rhythm. The isochronic lines were drawn by measuring the time delay between the intrinsic deflection of the epicardial lead to the reference point. To the right, the epicardial mapping was constructed by means of time measurements of the late potential when it exists. The image thus obtained indicates the sites of origin of abnormal excitation, i.e. the base of the right ventricular free wall, the middle zone of the left ventricular free wall and an area along the posterior interventricular groove. Those locations were also the sites of origin of ventricular tachycardic episodes

(paper thin right ventricle) but, in most cases, is limited to small zones which appear to be fibrotic and may show paradoxical movement.

According to this description, arrhythmogenic right ventricular dysplasia was found in four patients of our second group who were submitted to surgery. Leaving aside the case where the diagnosis of paper thin right ventricle was made before operation, it was seen in three instances where it appeared as a thinning of the right ventricular infundibular wall. In one instance, the syndrome was associated with abnormalities in the activation pattern of the free wall of the left ventricle, where late potentials were also recorded (Figure 24.6). This patient developed tachycardic episodes with QRS complexes originating either from the right or the left ventricle and therefore resembled some cases of Froment's series[61].Finally in one further instance, the apical muscle was remarkably thin.

The syndrome of 'arrhythmogenic right ventricular dysplasia' was also encountered in three non-operated cases where abnormalities were found at angiography either in the right ventricular infundibulum (two cases) or apex (one case). Those three patients could so far be successfully managed by antiarrhythmic agents only.

At the present time, the existence of this syndrome is, in our opinion, sufficiently well established to justify, whenever it is suspected, a right ventricular angiogram. This procedure will allow a firm diagnosis to be made.

As to the post-excitation syndrome itself, it remains to be further investigated especially with regard to its practical implications for the treatment of rhythm disturbances associated with ischaemic heart disease.

References

1. Lown, B., Fakhro, R., Hood, W. B. and Thorn, G. N. (1967). The coronary care unit. *J. Am. Med. Ass.*, **199,** 188

2. Hope, R. R., Williams, D. O., El-Sherif, N., Lazzara, R. and Scherlag, B. J. (1974). The efficacy of anti-arrhythmic agents during acute myocardial ischemia and the role of heart rate. *Circulation*, **50,** 507

3. Jelinek, M. V., Lohrbauer, L. and Lown, B. (1974). Antiarrhythmic drug therapy for sporadic ventricular ectopic arrhythmias. *Circulation*, **49,** 659

4. Moss, A. J. and Rivers, R. J. (1974). Termination and inhibition of recurrent tachycardias by implanted perivenous pacemakers. *Circulation*, **50,** 942

5. Wellens, H. J. J., Overdijk, A. D. and Durrer, D. (1974). Traitement d'une tachycardie ventriculaire itérative chronique par l'implantation d'un pacemaker. *Coeur med. Interne,* **13,** 683

6. Wellens, H. J. J., Durrer, D. R. and Lie, K. I. (1976). Observations on mechanisms of ventricular tachycardia in man. *Circulation,* **54,** 237

7. Fontaine, G., Beneton, H, Frank, R., Guiraudon, G., Grosgogeat, Y. and Facquet, J. (1975). Prévention de la tachycardie ventriculaire après infarctus du myocarde par pacemaker intracorporel. *Arch. Mal. Coeur Vaiss.,* **68,** 961

8. Gallagher, J., Oldham, H. N., Wallace, A. G., Peter, R. H. and Cassell, J. (1975). Ventricular aneurysm with ventricular tachycardia. Report of a case with epicardial mapping and successful resection. *Am. J. Cardiol.,* **35,** 696

9. Cough, O. A. (1959). Cardiac aneurysm with ventricular tachycardia and subsequent excision of aneurysm. *Circulation,* **20,** 251

10. Graham, A. F., Miller, D. C., Stinson, E. B., Daily, P. O., Fogarty, T. J. and Harrison, D. C. (1973). Surgical treatment of refractory life-threatening ventricular tachycardia. *Am. J. Cardiol.*, **32**, 909

11. Spurrell, R. A. J., Yates, A. K., Thornburn, C. W., Sowton, G. E. and Deuchar, D. C. (1975). Surgical treatment of ventricular tachycardia after epicardial mapping studies. *Br. Heart J.*, **37**, 115

12. Fontaine, G., Guiraudon, G., Frank, R., Vedel, J. and Coutte, R. (1976). Epicardial mapping and surgical treatment in 6 cases of resistant ventricular tachycardia not related to coronary artery disease. In: *The Conduction System of the Heart.* Wellens, Lie, Janse (eds.) (Leiden: Stenfert Kroese), p. 545

13. Froment, R., Gallavardin, L. and Cohen, P. (1953). Paroxysmal ventricular tachycardia; a clinical classification. *Br. Heart J.*, **15**, 172

14. Bouvrain, Y., Slama, R., Motte, G., Waynberger, M. and Crevelier, A. (1968). Les tachycardies ventriculaires: étiologie et évolution. A propos de 161 malades. *Arch. Mal. Coeur Vaiss.*, **61**, 909

15. Sebastien, Ph., Waynberger, M., Beaufils, Ph., Motte, G., Slama, R. and Bouvrain, Y. (1976). Les tachycardies ventriculaires isolées sana cardiopathie patente. *Arch. Mal. Coeur Vaiss.*, **69**, 910

16. Durrer, D., Van Lier, A. A. W. and Buller, J. (1964). Epicardial and intramural excitation in chronic myocardial infarction. *Am. Heart J.*, **68**, 765

17. Han, J., Detraglia, J., Millet, D. and Moe, G. K. (1966). Incidence of ectopic beats as a function of basic rate in the ventricle. *Am. Heart J.*, **72**, 632

18. Han, J., Millet, D., Chizzonitti, B. and Moe, G. K. (1966). Temporal dispersion of recovery of excitability in atrium and ventricle as a function of heart rate. *Am. Heart J.*, **71**, 481

19. Han, J. (1969). Mechanisms of ventricular arrhythmias associated with myocardial infarction. *Am. J. Cardiol.*, **24**, 800

20. Han, J., Goel, B. G. and Manson, C. S. (1970). Reentrant beats induced in the ventricle during coronary occlusion. *Am. Heart J.*, **80**, 778

21. Han, J. (1971). The concepts of reentrant activity responsible for ectopic rhythms. *Am. J. Cardiol.*, **28**, 253

22. Wit, A. L. and Bigger, Th. (1975). Possible electrophysiological mechanisms for lethal arrhythmias accompanying myocardial ischemia and infarction. *Circulation*, **52**, III-96

23. Scherlag, B. J., Hoper, R., Williams, D. O., El-Sherif, N. and Lazzara, R. (1976). Mechanisms of ectopic rhythm formation due to myocardial ischemia: effects of heart rate and ventricular premature beats. In: *The Conduction System of the Heart.* (Wellens, Lie, Janse (eds.) (Leiden: Stenfert Kroese), p. 633

24. Wellens, H. J. J., Schuilenburg, R. M. and Durrer, D. (1972). Electrical stimulation of the heart in patients with ventricular tachycardia. *Circulation*, **46**, 216

25. Wellens, H. J. J., Lie, K. I. and Durrer, D. (1974). Further observations on ventricular tachycardias as studied by electrical stimulation of the heart. *Circulation*, **49**, 647

26. Fontaine, G., Guiraudon, G., Frank, R., Gerbaux, A., Cousteau, J. P., Barillon, A., Gay, J., Cabrol, C. and Facquet, J. (1975). La cartographie épicardique et le traitement chirurgical par simple ventriculotomie de certaines tachycardies ventriculaires rebelles par réentrée. *Arch. Mal Coeur Vaiss.* **68**, 113

27. Fontaine, G., Frank, R., Vedel, J., Vachon, J. M., Guiraudon, G. Grosgogeat, Y. and Facquet, J. (1974). La genèse de certains troubles du rythme ventriculaire. *Nouv. Presse Med.*, **3**, 2321

28. Denes, P., Wu, D., Dhingra, R. C., Wyndham, C., Mautner, R. K. and Rosen, K. M. (1976). Electrophysiological studies in patients with chronic recurrent ventricular tachycardia. *Circulation*, **54**, 229

29. Durrer, D. (1968). Electrical aspects of human cardiac activity: a clinical physiological approach to excitation and stimulation. *Cardiovasc. Res.*, **2**, 1

30. Derrida, J. P. (1974). Intérêt des épreuves d'enregistrement et de stimulation endocavitaires dans l'étude des tachycardies ventriculaires. Thèse de Médecine, 1974, Paris VI

31. Cranefield, P. F. and Wit, A. L. (1974). Sustained rhythmicity in cardiac fibers with slow response activity triggered by propagated action potentials. *Circulation*, **50**, 97

32. Wellens, H. J. J., Schuilenburg, R. M. and Durrer, D. (1974). Electrical stimulation of the heart in patients with WPW syndrome type A. *Circulation*, **43**, 99

33. Spurrell, R. A. J., Sowton, E. and Deuchar, D. C. (1973). Ventricular tachycardia in 4 patients evaluated by programmed electrical stimulations of the heart and treated in 2 patients by surgical division of anterior radiation of left bundle branch. *Br. Heart J.*, **35**, 1014

34. Chadda, K. D., Banka, V. S. and Helfant, R. H. (1974). Rate dependent ventricular ectopia following acute coronary occlusion. The concept of an optimal anti-arrhythmic heart rate. *Circulation*, **49**, 654

35. Fontaine, G., Guiraudon, G., Frank, R., Vedel, J., Grosgogeat, Y. and Cabrol, C. Surgical treatment of resistant ventricular tachycardia (22 cases). Workshop on Sudden Death, Gent. (In press)

36. Kastor, J. A., Spear, J. F. and Moore, E. N. (1972). Localization of ventricular irritability by epicardial mapping: origin of digitalis-induced unifocal tachycardia, from the left ventricular Purkinje tissue. *Circulation*, **45**, 952

37. Fontaine, G., Frank, R., Bonnet, M., Cabrol, C. and Guiraudon, G. (1973). Méthode d'étude expérimentale et clinique des syndromes de Wolff–Parkinson–White et d'ischémie myocardique par cartographie de la dépolarisation ventriculaire épicardique. *Coeur et Méd. Intern.*, **12**, 105

38. Horowitz, L. N., Spear, J. F. and Moore, E. N. (1976). Subendocardial origin of ventricular arrhythmias in 24-hour old experimental myocardial infarction. *Circulation*, **53**, 56

39. Allessie, M. A., Bonke, F. I. M. and Schopman, F. J. H. (1973). Circus movement tachycardia in rabbit atrial muscle as a mechanism of tachycardia. *Circ. Res.*, **33**, 54

40. Allessie, M. A., Bonke, F. I. M. and Schopman, F. J. H. (1976). Observations on circus movement tachycardia in the isolated rabbit atrium. In: *The Conduction System of the Heart*. Wellens, Lie and Janse (eds). (Leiden: Stenfert Kroese)

41. Fontaine, G., Guiraudon, G., Frank, R., Vedel, J., Coutte, R., Dragodanne, C., Phan Thuc and Grosgogeat, Y. (1976). Cartographies épicardiques dans quatre cas de tachycardie ventriculaire par réentrée après infarctus du myocarde. 1. Origine de la tachycardie et attitude chirurgicale. *Arch. Mal. Coeur Vaiss.*, (in press)

42. Blanchot, P. and Warin, J. F. (1973). Un nouveau cas de tachycardie ventriculaire par réentrée. *Arch. Mal Coeur Vaiss.*, **66**, 915

43. Guérot, C., Valère, P. E., Castillo-Fenoy, A. and Tricot, R. (1976). Tachycardie par réentrée de branche à branche. *Arch. Mal. Coeur Vaiss.*, **67**, 1

44. Akhtar, M., Damato, A. N., Batsford, W. P., Ruskin, J N., Ogunkelu, J. B. and Vargas, G. (1974). Demonstration of reentry within the His–Purkinje system in man. *Circulation*, **50**, 1158

45. Touboul, P., Claveyrolas, R., Huerta, F., Porte, J. and Delahaye, J. P. (1975). Tachycardie ventriculaire induite par des battements supraventriculaires prématurés à complexe QRS normal. Analyse d'un cas. *Arch. Mal. Coeur Vaiss.*, **68**, 969

46. Touboul, P., Clement, C., Magrina, J., Tessier, Y. and Delahaye, J. P. (1972). Enregistrement de l'activité électrique du tissu de conduction auriculo-ventriculaire au cours des tachycardies ventriculaires. *Arch. Mal. Coeur Vaiss.*, **65**, 1409

47. Durrer, D., Van Dam, R. Th., Freud, G. E., Janse, M. J., Meijler, F. L. and Arzbaecher, R. C. (1970). Total excitation of the isolated human heart. *Circulation*, **41**, 899

48. Burchell, H. B. and Tuna, N. (1976). Initial vectors of ventricular premature beats and anterior fascicular conduction defects. *Eur. J. Cardiol.*, **4**, 71

49. Durrer, D., Formijne, P., Van Dam, R., Buller, J., Van Lier, A. and Meyler, F. (1961). Electrocardiogram in normal and some abnormal conditions. *Am. Heart J.*, **61**, 303

50. Kaiser, G. A., Waldo, A. L., Harris, P. D., Bowman, F. O., Hoffman, B. F. and Malm, J. R. (1969). New method to delineate myocardial damage at surgery. *Circulation, 39,* I 83

51. Kaiser, G. A., Waldo, A. L., Bowman, F. O., Hoffman, B. F. and Malm, J. R. (1970). The use of ventricular electrograms in operation for coronary artery disease and its complications. *Ann. Thor. Surg., 10,* 153

52. Durrer, D., Van Dam, R. Th., Freud, G. E., Meijler, F. L. and Roos, J. P. (1969). Excitation of the human heart. In: *Electrical Activity of the Heart.* (Springfield, Ill.: Charles C. Thomas), p. 53

53. Boineau, J. P. and Cox, J. L. (1973). Slow ventricular activation in acute myocardial infarction. A source of reentrant premature ventricular contractions. *Circulation, 48,* 702

54. Scherlag, B. J., El-Sherif, N., Hoper, R. and Lazzara, R. (1974). Characterization and localization of ventricular arrhythmias. Resulting from myocardial ischemia and infarction. *Circ. Res., 35,* 372

55. Williams, D. O., Scherlag, B. J., Hope, R. R., El-Sherif, N. and Lazzara, R. (1974). The pathophysiology of malignant ventricular arrhythmias during acute myocardial ischemia. *Circulation, 50,* 1163

56. Fontaine, G., Guiraudon, G. and Frank, R. (1977). Le syndrome de post-excitation. I. En rythme sinusal (in press)

57. Fontaine, G., Guiraudon, G. and Frank, R. (1977). Le syndrome de post-excitation. II. En tachycardie ventriculaire (in press)

58. Wit, A. L., Hoffman, B. F. and Cranefield, P. F. (1972). Slow conduction and reentry in the ventricular conducting system. Return extrasystole in canine Purkinje fibers. *Circ. Res., 30,* 1

59. Wit, A. L., Cranefield, P. F. and Hoffman, B. F. (1972). Slow conduction and reentry in the ventricular conducting system. Single and sustained circus movement in networks of canine and bovine Purkinje fibers. *Circ. Res., 30,* 11

60. Froment, R., Perrin, A., Loire, A. and Dalloz, C. (1968). Ventricule droit papyracé du jeune adulte par dystrophie congénitale. (A propos de deux cas anatomo-cliniques et de trois cas cliniques.) *Arch. Mal. Coeur Vaiss., 61,* 477

25

The Surgical Treatment of Arrhythmias

J. J. GALLAGHER, W. C. SEALY, R. W. ANDERSON, J. KASELL,
E. L. C. PRITCHETT, A. G. WALLACE and L. HARRISON

Departments of Medicine and Surgery, Medical Center
Duke University, Durham, North Carolina

PRE-EXCITATION SYNDROMES

Successful division of an accessory atrioventricular connection associated with the Wolff–Parkinson–White syndrome was first reported in 1968[1,2]. This operation was performed on a patient with a right lateral accessory pathway and involved an external dissection of the tricuspid annulus following mobilization of the right coronary artery from the AV groove. This approach had obvious limitations in terms of application to left-sided pathways where the presence of the coronary sinus and the large left coronary artery posed formidable technical barriers. In addition, because of the external approach, septal accessory pathways were clearly inaccessible. In 1974, Sealy and his co-workers reported an improved surgical approach utilizing an internal atriotomy at the level of the annulus, which has greatly simplified surgical approach to free wall accessory pathways and in some cases septal accessory pathways[3-5]. In addition to the improved surgical techniques[5,6], important advances have occurred in the manner of preoperative electrophysiological study[7-9]. Techniques are now available to localize the site of the accessory pathway and to implicate its participation in observed tachyarrhythmias. It is also possible to demonstrate the presence of multiple accessory pathways[10] as well as the presence of pathways with antegrade block and persistent retrograde conduction[11]. This allows preoperative differentiation of free wall from septal accessory pathways, a pivotal observation in selecting optimal candidates for surgery. Several centres have now reported varied success with epicardial mapping and attempted surgical division of accessory pathways. Our experience to date has attested to the value of this procedure in the management of selected patients with life-threatening or medically refractory dysrhythmias associated with the pre-excitation syndrome.

Surgical procedure for interruption of the accessory atrioventricular connection is divided into two steps: namely, the localization and subsequent interruption of the accessory pathway. The heart is exposed through a median sternotomy. The method used to localize the accessory pathway intraoperatively will be dictated by the preoperative studies and the haemodynamic state of the patient. Ideally, one should localize the site of antegrade pre-excitation during sinus rhythm or atrial pacing and the site of retrograde pre-excitation during reciprocating tachycardia or ventricular pacing[12]. Many patients will not tolerate extensive retrograde mapping during reciprocating tachycardia unless on cardiopulmonary bypass, and in this setting a ventricular pacing site near the presumed site of the accessory pathway should be used and a retrograde map obtained at the fastest ventricular rate attained without hypotension. It should be emphasized, however, that the presence of multiple accessory pathways can be easily obscured by the presence of an accessory pathway favoured by the site of pacing. If the results of the initial epicardial mapping indicate that the site of antegrade or retrograde pre-excitation overlies the anterior or posterior septal regions, more detailed localization may be necessary utilizing intracardiac mapping performed during cardiopulmonary bypass.

After the sites of the earliest ventricular and atrial activation have been determined, the site on the atrioventricular ring to be divided is approached from within the atrium. In the first ten cases of our series, we approached the ring from the epicardial side and divided the ventricle at its insertion into the annulus fibrosis. On the right side, this presented very little difficulty for the right coronary could be easily displaced down. However, on the left, the coronary sinus and coronary artery made this approach hazardous. It is now routine to divide the accessory connection on the atrial side of the annulus. For left-sided connections, the left atrioventricular ring is now exposed in the manner used for exposure of mitral valve replacements. The accessory pathway is divided by incising the atrium just above the annulus of the mitral valve, exposing the fat pad which surrounds the coronary artery and vein. It is technically possible to incise the mitral annulus in this manner from the left trigone (anterior insertion of the aorta into the fibrous skeleton of the heart) counterclockwise all the way around to the right trigone (the central fibrous body). Special care is taken to see that all of the fat around the coronary vessel is separated completely from the top of the ventricle and annulus with the dissection carried all the way to the epicardium. Using this approach, we have not injured either the mitral valve or the coronary vessels.

On the right side, the approach to the accessory pathway is again made with incisions just above the annulus fibrosis. The incisions can be made just above the annulus of the tricuspid valve beginning at the anterior aspect of the membranous ventricular septum clockwise all the way around the tricuspid circumference to almost the same point on the posterior aspect of the membranous septum.

One major and as yet not completely resolved problem has been in those patients with pre-excitation occurring posteriorly in the region of the crux[6]. Previously, attempts were made to divide such pathways by elevating the great coronary vein and dissecting this away from the top of the ventricular septum. The right atrial endocardium was then incised from above the annulus fibrosis beginning at the anterior lip of the coronary sinus and extending this to the middle of the free wall tricuspid ring. More recently, we have achieved success in interrupting septal accessory pathways which pre-excite the right side of the crux by incising the right atrial wall just beneath the orifice of the coronary sinus and dissecting the fat around the coronary vessels and in the triangular space above the posterior ventricular septum. This region is considered to be adequately dissected when the top of the ventricular septum and posteromedial left atrium can be viewed in the incision. If the left side of the crux is preexcited, a similar dissection of the posteromedial mitral annulus may be necessary. The single innovation most responsible for the increased rate of success appears to be the use of a nerve hook to thoroughly blunt dissect all possible connections between the atrium and ventricle coursing through the fat pads which fill the atrioventricular groove. The most superficial epicardial layer is generally left intact to minimize the chance of bleeding, but in two cases to date, pre-excitation was abolished only when the incision was carried completely through from endocardium to epicardium suggesting a superficial location of the accessory pathway in these cases. Proof that the pathway has been interrupted by the surgical procedure is obtained by repeating the sequence of atrial and ventricular activation during appropriate pacing using the methods employed before division. The postoperative check may consist of a preliminary survey while the patient is still on bypass, followed by a more detailed study after the heart has been closed.

The results of our experience to date with the pre-excitation syndrome are indicated in Tables 25.1 and 25.2. To date, we have studied 146 patients with the Wolff–Parkinson–White syndrome, of which 68 have been treated medically, eight have been paced, and 70 underwent attempted surgical interruption of the accessory pathway. There have been three postoperative deaths. The first occurred early in the series in a patient operated upon as an emergency. This patient was thought preoperatively to have the WPW syndrome, but because of

Table 25.1 WPW Surgery: 1968–1976

70 Patients operated
3 Deaths: 2 – Cardiomyopathy
 1 – Persistent SVT – ? WPW
48 Complete Corrections
8 His Bundle Ablations
11 Pre-excitation modified; Responsive to Medication
3 Pre-excitation unchanged; Persistent Arrhythmia

the urgent nature of her arrhythmia, she could not undergo electrophysiologic study. Epicardial mapping at the time of surgery failed to provide definitive evidence of pre-excitation. Division of the AV ring failed to abolish arrhythmia and she died several days postoperatively. The other two deaths occurred in patients who underwent successful division of the accessory pathway, but developed low output syndrome postoperatively. At autopsy, both had evidence of cardiomyopathy, but no residual connections were present. Five patients were documented to have two distinct accessory atrioventricular connections. Attempts were made to divide the accessory connection in 72 instances. In the group with accessory connections between the free wall portions of the right atrium and right ventricle, 13 of 15 pathways were successfully divided. In one of these failures the patient had presented with ventricular fibrillation. Surgery was successful in abolishing evidence of antegrade pre-excitation and resulted in a normal ventricular response during atrial fibrillation. However, the postoperative study indicated intact retrograde conduction over an accessory pathway in the same region of the heart. Subsequent occasional attacks of reciprocating tachycardia in this patient have been easily managed with medical therapy. The other failure was that of the patient who died postoperatively from cardiomyopathy. In the group with septal accessory con-

Table 25.2   Successful Interruption of Accessory Pathway

RV	Septal	LV
13/15	12/22	28/35

nections 12 of 22 were successfully divided. In this group, it is of note that the last seven septal accessory pathways operated on have been successfully divided. Finally, in the group with accessory pathways between the free wall portion of the left atrium and left ventricle, 28 of 35 pathways were divided. Two of these failures occurred in the patients who underwent successful division of the accessory pathway but died postoperatively in low output failure. Both had cardiomyopathy. (One of these was listed in the group of right sided pathways since he had two accessory pathways.) In one of the five remaining failures, the patient had presented with ventricular fibrillation. Again, all antegrade evidence of pre-excitation was abolished as was the rapid ventricular response during atrial fibrillation. However, retrograde conduction over the accessory pathway recurred postoperatively.

In this group of 70 patients, therefore, there were 48 survivors in whom complete correction of pre-excitation was achieved. Eight patients required division of the His bundle. In eleven patients, the accessory pathway was modified and the associated arrhythmias now became responsive to medication. Three patients have continued to have recurrent arrhythmia despite drug therapy postoperatively. Sixty-four of the 67 survivors are now free of arrhythmia.

ACCESSORY ATRIOVENTRICULAR CONNECTIONS CAPABLE OF ONLY RETROGRADE CONDUCTION

It has now been demonstrated by several groups that patients who appear to have paroxysmal atrial tachycardia due to re-entry in the AV node may, in fact, be utilizing an accessory atrioventricular connection in the retrograde direction during tachycardia. In such patients, no overt evidence of pre-excitation is seen during sinus rhythm or with right or left atrial pacing[11,13]. To date, we have studied 24 patients with reciprocating tachycardia and no overt evidence of pre-excitation. In eleven of these, participation of an accessory atrioventricular connection capable of only retrograde conduction in the re-entry circuit was documented. These are summarized in Table 25.3. While selection is present in any referral series, the incidence noted in this series and by others[14] suggests the value of performing electrophysiologic studies in patients with supraventricular tachycardias refractory to medical management in an attempt to define a surgically remediable cause. Three of our patients were managed successfully on medical regimens. Eight patients were subjected to surgery and the accessory pathway was localized and divided in six of seven patients. In one patient, we failed to completely divide the accessory pathway and on reopera-

Table 25.3   Accessory A–V Connections Capable of only Retrograde Conduction

Site	Associated Anomaly	Intervention	Comment
1. Left Lateral FW	None	Quinidine	RT abolished
2. Left Lateral FW	None	Digoxin & Propranolol	RT abolished
3. Left Lateral FW	LGL syndrome	Propranolol	RT abolished
4. Left Lateral FW	None	Surgery – AP divided	RT abolished
5. Left Lateral FW	None	Surgery – AP divided	RT abolished
6. Left Lateral FW	EAVN	Surgery – AP divided	RT abolished
7. Septal	Cardiomyopathy	Surgery – A–V node His section	Incomplete interruption of A–V node His bundle; slow RT 125/min
8. Septal	EAVN	Surgery – AP frozen	RT abolished
9. Right posterior FW	Ebsteins	Surgery – AP divided Porcine Tricuspid Valve	RT abolished
10 Left Anterior Paraseptal	EAVN	Surgery – AP not divided; His Frozen	RT abolished
11 Septal	? Balloon	Surgery – AP and His (Contiguous) Frozen	RT abolished
Secondary			
12 Right Lateral FW	Ebstein	Surgery – Antegrade Function of AP Abolished; Retrograde Conduction in AP returned	Presented with VF; rare RT due to persistent retrograde function of AP managed medically
13 Right Anterior FW	History of small VSD	Surgery – AP divided	Postoperative return of retrograde function of AP; AP completely divided on reoperation

FW = Free Wall; AP = Accessory Pathway; RT = Reciprocating Tachycardia (SVT); EAVN = Enhanced A–V node conduction

tion elected to ablate the His bundle. In the remaining surgical patient, severe cardiomyopathy was present. The accessory pathway had been localized preoperatively to the septum. In an attempt to limit the duration of cardiopulmonary bypass, no attempt was made to divide the accessory pathway and instead the His bundle was ablated. Two additional patients with classic Wolff–Parkinson–White syndrome are included (secondary group.) Following an operative attempt to divide the accessory pathway, retrograde function of an accessory pathway returned postoperatively at a site indistinguishable from the original accessory pathway. One of these patients was reoperated on successfully, while the other patient elected to pursue medical management with good result.

CRYOSURGICAL ABLATION OF THE AV NODE–HIS BUNDLE: A METHOD FOR PRODUCING AV BLOCK

Previously reported efforts to produce AV block in man have advocated cautery, suture ligation, and incision of the AV node–His bundle area. The use of cautery has some obvious disadvantages in that heat denatures collagen, destroys fibroblasts, and cannot be applied to effect a reproducible and irreversible state of dysfunction. Methods of suture ligation have been associated with a high incidence of return to normal sinus rhythm in both experimental and clinical studies. Suture ligation, incision, and cautery are all associated with risk of inducing tricuspid insufficiency, septal defects, and aneurysms and fistulae of the aortic sinuses of Valsalva. We therefore devised a cryosurgical unit to effect reversible or permanent atrioventricular block[15]. The instrument employed utilized expanding nitrous oxide as the coolant. Expansion of the gas within the tip (5 mm diameter) of a hand-held probe resulted in cooling. The probe tip temperature was monitored on a console via a thermocouple in the tip and temperature could be varied from room temperature to $-60°C$ ($\pm 5°C$) by controlling the back pressure on the escaping gas. The instrument was designed so that controlled cooling to $0\ °C$ could be delivered to an area, resulting in cessation of physiological function and return of normal function of rewarming. In this manner, the result of cooling an area of tissue suspected of containing conduction tissue could be examined in a reversible manner before trying an irreversible freeze. Once the area to be frozen was located, the instrument had the capacity to produce an iceball 15 mm in diameter at a temperature of $-60\ °C$. The procedure was initially carried out in 20 dogs. After documenting the safety and feasibility (Figure 25.1) of this approach, we have used the technique in seven patients with complete success in six. Two patients had reciprocating tachycardia due to accessory pathways capable of conducting only retrogradely. Both were in locations difficult to approach and both required open-heart surgery for other reasons. To minimize their cardiopulmonary bypass time, it was elected to ablate their His bundles. Four of the remaining five patients demonstrated abnormally enhanced conduction in their AV node, which in concert with various atrial tachyarrhythmias resulted in

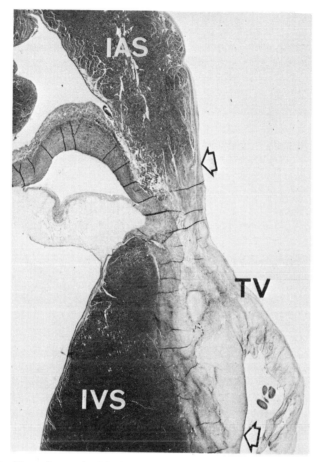

Figure 25.1 Photomicrograph of the lesion in atrioventricular conduction tissue of the dog one month after cryoablation. The arrows point to the margins of the scarred area. The conduction fibres have been replaced by collagen. Masson's stain, IAS = interatrial septum, TV = tricuspid valve, IVS = interventricular septum

debilitating ventricular responses refractory to medical management. The remaining patient had a sick sinus syndrome with bradycardia–tachycardia. He was scheduled for implantation of a permanent ventricular pacemaker and because of poor tolerance of antiarrhythmic agents it was elected to ablate the His bundle. In the six successful cases, a well-defined His bundle deflection could be localized by intracardiac mapping on cardiopulmonary bypass. When the temperature of the His bundle area was lowered to 0 °C, complete heart block occurred in each of these with return of normal conduction on rewarming. In the one failure, a convincing His deflection could never be localized. After convalescence, all the patients were restudied. In every instance, inhibition of the pacemaker resulted in prompt appearance of a junctional escape rhythm at rates of 45–60/min associated with a

QRS configuration identical to that observed preoperatively during sinus rhythm. The response of this pacemaker to atropine was minimal but acceleration of the pacemaker occurred with administration of isuprel (isoproterenol). These results were felt to be consistent with the location of a stable subsidiary pacemaker in the distal His bundle. Several of the patients in this series have now been followed for over 6 months with no return of conduction.

An illustrative example is shown in Figures 25.2–25.4. The patient was a 52-year-old man with a history of rheumatic valvular heart disease and disabling ventricular responses secondary to atrial flutter and atrial fibrillation. No control had been obtained by the use of large doses of propranolol, procaine amide

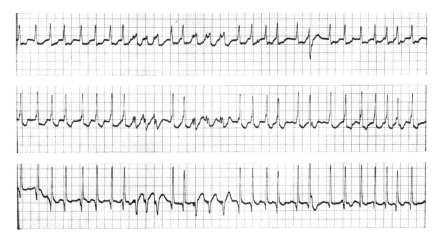

Figure 25.2   Rapid ventricular response during atrial flutter-fibrillation due to enhanced conduction in the AV node.

Recordings from above down are standard ECG leads I, II and III. A rapid ventricular response is present with runs of left bundle branch block aberration. See text for discussion

and digoxin. In sinus rhythm, he had a normal P–R interval and a non-specific interventricular conduction defect. On electrophysiological study, he was shown to have a P–A interval of 40 msec, an A–H interval of 50 msec, and an H–V interval of 65 msec. There was evidence of enhanced AV nodal conduction evidenced by his ability to conduct 1 : 1 in the antegrade direction to cycle length as short as 230 msec. There was cycle length related right bundle branch block and left bundle branch block. Atrial fibrillation was accompanied by a rapid ventricular response with R–R intervals frequently as short as 225 msec (Figure 25.1). Intracavitary recordings revealed that all complexes were preceded by a His deflection at an H–V equal to or greater than that present in sinus rhythm (Figure 25.3). Postoperatively he was paced at a rate of 70/min.

ATRIAL FLUTTER

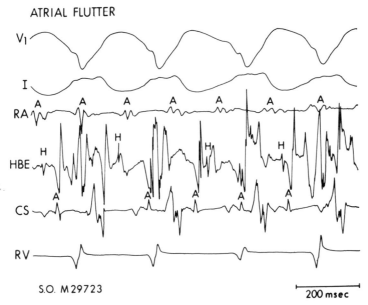

S.O. M29723

200 msec

Figure 25.3 Intracavitary recording during atrial flutter.

Recordings from above down are standard ECG leads V_1, I and bipolar electrogram recorded from the right atrium (RA), the His bundle electrogram (HBE), the coronary sinus (CS), and the right ventricle (RV).

Atrial flutter is present with a rapid ventricular response. All ventricular responses are preceded by a His deflection with a prolonged H–V interval indicating supraventricular origin with bundle branch block aberration

On inhibition of his pacemaker, an escape rhythm with a relatively narrow QRS identical to that present in sinus rhythm readily appeared (Figure 25.4).

The initial lesions produced by this technique are reversible. The permanent lesions induced by irreversible freezing are homogeneous (Figure 25.5) and demarcated without tendency to rupture, aneurysm formation or intracardiac thrombosis. Particularly attractive is the marked resistance of vascular elements, collagen, and fibroblasts to hypothermal injury.

CRYOABLATION OF ACCESSORY ATRIOVENTRICULAR CONNECTIONS

The technique of cryothermia has now been applied in four patients with the pre-excitation syndrome[16]. The first patient presented with a normal P–R interval with a delta wave and reciprocating tachycardia. Preoperative electrophysiologic study suggested a free wall atrioventricular connection at the left posterior AV groove. At surgery, epicardial mapping confirmed the site of pre-excitation on the posterior LV wall (Figure 25.6). An electrogram arising from

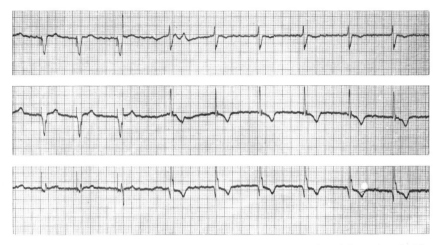

Figure 25.4   Demonstration of escape rhythm following cryoablation of the His bundle. The recordings from above down are standard ECG leads I, II and III. Atrial fibrillation is present with complete heart block. The paced ventricular rhythm is initially present in the first three complexes. Following this, the pacemaker is inhibited and a spontaneous escape rhythm appears associated with a relatively narrow QRS. See text for discussion

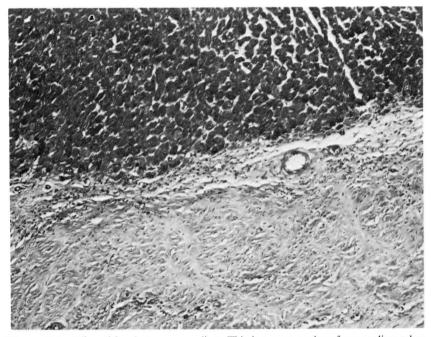

Figure 25.5   Effect of freezing on myocardium. This is a cross-section of myocardium taken from the margin of a lesion induced by applying the freezing probe to the surface epicardium of a dog. The section was taken one month after induction of the lesion. Note the sharp demarcation between normal myocardial tissue above and the area replaced by homogeneous fibrosis below

LA PACING CL 500 msec

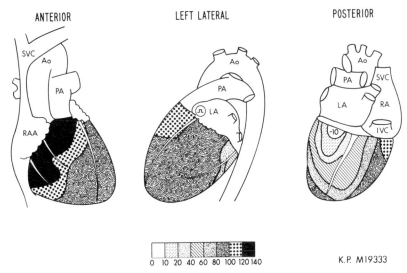

Figure 25.6 Epicardial mapping of a patient with a variant form of pre-excitation.

The epicardial map was performed during pacing of the left atrial appendage at a cycle length of 500 msec. Pre-excitation is noted on the posterior left ventricle with no evidence of fusion

the accessory pathway was recorded at the site of earliest ventricular activation (Figure 25.7). This electrogram could be recorded a full 1 cm distal to the AV ring, a site that was unquestionably on the ventricle. As the probe was moved from AV ring toward the apex, the interval from the accessory pathway electrogram to the ventricular electrogram gradually shortened until the two merged approximately 1 cm distal to the AV ring (Figure 25.8). We thought it unlikely that this electrogram represented atrial depolarization since this electrogram: (a) occurred after inscription of all contiguous atrial sites; (b) was recorded from the ventricle below the AV groove and merged distally with the local ventricular electrogram; and (c) could no longer be recorded after freezing the site of ventricular pre-excitation. Local pressure in the region of the accessory pathway electrogram during antegrade pre-excitation resulted in normalization of the QRS complex. A lesion was induced by cooling at $-60\,°C$ for 90 sec. The diameter of this lesion was 8 mm. A contiguous area along the course of the electrogram was also cooled to $-60\,°C$ for 90 sec. After freezing, the accessory pathway electrogram could no longer be recorded. Pre-excitation was gone, and no arrhythmias could be provoked. Repeat epicardial mapping during left atrial pacing showed a normal sequence of ventricular activation (Figure 25.9). He was completely restudied nine days postoperatively and showed no evidence of antegrade or retrograde pre-excitation and no arrhythmias could be produced.

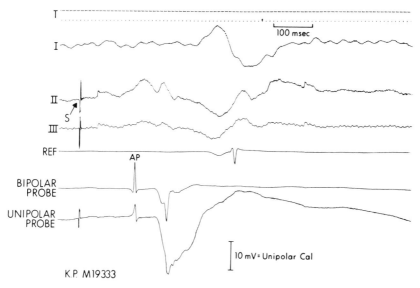

Figure 25.7 Epicardial recording from the area of pre-excitation during left atrial pacing. Recordings from above down are standard ECG leads I, II and III, a bipolar ventricular reference and bipolar and unipolar recordings from the mapping probe. This recording was obtained when the probe was on the ventricle and records an electrogram thought to arise from the accessory pathway. Note the QS morphology of the unipolar recording from the earliest area of pre-excitation. See text for discussion

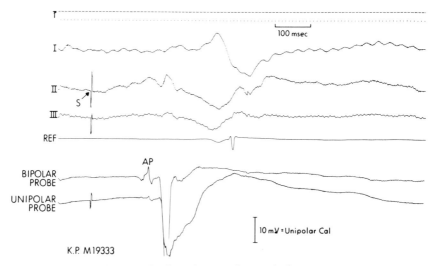

Figure 25.8 Epicardial recording from the area of pre-excitation.
This recording was obtained from an area 1 cm distal to the site at which the recording shown in Figure 25.7 was obtained. The previously noted electrogram has now merged with the ventricular electrogram

POST-FREEZE

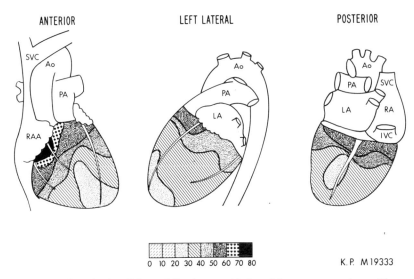

ANTERIOR   LEFT LATERAL   POSTERIOR

0 10 20 30 40 50 60 70 80

K. P. M 19333

Figure 25.9 Normal epicardial map following cryoablation of the accessory pathway. The map was obtained during left atrial pacing. The ventricular data is referenced to the onset of the QRS in the surface ECG leads. The previously noted area of pre-excitation is absent and the epicardial map shows a normal sequence of ventricular activation

The second patient presented with a refractory reciprocating tachycardia and was found to have an accessory pathway in the septum capable of only retrograde conduction. Retrograde conduction was abolished by applying a temperature of 0 °C to the annulus at this site during tachycardia while on cardiopulmonary bypass. Conduction over the accessory pathway and reciprocating tachycardia returned with rewarming. Ablation of the accessory pathway was obtained by applying a temperature of −60 °C for 90 sec on two occasions to the same area. The His bundle was not injured. On restudy nine days postoperatively, ventricular pacing was performed and retrograde conduction to the atria was not possible. No reciprocating tachycardia could be induced and antegrade conduction remained intact.

The third patient also presented with reciprocating tachycardia which required participation of an accessory pathway in the septum capable of only retrograde conduction. Retrograde atrial pre-excitation following premature ventricular beats introduced during reciprocating tachycardia was clearly demonstrated preoperatively. At surgery, the accessory pathway was found to be contiguous with the His bundle and application of cooling in this area resulted in block of both the accessory pathway and the His bundle. An irreversible lesion was caused by applying a temperature of −60 °C for 90 sec on two occasions. Retrograde conduction was no longer possible and no further episodes of reciprocating tachycardia were observed. The final patient was a 9-month-old infant with a ventricular septal defect and reciprocating tachycardia involving a free-wall accessory connection in the right posterior AV groove. The accessory pathway was ablated by external freezing and the ventricular septal defect repaired. She has remained free of arrhythmia in follow-up.

The use of cryothermia thus appears to be a useful adjunct to the surgical approach for ablation of accessory pathways.

CRYOSURGERY FOR VENTRICULAR TACHYCARDIA

Our initial experience with cryothermia for ablation of the His bundle and accessory connections suggested its possible utility for ablating sites of dysrhythmia due to ectopy or re-entry at other sites.

A 37-year-old man presented with a history of ventricular tachycardia for four months. His past history was of significance in that he had suffered from the CRST syndrome (calcinosis circumscripta, Raynaud's phenomenon sclerodactyly, and telangiectasia). He presented with right heart failure and persistent ventricular tachycardia at a rate of 150 min. On angiography he was noted to have normal coronaries and a normal left ventricle. His right ventricle was dilated and contracted poorly but his pulmonary pressures were normal. On electrophysiologic study, he appeared to have an ectopic focus arising in the anterior area of the right ventricle. His tachycardia proved resistant to all antiarrhythmic agents, as well as attempts at overdrive pacing from the atrium and ventricle. He was therefore taken to surgery where epicardial mapping demonstrated earliest activation occurring on the anterior right ventricle near the outflow tract. This focus was cooled to 0 °C with a surface probe resulting in immediate cessation of tachycardia and return to normal sinus rhythm. On rewarming, the ventricular tachycardia reappeared. The area was therefore frozen at −60 °C for 90 sec on three separate occasions. He has remained completely free of arrhythmia in 2.5 months of follow-up, on no medication except maintenance digoxin.

Initial results obtained with cryothermia appear promising, but long term follow-up of these patients will be necessary before the procedure can be considered established. Work is presently underway to explore the applicability of this method to ablation of other ectopic and re-entrant sites of supraventricular and ventricular dysrhythmias.

Acknowledgement
The authors wish to express their gratitude to the many Cardiology Fellows who participated in these studies; to Laura Cook, R.N., and to Donald Kopp, L.P.N., the staff of the Electrophysiology Laboratory; to Don Powell, David Huggett, Jim Rogers and Tommie McLain, who prepared the illustrations; and to Sharon Christensen for coordinating patient care and preparing the manuscript.

This work was supported in part by grants from the USPHS HL–15190, HL–17670 and HL–13290, and by a grant from the General Clinical Research Centers Program of the Division of Research Resources, NIH RR–30. This work was done during the tenure of an Established Investigatorship of the American Heart Association of Dr. John J. Gallagher and during the tenure of an NIH Research Career Development Award (HL–70455) from the USPHS of Dr. Robert W. Anderson. This work was also supported by the Joseph Barham Cardiovascular Research Fund.

References

1. Cobb, F. R., Blumenschein, S. D., Sealy, W. C., Boineau, J. P., Wagner, G. S. and Wallace, A. G. (1968). Successful surgical interruption of the bundle of Kent in a patient with Wolff–Parkinson–White syndrome. *Circulation,* **38,** 1018

2. Sealy, W. C., Hattler, B. C., Blumenschein, S. D. and Cobb, F. R. (1969). Surgical treatment of Wolff–Parkinson–White syndrome. *Ann. Thorac. Surg.,* **8,** 1

3. Wallace, A. G., Sealy, W. C., Gallagher, J. J., Svenson, R. H., Strauss, H. C. and Kasell, J. (1974). Surgical correction of anomalous left ventricular preexcitation: Wolff–Parkinson–White (Type A). *Circulation,* **49,** 206

4. Sealy, W. C. and Wallace, A. G. (1974). Surgical treatment of Wolff–Parkinson–White syndrome. *J. Thorac. Cardiovasc. Surg.,* **68,** 757

5. Sealy, W. C., Wallace, A. G., Ramming K. P., Gallagher, J. J. and Svenson, R. H. (1974). An improved operation for the definitive treatment of the Wolff–Parkinson–White syndrome. *Ann. Thorac. Surg.,* **17,** 107

6. Sealy, W. C., Gallagher, J. J. and Wallace, A. G. (1976). The surgical treatment of the Wolff–Parkinson–White syndrome; evaluation of the improved methods of identification and interruption of the Kent bundle. *Ann. Thorac. Surg.,* **22,** 443

7. Gallagher, J. J., Gilbert, M., Svenson, R. H., Sealy, W. C., Kasell, J. and Wallace A. G. (1975). Wolff–Parkinson–White syndrome: the problem, evaluation and surgical correction. *Circulation,* **51,** 767

8. Gallagher, J. J., Svenson, R. H., Sealy, W. C. and Wallace, A. G. (1976). The Wolff–Parkinson–White syndrome and the preexcitation dysrhythmias. *Med. Clin. N. Am.,* **60,** 101

9. Gallagher, J. J., Sealy, W. C., Wallace, A. G. and Kasell, J. (1976). Correlation between catheter electrophysiologic studies and findings on mapping of ventricular excitation in the WPW syndrome. In: *The Conduction System of the Heart,* Wellens, Lie and Janse (eds.), Amsterdam, HE Stenfert Kroese BV

10. Gallagher, J. J., Sealy, W. C., Kasell, J. and Wallace, A. G. (1976). Multiple accessory pathways in patients with the preexcitation syndrome. *Circulation* (in press)

11. Pritchett, E. L. C., Gallagher, J. J., Sealy, W. C., Campbell, R. W. F., Sellers, T. D. and Wallace, A. G. Primary and secondary unidirectional (retrograde) accessory pathways. (Submitted for publication.)

12. Gallagher, J. J. and Kasell, J. Epicardial mapping in the Wolff–Parkinson–White syndrome. *Cardiology* (in press)

13. Tonkin, A. M., Gallagher, J. J., Svenson, R. H., Wallace, A. G. and Sealy, W. C. (1975). Anterograde block in accessory pathways with retrograde conduction in reciprocating tachycardia. *Eur. J. Cardiol.,* **3,** 143

14. Coumel, P., Attuel, P. and Flammang, D. (1976). The role of the conduction system in supraventricular tachycardia. In: *The Conduction System of the Heart,* Wellens, Lie and Janse (eds.). Amsterdam, H. E. Stenfert Kroese BV

15. Harrison, L., Gallagher, J. J., Kasell, J., Anderson, R. W., Mikat, E., Hackel, D. B. and

Wallace, A. G. (1977). Cryosurgical ablation of the A–V node-His bundle: a new method for producing A–V block. *Circulation* (in press)

16. Gallagher, J. J., Sealy, W. C., Anderson, R. W., Kasell, J., Millar, R., Campbell, R. W. F., Harrison, L., Pritchett, E. L. C. and Wallace, A. G. (1977). Cryoablation of accessory atrioventricular connections: a new technique for correction of the preexcitation syndrome. *Circulation* (in press)

Index